THE INTERPRETATION OF DREAMS AND OF JOKES

The Interpretation of Dreams and of Jokes provides a unique and integrative introduction to dream science. It addresses a notable gap in cognitive psychology on the subject of dreams and explores significant overlaps between the phenomena of dreams and jokes.

Bringing together extensive research from cognitive psychology, neuroscience, and psychoanalysis, the book provides a coherent approach to dream science that is underpinned by experimental and theoretical research. It considers the significance of dreams and their relationships to jokes, examining how both require an understanding of latent contents in which context plays a crucial role. The book outlines a history of dream research and dream science and introduces several original dreams, along with some well-known classic ones, for analysis. The book's chapters explore how we can interpret meaning in dreams, how dreams might be indicators of inner psychological and somatic states, whether dreams can predict significant future events, whether dreams can be used in problem-solving, and the relationship between dreams, aphasia, memory, and waking consciousness in general.

This groundbreaking book will be essential reading for researchers and students from psychological and psychoanalytic backgrounds who are interested in the analysis and science of dreams.

Matthew Hugh Erdelyi is Professor Emeritus of Psychology and Formerly Stern Professor of Humor at Brooklyn College, CUNY, USA.

THE INTERPRETATION OF DREAMS AND OF JOKES

The Art and the Science

Matthew Hugh Erdelyi

Routledge
Taylor & Francis Group
NEW YORK AND LONDON

Designed cover image: © 2022 Estate of Pablo Picasso / Artists Rights Society (ARS), New York

First published 2023
by Routledge
605 Third Avenue, New York, NY 10158

and by Routledge
4 Park Square, Milton Park, Abingdon, Oxon, OX14 4RN

Routledge is an imprint of the Taylor & Francis Group, an informa business

ISBN: 9781032292229 (hbk)
ISBN: 9781032292212 (pbk)
ISBN: 9781003300441 (ebk)

DOI: 10.4324/9781003300441

Typeset in Bembo
by Newgen Publishing UK

To the Cica
Who knows the meaning of words
My wise woman who knows the meaning of dreams
With appreciation and love

CONTENTS

ACKNOWLEDGMENTS

I am pleased to acknowledge my immense debt of gratitude to my wife, Diane Zizak, for her help with my book, from beginning to end. As an experimental psychologist with whom I have actually published work in the past, she was able to provide expert suggestions and criticisms throughout the life of the project; as a student of Chinese since her college days, she was also able to contribute an original section to the book, "Freud Dreams Chinese Poetry," which brings important ideas—both theoretical and methodological—to dream science. I thank my friend, the dream psychologist, David Jenkins, for his serious readings of the developing manuscript and his real understanding of what I was trying to accomplish in some sections, especially my whimsical "*N*, the Magician." I thank the neuroscientist Peter Brugger, of Zurich, for his helpful comments and also for his short but important review article on the incorporation of drastic body-events in dreams which advanced my understanding of aphasic dream memory. I wish to acknowledge the memory scholar, Richard Schweickert, whom I met at an international dream conference in a former abbey at Rolduc, The Netherlands. He gave me helpful feedback on portions of my book and contributed his two beautiful network figures of the dreams of "Arlie" and "The Natural Scientist." I also wish to thank Bill Domhoff for his help with my project. He was generous in sharing his expertise and reprints when I started my book about a decade ago, even if he no doubt felt I went astray once I found my footing in the field. Even though I have sometimes been critical of his ideas, I acknowledge Bill Domhoff's contribution to my book—and dream science in general—especially for his decisive refutation with quantitative content-analysis, of popular misconceptions about the meaninglessness of dreams. Finally, I wish to thank my steadying and patient editors at Routledge, Emilie Coin and Khyati Sanger, for helping me bring my project to the light of day.

SYNOPSIS OF BOOK

When behaviorism finally began to lose its hold on psychology in the late 1950s and "cognitive psychology"—the psychology of the very topics that had been consigned to behaviorism's forbidden "black box"—displaced it as the basic orientation of the field, it seemed natural that a great efflorescence of cognitive research would ensue, which it did. Nevertheless, more than half a century after the much celebrated "cognitive revolution," cognitive psychology has remained preternaturally silent on the subject of dreams. There has been important neuroscience work on dreaming—for example, what does the brain do and not do while we are dreaming—but, except for an extensive literature on the quantitative content-analysis of dreams, there has been virtually no work on the classic issues of dreams: What do dreams mean—if they mean anything? How do we interpret their deep ("latent") meanings—if they have deep meanings? Are dreams sensitive indicators of inner psychological and somatic states, and can they predict future psychological or somatic developments? Are dreams hypermnesic—do they contact memories inaccessible to waking consciousness? Can dreams uniquely solve problems, from brainteasers to scientific and artistic puzzles to life-and-death conundrums? What is the relation between dreams and other release phenomena such as jokes and aphasia? This book seeks to remedy academic psychology's silence and move toward a scientific resolution of the riddle of dreams. In a technical appendix, Signal Detection Theory is introduced to dream science, along with an original technique for controlling response criteria in dream narratives which can be implemented retroactively to already collected—or published—dreams.

BRIEF INTRODUCTION

This work is a broadly integrative project that seeks to lay the scientific foundations for the extraction of meaning from dreams, jokes, and other *release phenomena*—forms of cognition that are released as a result of diminished inhibition and regulation by higher-order systems. The subject has many moving parts, historically and conceptually, and involves the weaving of an extensive tapestry from quite disparate threads. To ensure that the handful of basic points are not lost in developing the comprehensive picture, the essential ideas are highlighted in this purposely brief introduction.

First and foremost, it will be shown that, notwithstanding some background skepticism in academic psychology, dreams indeed have meaning, and not at just at one level. Both the *manifest* (surface) and *latent* (deeper) contents of dreams are rich in meanings. *Quantitative content-analysis* has decisively shown that the experiences and concerns of waking-life are substantially (and positively) correlated with the content of dreams, so much so that the rough *continuity* between dream-life and awake-life has become the received view.

Dreams are "paradoxical" phenomena characterized by the simultaneous *deactivation* of executive control systems (the "ego" in Freud's terminology, "reason" in Plato's, "prefrontal cortical areas" in modern neuroscience) and the *hyperactivation* of more primitive systems (the "id," the "beast," the "reptilian brain," the "limbic system"). Modern research shows that these heightened activation–deactivation states, which are associated with dreaming, occur cyclically several times a night in adults and can readily account for the release from organization and control observed in dreams. The basic neurological hardware supporting some of the prominent psychological phenomena is elaborated in a dedicated chapter.

Universal symbols (biologically prepared meanings which, in the case of Freudian sexual symbols, involve concretistic representations in which symbols physically

DOI: 10.4324/9781003300441-1

resemble their referents) play a role in interpretation. The essential factor in the extraction of latent contents from manifest contents, however, is the *context* that embeds the manifest contents. A formal definition of latent contents is proposed that treats latent contents as *interactions* of manifest contents with context. These kinds of interactions are evident in the extraction of depth in domains outside of dreams—for example, in Helmholtz's "unconscious inferences," which yield 3-D percepts from shifting surface 2-D displays and the consequent perceptual constancies and illusions that result.

A proposal developed in a chapter of the book is that *dreaming is a form of noisy remembering* and that, as will be shown unambiguously, the distortions found in dreams and in recollections of complex narratives (like the famous "War of the Ghosts" story introduced into psychology by Bartlett) are *identical.* The dozen or so distortions Freud documents in his writings on dreams, clinical case histories, jokes, and the parapraxes (Freudian slips) were recapitulated three decades later by Bartlett in his laboratory work on perceptual and memory "reconstructions." The striking overlaps suggest that not just a class of dream symbols but also a class of distortions may be "universal." Bartlettian and Freudian distortions, in any case, are the same, even if the explanation given for the distortions are different—defense in the case of Freud, cognitive "schematization" in the case of Bartlett. It is a cinch that we are not dealing with an either-or reality and that both explanations tell part of the story.

A leitmotiv of the book is that dreams comprise but one dialect among a broader class of release phenomena—the aphasias, daydreams and fantasy, subliminal percepts, jokes, parapraxes, psychotic thinking, poetry, fairy-tales—which points to an underlying unity among a sweep of superficially disparate psychological realms. The similarities can be striking but the differences among the dialects can also be critical, yielding significant theoretical and methodological opportunities, for what is refractory in one domain may be simple, even obvious, in another. Physics and mathematics abound in apposite examples.

Jokes are a case in point for dreams. Freud published his joke book, *Jokes and their relation to the unconscious*, in 1905, just a few years after the appearance of *The interpretation of dreams*, and showed the existence of significant homologies between jokes and dreams. Neither psychoanalysts nor academic psychologists have made much of jokes—it is as if jokes lacked the necessary gravitas to be taken seriously—even though it turns out that jokes are Goldilocks stimuli for psychology: They are not too simple like nonsense syllables or word-strings; they are not too complex like case-histories or full-fledged dream samples; they are just right.

Using jokes as a model of dreams, for example, renders the distinction between manifest and latent contents (rejected for dreams in some quarters) not only true but obvious. When asked if we "got" a joke, we are being asked, in effect, if we managed to interpret the latent content of the joke. Tests have shown that jokes that subjects claim to have "gotten" yield highly concordant interpretations (in the order of 90% agreement). Interpretation, obviously, can be highly reliable. Not only are latent contents real but it also is possible to measure "sensitivity" to latent contents using Signal Detection Theory techniques (elaborated in a substantive APPENDIX) which show that significant individual differences exist in sensitivity to latent contents, some individuals being more sensitive than others. Jokes also reveal plainly the operation of *defense* in connection with emotionally fraught (sexual, aggressive) contents, which are demonstrably relegated to latent contents and largely omitted from manifest contents. This is a controversial claim made for dreams that is obvious in jokes.

Another powerful model of dreams that is examined in some detail is aphasia. It is typically ignored in neuroscience approaches to dreams, although aphasic errors (*paraphasias*), like jokes, often reveal meanings ensconced in garbled manifest contents that can be reliably interpreted.

The issue of dream *sensitivity* to inaccessible contents—the "X-ray" aspect of dreams—is important both theoretically and clinically. Because they are disinhibited, dreams often reveal psychological contents not readily accessible to consciousness. Like a tipsy friend, dreams can be simultaneously confusing and honest, and for the same reason: They can be confusing because of the dreamer's loss of executive control and they are honest because of the dreamer's loss of executive control. Thus, dreams may be important sources of information about current psychological and somatic states and, also, knowledge about emotional and cognitive trends in the individual which, because of wakeful inhibitions, remain hidden for some time until the dissipation of inhibition. There already exist lines of research evidence, probed in the book, supporting these claims, but a great deal of confirmatory work remains to be done.

If it could be decisively demonstrated that dreams can contact pathological conditions or future psychological and somatic developments, the practical implications would render the interpretation of dreams not a matter of theoretical predilection but an outright necessity for both psychology and medicine. Experimental psychologists now have statistical tools which classic theorists such as Freud or Jung—or Aristotle or Galen—did not, to evaluate the empirical status of dreams as sensitive indicators of current and future psychological and somatic events. Some of the potential payoffs could be game changers.

1

HISTORICAL FORESHADOWINGS

Across time and across cultures, dreams have fascinated human beings. One is tempted to assert that this fascination extends back to the dawn of humankind but here we must contend with the fact that we do not really have the data since written language is a very new achievement of civilization, spanning no more than a few thousand years.

Interestingly, what holds for the history of humankind holds also for every living human being, for, despite major modern breakthroughs in objectively gauging the occurrence of dreams in sleep, we really do not know how far back dreams extend in the life of a human being. One could argue from the scientific literature that the younger we are, the more time we spend in the dream state, with the fetus occupied with dreaming more than at any future time; or, we could also argue—again from modern scientific research—that notwithstanding the objective indications of dreaming, most of us do not really engage in dreaming until we are about seven years of age and do not hit our dreaming stride until around puberty. Dreaming, as we shall see, is not only fascinating but is also tricky.

4,000 Years Ago: The Dream of Dumuzi and the Interpretation of Geshitinanna

If we were to consider the past 3,000 years, we would have more data than we could easily handle in any brief historical introduction. But, if we strained further back, even a little, the written history of dreaming precipitously drops off. Perhaps the earliest dream recorded in writing (on clay tablets) goes back some 4,000 years. It is a nightmare reported by the Sumerian shepherd-king, Dumuzi, to Geshitinanna, "My sister who knows the meaning of words, my wise woman who knows the meaning of dreams" (Wolkstein & Kramer, 1983, p. 75):

DOI: 10.4324/9781003300441-2

My sister, listen to my dream:
Rushes grow thick about me.
A single growing reed trembles for me.
From a double-growing reed, first one, then the other, is removed.
In a wooded grove, the terror of tall trees rises about me. . . .
Water is poured over my holy hearth.
My shepherd's crook has disappeared.
An eagle seizes a lamb from the sheepfold.
A falcon catches a sparrow on the reed fence.
My sister, your goats drag their lapis beards in the dust.
Your sheep scratch the earth with bent feet.
The churn lies silent; no milk is poured.
The cup lies shattered; Dumuzi is no more.
The sheepfold is given to the winds.

(Wolkstein & Kramer, 1983, pp. 75–76)
[Reprinted with the permission of Rachel Zucker, Estate Administrator]

Because of its terrible meaning, Geshitinanna wishes her brother had not shared his dream ("My brother, do not tell me your dream/ Dumuzi, do not tell me such a dream" [p. 75], but she proceeds to give a symbolic interpretation of the dream (e.g., the "single growing reed" represents their mother; the "double-growing reed," Dumuzi and Geshitinanna), with the overall gloom-drenched dream foretelling the impending death of the family.

This ancient dream makes contact with several issues in modern dream psychology. Dumuzi's dream, for example, seems to have nothing to do with wish-fulfillment, as Freud would have it; it is a negative, upsetting dream, which, as research shows, characterizes the majority of dreams. Some dreams, of course, are positive, even wish-fulfilling (we will presently encounter several of these) but most dreams are not wish-fulfilling. Despite the contraveiling evidence, Freud obstinately tried to hold on to his wish-fulfillment theory of dreaming (arguing, e.g., that what seems to be negative on the surface might be wish-fulfilling at a deeper level, or that a negative dream might represent a guilt-based wish to punish oneself) but, because of the trauma-related nightmares observed on a massive scale in the dreams of traumatized soldiers in WWI, Freud eventually was forced to acknowledge that dreams, after all, were not necessarily wish-fulfilling.

Geshitinanna's interpretation of the dream does resonate with Freud's emphasis of psychological depth and the necessity of distinguishing *manifest* (surface) from *latent* (deeper) *content*. The semantic action in Geshitinanna's interpretation of Dumuzi's dream lies in the latent (deeper) content. Except for the concluding fragment ("Dumuzi is no more ..."), a quantitative *content-analysis* of the manifest content would mostly yield a count of fauna and animals (rushes, reeds, groves, tall trees, goats, sheep, eagles, lambs, falcons). As will be elaborated in more detail in Chapters 2 and 5, many modern dream researchers have limited themselves, essentially, to such counts of surface semantic contents. The neuroscientist and psychiatrist, Allan Hobson, perhaps the most influential dream theorist since Freud (and, also, a severe critic of Freud), actually denied the existence of latent contents and insisted on the "transparency" of dreams. As we shall see, this denial of depth is not viable. *Both* surface and deep semantic contents exist in meaningful communications and both need to be assessed for a full assay of dream content.

Finally, it may be noted that Dumuzi's dream anticipates the *continuity principle* widely espoused by modern dream scientists, which holds that there is a rough continuity between the events and concerns of waking life and the events and concerns of dreaming life. The fauna and animals in Dumuzi's dream obviously reflect the contents of Dumuzi's world. We do not know, however, what specific concerns and anxieties from his waking life animated the scary content in Dumuzi's dream.

It is possible that with some effort we might find another written dream report that antedates Dumuzi's but, because of the disappearance of written language as we go back in time, it is not likely to be much older. As noted, the historical fact of the evanescence of language has a counterpart in the dreams of contemporary living human beings. Freud made much of the problem of "representability" in dreams since dreams do not (usually) have abstract linguistic representations available to them and express themselves mostly in concretistic terms, especially in visual imagery and behavioral enactments ("dramatizations"). When we report a dream we (like Dumuzi) tend to report images of scenes, people, actions, and not abstract propositions such as would be found in a legal brief or a mathematical proof.

Here, there is substantial convergence between psychological observation and modern neuroscience research. Dreams are *paradoxical states* in which the advanced executive systems of the mind or brain responsible for logical, abstract thinking (the "ego" in Freud's system, "reason" in Plato's, "prefrontal cortical areas" in neuroscience) are substantially deactivated while, simultaneously, phylogenetically more primitive systems, such as the "reptilian brain" and the *limbic system*, as well as the more posterior imagery areas in the neocortex, are highly activated. Thus, dreams, as Freud stressed more than a century ago, are "regressive" in content and form, a notion that Freud adapted from his favorite neuroscientist, Hughlings Jackson, who had proposed that brain damage results in a phylogenetic "retrogression" in function, from more advanced to more primitive. Actually, it might not be unreasonable to consider dreaming as reflecting, in some sense, transitory episodes of brain "damage" in which certain brain areas are effectively knocked out, even if temporarily.

Cro-Magnon Cave Painting of a Dream: Jouvet's Interpretation

Even if ancient humans experienced dreams as abundantly as modern humans, they would not have been able, because of the absence of written language, to leave records of their dreams except, perhaps, for concrete depictions in the form of paintings or petroglyphs. In fact, there are some, although very few, cases of ancient dream representations found in cave paintings, the oldest of which is a Cro-Magnon cave-painting going back some 18,000 years. It was introduced into the

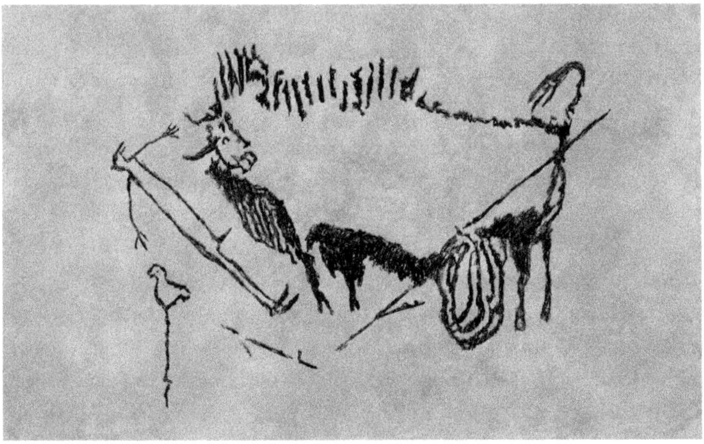

FIGURE 1.1 Cro-Magnon cave painting in Lascaux, France, of a dream from some 18,000 years ago. (Ellie Lacourt, rendering artist).

psychological literature and interpreted by the great dream neuroscientist Michel Jouvet, who originally designated dreams as "paradoxical sleep." This pictorial report of a dream, which Jouvet used as the cover of his 1999 book (*The Paradox of sleep: The story of dreaming*) is rendered above (in Figure 1.1) because, like Dumuzi's dream, it links up with important themes in modern dream psychology and is a good conduit for introducing some key players in modern dream science.

A notable fact about Jouvet's interpretation of the cave painting is that it is the only interpretation in the whole book. Jouvet courses over a wide terrain–dreaming in cats, rapid eye-movement (REM) in sleep, electroencephalograms (EEG's), genetic reprogramming during dreaming, muscle inhibition, the pons and the medulla in the brainstem, dreaming in dolphins—but, like many biologists dealing with dreams, he focuses on *mechanisms* and *functions*, and not on the *meaning* of dreams. Unlike Hobson, who was a psychiatrist with a knowledge of psychoanalysis and whose anti-psychoanalytic vehemence was (as he sometimes noted) partly a reaction to the excesses of the psychoanalytic establishment in Boston (where he got his psychiatric training), Jouvet was not conversant with psychoanalysis. Nevertheless, Jouvet devoted many pages of his book to criticisms of psychoanalysis which, as he acknowledged, he took wholesale from Hobson, who had spent a fraught year away from Harvard doing research with Jouvet in France, at Lyon. Jouvet did form a friendly relationship with Charles Fisher, a noted psychoanalyst visiting France from New York City, who figures prominently in our story, but, although he regarded Fisher as a "great physiologist" and "one of the founding fathers of the modern neurobiology of dreaming" (p. 122), Jouvet found it difficult to reconcile his admiration for Fisher with Fisher's devotion to psychoanalysis.

It is only when Jouvet is obliged to deal with a semantic phenomenon—the meaning of the Cro-Magnon artist's dream—that he resorts to dream interpretation.

But why, in the first place, is the cave-painting considered a dream? This in itself turns out to be an interpretation based on the discovery by Charles Fisher and others (Fisher, Gross, & Zuch, 1965; Ohlmeyer, Brilmeyer, & Hüllstrung, 1944) that dreaming in men is highly correlated with the occurrence of penile erections. Penile erections thus join several other objective indicators of dreaming discovered or codified at the University of Chicago in the 1950s by, among others, Nathaniel Kleitman, Eugene Aserinsky, and William Dement (Aserinsky & Kleitman, 1953; Dement & Kleitman, 1957). (An obvious question about penile erections, resolved later on, is whether women experience similar behavioral arousal while dreaming. The answer is, yes, as dreaming in women is found to be highly correlated with clitoral engorgement and vaginal lubrication. What is not resolved is whether such unambiguous behavioral arousal in sexual organs can be considered sexual since verbal reports by both men and women during these periods of dream arousals are not typically about sex.)

Jouvet's interpretation of the cave painting of the slumbering man next to the mortally wounded bison (note the bison's entrails are hanging out; the spear has gone through the animal and a broken piece of the spear lies on the ground) was that the sleeping man was dreaming—wishfully dreaming—about a successful hunt. The fact that he was dreaming was evidenced by the man's erection (which we now know almost invariably indicates dreaming in a sleeping man). The bird in the manifest content was linked to shamanic notions of the period but was left undeveloped.

Semantic Depth: Manifest vs. Latent Content

Jouvet's interpretation of the dream points to a key notion about dream interpretation that will be a leitmotif of the present work: The latent content of a dream is the interaction of the manifest content with context, namely, additional information (external or internal). When we are dealing with a dream text we are in effect dealing not with one but with at least two different stimuli: (1) the *manifest content* and (2) the *interaction* of the manifest content with context, which constitutes the *latent content*. Research psychologists familiar with standard statistics, as they must be in order to publish their work in scientific journals, have been trained to report not only *main effects* but also *interactions*, and are cognizant of the fact that important findings are often found not in the main effects but in the interactions. Similarly, in dreams—and in jokes—the action often resides in the interaction of manifest content with context, i.e., in the latent content. Now, context in a given situation may be insufficient and only with additional contextual information can a definite interpretation be achieved. The addition of more context may alter the preliminary interpretation extracted. This is obvious to anyone working on a cross-word puzzle. In the present case, Jouvet's interpretation, although reasonable, may be premature. Further context may lead elsewhere. For example, it is relevant information that a recently dead man may develop an erection, sometimes referred to as "angel lust." Thus, an alternative hypothesis (interpretation) is that the reclining man is actually dead, perhaps killed by the wounded bison, and is evidencing angel lust. Further context, however, would side with Jouvet's interpretation, as postmortem erections usually occur when the man dies vertically or face-down and remains so.

The moral here is not that interpretation is invariably doomed to uncertainty but that reliable interpretation may require more information. In a "semantic algebra game," to be elaborated later on in Chapter 2, in which a semantic x is embedded in a succession of additional contextual frames, it can be shown (and has been shown) that, with sufficient additional contextual cues, tentative interpretations change with more context but eventually settle on a reliable, fixed meaning.

Repression of Dreams

If the Cro-Magnon artist already knew the relationship between dreams and penile erections then, as Jouvet notes, this information, which we have adduced to a discovery of the 20th century, must have been known and then forgotten for a long time. Further, introducing a surprising (but unacknowledged) Freudian note, Jouvet suggests that this forgetting may have been tendentious: "I have no valid explanation for the disappearance of interest in dream erection for thousands of years. Certainly, the three great Monotheistic religions tended to censor the phenomenon. Dreams were divine messages to dreamers, but if they were accompanied by an erection it might suggest some influence from the devil!" (pp. 171–172).

Censorship of dreams, which tend to be too honest (because they are disinhibited), is an old story. For example, St. Augustine (354–430 AD), from whom Carl Gustav Jung adopted the term *archetype*, was an ardent convert to Christianity from paganism but found himself vexed by the flagrantly pagan content of some of his dreams and worried about his moral responsibility for his immoral mental life of the night. Eventually he came to terms with his pagan dreams by concluding that we are not morally responsible for the contents of our dreams. St. Jerome (347–419 AD), another influential Church father, who first translated the Hebrew Bible into Latin, did not make his peace with dreams and tendentiously mistranslated "dream interpretation" (more generally, *observo somnia*, or, the "observation of dreams") as "witchcraft," thereby rendering the subject blasphemous, and therefore potentially dangerous to those attracted to the subject.

Dreams in Religion, Philosophy, Medicine, and War

With the efflorescence of written language a few thousand years ago, dreams widely permeated human culture, high and low. Every major religion—Judaism, Christianity, Islam, Hinduism, Buddhism—was touched, to a larger or lesser extent, by dreams. (For an excellent historical overview, see the late Robert Van De Castle's [1994], *Our dreaming mind*.) One interesting fact, which will be later taken up in our effort to understand *universal symbols* and *archetypes*, is the miracle of the "virgin birth" which crops up in two very different major religious traditions, Christianity and Buddhism.

The Christian story is well known in the Western world. Mary, the future mother of Jesus, is betrothed to Joseph. A terrible problem—and a dangerous one in those days—crops up. Mary is pregnant before the marriage. Joseph, who is described as a "just man," considers "to divorce her quietly," but an angel appears to Joseph in a dream and assures him that Mary is pure, explaining "that what is conceived in her is of the Holy Spirit" (Matthew, 2:18), and that the resulting child would be a son, to be called Jesus, who would save his people from their sins and would be called, among other names, the "Son of God" (Luke 1:35). Why is it important for Christians to have their savior be conceived "without sin" (i.e., without sex)? Here Freud might have some things to say on the subject.

The Buddhist version of the Buddha's virginal conception is also quite Freudian, but with a different slant. Queen Maya, the future mother of the Buddha, had a dream in which she was transported to a golden palace on a high Himalayan peak. A magnificent white elephant with six shining tusks appears and circles her several times and, finally, painlessly pierces her side with one of his tusks. She awoke to the song of a bird and realized that she had conceived a child who would be a universal monarch. The child, Siddhartha Gautama, grew up in royal opulence but, abandoning his home and his family, and subjecting himself to years of grueling spiritual struggles, achieves enlightenment and becomes the Buddha, the Awakened One. There is more Freud in the Buddha conception story but, perhaps, we need not belabor the subject any further.

Not only the religious intelligentsia but also the great philosophers and physicians of antiquity were touched by dreams and contributed to our understanding of dreams. Both Hippocrates (469–391 BC), the putative father of medicine, and Aristotle (384–322 BC), Plato's student, published works on dreams (Aristotle actually published three works on the subject, including *On dreams*). Aristotle had a very modern—and possibly correct—theory of why dreams might be especially sensitive indicators of current body states. His theory was that because of the absence of interference by external stimuli during sleep, greater attention can be focused on subtle internal sensations expressed in dreams and therefore significant patterns detected that otherwise might have been missed.

Aristotle also scoops, by more than two thousand years, the recently published proposal by the author (Erdelyi, 2014), that universal symbols are universal by dint of the universality of their referents. The proposal applies to *concretistic symbols*, that is, ones which analogically represent referents by physical or functional resemblances (semioticists prefer to call these "signs," but to avoid undue proliferation of terms, we shall contrapose concretistic with abstract representations). Abstract symbols, unlike their concretistic counterparts, represent referents arbitrarily. Thus, the Hungarian word *három* represents "three," but only by arbitrary convention, whereas the Roman numeral "III" or the Chinese "三" concretistically represent the number *three* because three sticks are involved. This approach readily explains Freud's universal sex symbols: A penis is universally a penis across the world, and so any primitive symbol that resembles the universal referent—a spear, a gun, a rocket, an elephant's trunk—can be treated as a universal phallic symbol.

Could the reader readily conjecture why "three" (or a "triangle," or a "fleur-de-lis") might be, as Freud claims, a universal symbol for the male genitalia, or why a "box" or a "nest" symbolize the female sex organ? Aristotle had proposed that "the most skillful interpreter of dreams is he who has the faculty of observing resemblances" such as shape, colors, textures, activities, or sounds (as in puns). The subject is potentially critical for dream interpretation, for, if we can read the universal symbols in dreams, we will have taken a major step toward interpreting dreams. The subject will be taken up in more detail later on.

Claudius Galen (approximately, 131 AD–201 AD), the personal physician of the philosopher emperor, Marcus Aurelius, and the last great scientific physician before the Dark Ages in Europe, emphasized along with other thinkers (including Aristotle) that dreams might have special diagnostic utility, revealing the problem and location requiring medical intervention. This "X-ray" aspect of dreams (Van De Castle, 1994, p. XXV), on which there is some, though not yet enough research, is a crucial issue for dream psychology and will be examined critically later on in our book.

We might briefly note the important contributions to dream interpretation of a contemporary of Galen's, Artemidorus of Daldis (who was, actually, born in the ancient city of Ephesus, but chose the inconsequential town of Daldis for his name to memorialize his mother, who was born in Daldis). His great dream book, *Oneirocritica*, usually translated as *The interpretation of dreams*, scoops, in this case, and by some 1800 years, the title of Sigmund Freud's 1900 masterwork, *The interpretation of dreams.* (Just as Artemidorus was from Ephesus and not from Daldis, Sigmund Freud's famous book appeared in 1899 and not, as is officially rendered, 1900. We shall go along with both of these trifling artifices and continue to treat Artemidorus as from Daldis and to give the date of Freud's book as 1900.) Artemidorus's work, which was immensely influential around the civilized world, including the Islamic world, was divided into five books, the last two of which were kept secret to give Artemidorus's apprentice son a leg up in the interpretation business. Like Aristotle, Artemidorus placed considerable emphasis on analogic resemblances in dream interpretation. Thus: Dreams of tools that cut or divide, signify disagreements or injuries; tools that smooth surfaces, predict the smoothing of relationships; a wolf in a dream signifies a violent enemy, while a fox signifies a cunning, wily adversary. In significant ways Artemidorus's *Oneirocritica* anticipates Freudian and Jungian techniques. The interpreter needs to acquire detailed information on the dreamer's identity, occupation, age, finances, health, and the local customs of his world. Furthermore, the interpreter needs to make it his business to know every detail of the dream and the dreamer's attitude to each detail. According to our approach, this information constitutes some of the critical context needed for interpretation. Thus, for Artemidorus, it is not just a question of mechanically plugging in meanings for given dream contents. Artemidorus also anticipates the importance of *symbolism*, *metaphor*, and *puns*, which form such critical aspects of the Freudian approach and which only now are beginning to be rediscovered by quantitative content-analysts—of this, more later.

Apart from the thinking classes—religious thinkers, philosophers, physicians—dream interpretation was also a serious preoccupation of great men of action. Alexander the Great (356–323 BC) had been stymied in his efforts to conquer Tyre and was considering retreating from the siege of the mighty city. He then had a fateful dream (fateful and terrible for the poor people of Tyre). In the dream a satyr appeared and mocked Alexander. Alexander tried to catch the insolent satyr who, after much chasing, fell into his hands. The dream interpreter used a very contemporary Freudian word-play technique: The Greek word for satyr, *satyros*, can be divided into two parts, *sa* ("yours") and *tyros* (Tyre)—hence, *Tyre is yours.* (Of course, the capture of the difficult satyr is quite suggestive in itself.) Alexander redoubled his siege of the city and finally prevailed. The story, of course, proves nothing. Alexander might have conquered Tyre, with or without the dream, but Alexander took the matter of dream interpretation seriously and throughout his arc of conquests of the Persian empire, had the interpreter, Aristander of Telmessos, accompany him to provide him a handy conduit to the wisdom of dreams.

Bias in Interpretation

Aside from the empirical question of whether dreams can predict future events, which will be an issue in our later discussions, an important methodological problem concerns the possible biases, or even agendas, of the interpreter. We see this in a work of that great methodologist, William Shakespeare, who in his play, *Julius Caesar*, poses the problem of two contradictory interpretations being rendered for the same dream. The dream was dreamt by Caesars's wife, Calpurnia, who was terrified by the dream and begged her husband not to go to the Forum, lest he be assassinated there by the Senators of Rome. Caesar describes his wife's dream as follows:

> She dream'd tonight she saw my statue,
> Which, like a fountain with a hundred
> spouts,
> Did run pure blood; and many lusty Romans
> came smiling,
> and did bathe their hands in it:
> And these does she apply for warnings and
> portents
> and evils imminent; and on her knee
> Hath begg'd that I will stay at home today.

But Decius, one of the Senate conspirators who has come to fetch Caesar to the Forum, disarms Caesar with a different (and fatal) interpretation:

> This dream is all amiss interpreted:
> It was a vision fair and fortunate:

> Your statue spouting blood in many pipes,
> In which so many smiling Romans bath'd,
> Signifies that from you great Rome shall
> suck
> Reviving blood; and that great men shall
> press
> For tinctures, stains, relics, and cognizance.
> This by Calpurnia's dream is signified.

If we are to lay the foundations for a science of dream interpretation, which is the goal of the present work, it will be essential to develop techniques that yield unbiased outcomes. The interpretation of a dream should be as unbiased as, say, the interpretation of a pregnancy test. Whether the woman is desperate for a positive result or desperate for a negative result, the test should be honest, yielding not what is desired but what is true.

The great Roman orator, Cicero (104–8 BC), who was a sharp-tongued intellect of ancient times who held no brief for dreams, in part because of the problem of the same dream yielding different interpretations, actually wrote a treatise, "Argument Against Taking Dreams Seriously," which prefigures, as we will see, much of modern academic psychology's attitude toward dreams. Cicero's disdain for dreams was scathing and ad hominem:

> Even if true interpretations of dreams could exist, it is certainly not in the possession of those who profess it, for these people are the lowest and most ignorant of the people. . . . Let us reject, therefore, this divination of dreams, as well as all other kinds. For, to speak truly, that superstition has extended itself through all nations, and has oppressed the intellectual energies of all men, and has betrayed them into endless imbecilities. (Cicero. "Argument Against Taking Dreams Seriously."
>
> In R. L. Woods (Ed.). *The World of Dreams.* NY: Random House, 1947, p. 199.)

We should not argue with Cicero's scathing dismissal of dream interpretation. Rather, we should treat his assertion as our null-hypothesis and, as experimental psychologists are trained to do, prove the null hypothesis to be empirically false. Modern psychology, although it has not been as explicit as Cicero, has by and large taken the same position, and has, basically, gone to sleep on dreams for some half a century. Allan Hobson, who is often credited with modern psychology's widespread dismissal of the meaningfulness of dreams, began to back down on the basis of developing and irrefutable research data. Although Hobson continued to assert the transparency of dreams and to deny the reality of latent contents, more recently he complained about having been "misunderstood" with respect to dream meaning. But, as we shall see, the meaning of dreams that Hobson was willing to concede (in what he calls the "formalistic" approach) is a generic take on dream meaning and not the personal insights involving the individual dreamer that often are hidden from the dreamer and which could be life-changing for the dreamer.

Behaviorism and the Eclipse of Dreams in Modern Psychology

Perhaps the eclipse of dreams in modern psychology has a wider ambit than Hobson's work and is more broadly a function of the "cognitive revolution" against behaviorism not yet fully asserting itself in dream science. (Hobson, actually, was the recipient of the brain waves of his late colleague at Harvard, B. F. Skinner, the avatar of radical behaviorism, who made a gift of a record of his EEG waves to Hobson).

Two problems of behaviorism are especially germane for dream science: (1) behaviorism's superficialism (only the palpable surface content of stimuli or behaviors can be regarded as scientific, and not the deeper inferred contents), an issue, as will be seen, that still smolders in modern quantitative analytic approaches to dreams; and (2) behaviorism's extreme empiricist stance—the mind is a *tabula rasa* (a blank slate) on which experience writes; what we known is only what we learn. Both of these guiding stances of behaviorism have been widely falsified, in one important case by two students of Skinner.

Behaviorism's untrammeled embrace of empiricism led to its absolutist stance on the "nurture" side of the *Nature vs. Nurture* controversy. The classic contraposition was introduced into psychology over a hundred years ago by Sir Francis Galton (a half-cousin of Darwin's), but was already anticipated by none other than Shakespeare. In his strange, last play, *The Tempest*, Shakespeare has Prospero despair of his efforts to nurture Caliban, his charge: "A devil, a born devil, on whose nature/ Nurture can never stick; on whom my pains, / Humanely taken, all, all lost, quite lost . . . . (*The Tempest*, IV, 1).

To the contrary, John B. Watson, the father of behaviorism, made the strong claim that nurture, properly applied, can override nature:

> Give me a dozen healthy infants, well formed, and my own specified world to bring them up in and I'll guarantee to take any at random and to train him to become any type of specialist I might select—doctor, lawyer, artist, merchant chief, and yes, even beggar-man and thief, regardless of the talents, penchants, tendencies, abilities, vocations, and race of his ancestors.
>
> *(1930, p. 104)*

Thus, according to Watson, we are what we learn—and *conditioning* (mostly classical, or Pavlovian conditioning in Watson's treatment), is the major conduit for this learning. Watson's view led to one of the most celebrated experimental studies in psychology, "The Case of Little Albert," carried out by Watson and his research assistant, Rosalie Rayner (published in 1920), in which it was demonstrated that an irrational fear, such as the fear of a small, unthreatening animal, was the result of Pavlovian conditioning and not a symbolic expression of some unconscious fear of, for example, castration (as claimed by Freud (1909a/1955) for "Little Hans," who was terrified of horses).

Conditioning and Instinctive Drift

Watson and Rayner's technique for training the (presumably) all-malleable infant, Albert, an 11-month-old child, was the same as the one used by Pavlov to train his dogs to salivate to an initially neutral stimulus, such as a bell. In the Watson and Rayner study, Little Albert was trained to develop a fear of an albino rat, which he had originally liked (he smiled at the rat, reached out to it, called it "doggie"), through the pairing of a startling loud noise with the rat. After a few such pairings, Little Albert was scared of the rat, cried on its sight, and tried to crawl away from it. He had, in short, learned a phobia through classical conditioning.

The study was not without its problems. How could it account for phobias for which no unpleasant associated events could be remembered (forgetting, perhaps)? And, most critically, are the data reliable? It is clear from subsequent experimental work (see Dollard & Miller, 1950) and the literatures on "traumatic conditioning" that fear can be classically conditioned (and lead to "traumatic neurosis," or, to symptoms of what is called these days, "post-traumatic-stress-disorder"), but what of cases where classical conditioning does not work as intended? It is in their failures that conditioning studies open the door to biological biases in cognition—and, therefore, in dreams.

There was, in fact, an important failure to replicate the Little Albert results by Elsie Bregman (1934), a graduate student of Louis Thorndike, who along with B. F. Skinner, developed the second principal modality of conditioning, *instrumental conditioning* (Thorndike's term), or *operant conditioning* (Skinner's). Bregman tried to replicate the Watson and Reyner study with inanimate stimuli rather than a rat, for example, a wood block or pieces of cloth, but got nothing—neither conditioning, nor recognition in the field for her non-replication. Watson, after all, was a world famous psychologist and the neophyte Bregman might not have been up to the task. Only decades later, when similar negative findings began to churn the other conditioning literatures, did it become clear that biological biases had to be considered in conditioning—the mind was not a *tabula rasa*, after all—and an interpretation of the non-replication became possible. As with a dream, additional information had to be applied to the phenomenon—in this case, the failure by Bregman to replicate Watson and Rayner—to extract its meaning.

There was no long-term follow-up in Watson's laboratory. One reason for this was that, notwithstanding Watson's international fame and his professorship at The Johns Hopkins University, he was canned from his job for creating a sex scandal that was much ballyhooed in the local press: Watson, a married man—and married to a wife with a powerful family—was discovered to be having a sexual affair with his research assistant, Rosalie Rayner. Watson sent out some 300 letters of application to other universities, but he was blackballed from academia and eventually had to find employment in the real world outside. He was a resourceful man, famous not for no reason, and finally took a position at the J. Walter Thompson advertising agency, of which, within three years, he became vice president. (For sentimental, old-fashioned readers, it might be added that the gentleman married the lady, with whom he was to have two children, and that they actually lived happily ever after until her death at a young age.)

Decades later, two students of B. F. Skinner's at Harvard, Keller Breland and Marian Breland, who after graduating sought to capitalize on their expertise in animal learning by starting a business for training animals, discovered that animals outside of the rarified confines of the Harvard Psychology Department did not behave according to expectations. In their 1961 paper in the *American Psychologist*, "The Misbehavior of Organisms," they highlighted the notion of *instinctive drift*, by which they meant biological biases that demonstrably intrude into straightforward operant conditioning. Although the title of their paper was not without meaning, it bears some interpretation: The crucial context is that Skinner's (1938) magnum opus was titled, *The behavior of organisms.* Clearly, what was intended by Breland and Breland was that in the real world, animals did not necessarily follow the simple precepts of operant conditioning laid down by their famous professor.

A few examples illustrate the point. In an effort to train pigeons to play baseball, pigeons were successfully conditioned to hit with their beak a ball that was pitched to them (it was not a Tom Seaver hard ball but a gently lobbed ping-pong ball). Success required some sensory-motor coordination, but the pigeons mastered the task, with hits "reinforced" with a grain of maize. With this difficult part out of the way, the second easy step was to condition the pigeons to run or hop to first base after getting a hit. But the pigeons could not master this simple task. Instead, after getting a hit, they seemed to be overcome by an invincible urge to chase the bouncing ball they had hit. It was as if there already was a stamped-in, deeper program in the pigeon: Chase the bobbing stimulus (for it might be a delectable morsel of food). Thus, not all the action is at the surface and under the convenient control of the experimenter.

Here are a few, even simpler examples (not drawn from Breland & Breland): As Skinner famously showed, a pigeon could be reliably conditioned to peck at a disk to get some food reinforcement. Yet, strangely, pigeons could not learn *not-to-peck* to get reinforcement (Williams & Williams, 1969). Nor could they learn to escape a shock by pecking at a disk (Hineline & Rachlin, 1969), though they could learn to flap their wings or hop to escape.

Essentially equivalent findings have been reported for *imitation* learning (Miller & Dollard, 1941), or *observational learning* (Bandura, 1977; Bandura, Ross, & Ross, 1963)—basically, "monkey-see-monkey-do" learning. An untrained monkey who was not afraid of snakes is made to watch a film in which another monkey is startled by a snake and reacts with much fear. The observer monkey thereafter reacts with fear to a picture of a snake. Interestingly, if the snake is spliced out of the film and a neutral stimulus, such as a flower, is substituted for it, the observation of a monkey showing fear to the flower does not yield observational learning. Apparently, there is biological preparation for learning to fear a snake, but not for learning to fear a flower. (For an excellent overview, see Mineka & Zinbarg (2006).)

In sum, a superficialist approach, focusing only on surface stimuli and responses, is insufficient. Nature plays a role also. In reality, it is not "Nature vs. Nurture" but "Nature *and* Nurture." Modern research on *heritability* (h^2), a mathematical index of the extent to which genetic factors are involved in some psychological trait (from 0% to 100%), shows that for virtually every personality trait studied, normal or abnormal—neuroticism, extraversion, agreeableness, conscientiousness, hypnotizability, IQ, homosexuality, religiosity, schizophrenia—heritability is around 50%. Biological biases should therefore be taken into account in dream interpretation. Universal symbols or more complex cognitive schemas may have a partly biological foundation; we may be predisposed to dream of certain things and in certain ways.

Dreams and Darwin

The breakdown of the extreme empiricist position has been a great shock to social scientists, and not just to behaviorists. Empiricism was an almost axiomatic starting point for major segments of the field. Even William James (1890), in his classic *Principles of psychology*, asserted that we have to learn to see meaningfully, stating that the visual world of the infant is "one great booming, buzzing confusion" (p. 488). Not so. Newly born infants may perhaps not see as well as older children (they tend, for example, to be near-sighted) but they do see a meaningful world around them. They can even perceive "beauty" in humans, which is not, as sometimes asserted, all a cultural artifact, as newborns selectively gaze more at attractive humans and less at unattractive ones. As unpalatable as the Nature position has been to social scientists, the importance of genetic factors for psychology has moved from argument to solid consensus. The best summary conclusion is that heritability, h^2, is 50% ± 20% for psychological traits (the ± 20% reflecting variability in the data reported in the research literature). Even at its lower range (around 30%), genetic factors are hugely significant and can no longer be dismissed by psychological scientists. Dream science cannot be an exception. Nature may play a guiding role in the content and style of our dreams.

We might stop here and declare the fact a fact. But we could choose to probe further and ask how Nature stamped itself so indelibly upon our minds. Here Charles Darwin's theory of evolution may provide a bridging answer: We have evolved, over endless generations, to be the way we are physically. This is almost universally accepted among scientists. If so, why restrict ourselves to the physical? We may assume that we have analogously evolved psychologically. Actually, Darwin himself explicitly pointed in this direction in his epochal book, *The origin of species* (1859). He had tried, in this early work, to avoid dealing with humans for fear, quite justified as it turned out, of provoking the opprobrium of religious people (including his wife) for propounding a theory that upended a literalistic interpretation of creation in the *Bible*. Yet, toward the conclusion of his book, Darwin presciently predicted that his theory of evolution would lay a new foundation for psychology.

Psychologists have for a long time attempted to incorporate Darwin into their conceptual framework but only in the last generation has Darwinian psychology, most commonly called *evolutionary psychology*, seriously penetrated the discipline.

Even dream theory has begun to be influenced. Importantly for our purposes, Darwinian psychology provides a framework for psychological universals, including dream symbols or more complex dream schemas (*archetypes of the collective unconscious*, in Jung's language). Jung, indeed, may be regarded as the earliest proponent of evolutionary psychology:

> Our mind has its history, just as the body has its history. . . . Our unconscious mind, like our body, is a storehouse of relics and memories of the past. A study of the unconscious collective mind would reveal the same discoveries as you make in comparative anatomy. . . . [At birth our] mind is not a *tabula rasa.*
>
> *(Jung, 1968, pp. 44–45)*

Thus, we are biologically programmed to think—to fantasize, to dream, to hallucinate—in certain standard ways. The collective unconscious, made up of archetypes, is therefore a transpersonal unconscious that we all more or less share as a result of our common biological ancestry.

In his book, *The expression of the emotions in man and animal*, Darwin (1872/1879) showed clearly that animal expressions follow universal rules. For example, the face of a threatening dog (Figure 1.2) is unambiguous; Cicero would not have cared to pet this pooch. Further, not only do animals emit standard communicative expressions, but they are also excellent interpreters of them—their lives depend on it! Thus, there are not only biologically prepared meanings in animal expressions, but also, as Darwin noted (1872/1879, p. 1471), biologically prepared mechanisms for interpreting such expressions.

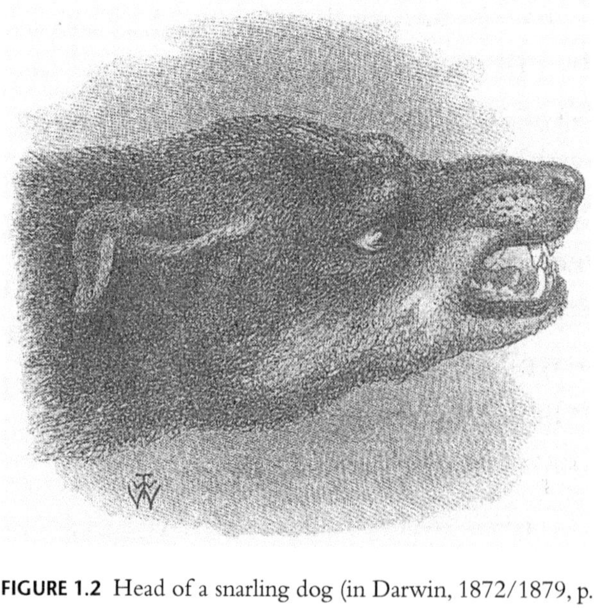

FIGURE 1.2 Head of a snarling dog (in Darwin, 1872/1879, p. 1327).

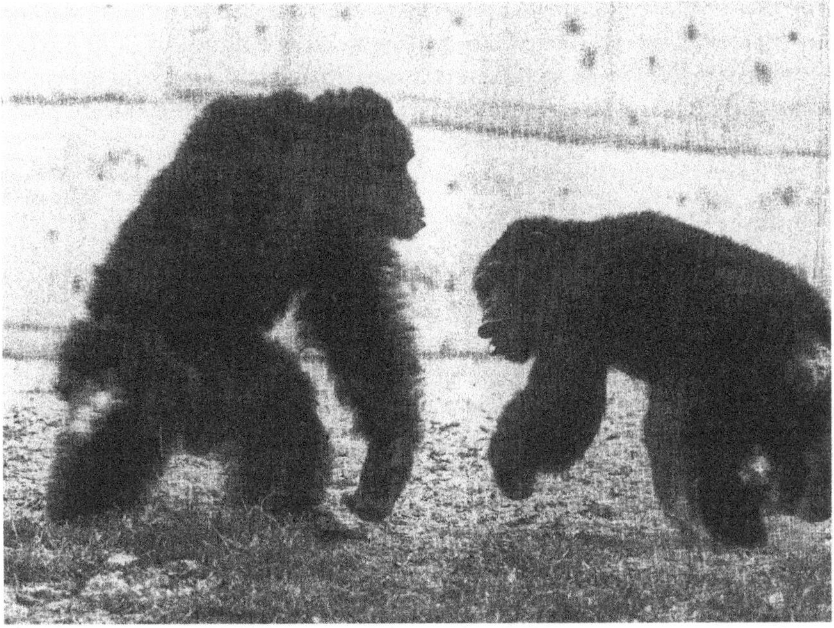

FIGURE 1.3 Nikkie (left) looks larger, walking upright with bristling hair, while the shrinking Luit avoids him with "greeting" sounds." (Frans De Waal (2007). *Chimpanzee politics: Power and sex among apes*. Baltimore: Johns Hopins University Press) (p. 130.) [Reproduced with permission, The Johns Hopkins University Press.]

In his book, *Chimpanzee politics: Power and sex among apes*, Frans De Waal (2007) presents a photo, meaningful to us humans, of a dominant male chimpanzee, Nikkie, assuming a dominant, threatening posture (the bristling hair is standard in such meaningful displays) toward his opponent, Luit, who obviously knows body language for submission (see Figure 1.3). Animals, as De Waal shows, are more sensitive interpreters of the body language of their conspecifics than humans and anticipate interpersonal developments that are not obvious to the human expert for weeks. Thus, we might profitably invest some research effort to discovering some universal themes in human dreams. Jung has already suggested standard motifs which are archetypal (the mandala, the wise old man, the monster, the hero) but experimental psychology has not engaged this facet of dreams and Jung's proposed archetypes await validation.

Darwin devotes considerable attention to the question of the universal expression of emotions by humans—fear, grief, dejection, anger, disgust, surprise, joy—which modern research shows are more or less universally interpreted across cultures (Ekman & Friesen, 1975). Thus, observers from five countries—the United States, Brazil, Chile, Argentina, and Japan—tend to reliably recognize the expressions of *fear*, *disgust*, *happiness*, and *anger*. Even these "universal" facial expressions are not, however, perfectly interpreted by humans. The recognition of "happiness" comes closest to unanimity (for observers from the five countries, concordance rates were,

97%, 95%, 95%, 98%, and 100%, respectively). The recognition of "fear" was the least concordant among interpreters, ranging from 54% in Argentina to 85% in the United States. The point here is that even when interpretation is extremely accurate, we cannot expect perfect performance, and must be satisfied with probabilities (which are impressive in these cases).

Helmholtz's "Unconscious Inferences": Interpreting Depth and Constancies from Shifting 2-D Displays

The interpretation of complex visual patterns has been a classic issue in visual perception. The great 19th-century physicist–physiologist–psychologist, Hermann Von Helmholtz, introduced the influential notion of *unconscious inference* to explain how humans are able to perceive distance and make adjustments for distance in extracting *constancy* (of size, shape) from the chaotically varying objective stimuli impinging upon our retinas. This is a truly remarkable interpretative achievement, involving the magical extraction of 3-D perception from 2-D displays, a feat that goes largely unappreciated because all of us (and animals, too) do it so effortlessly. Size-constancy (our ability to see objects as retaining their constant size notwithstanding changes of the objective size of the images subtended on our retinas), involves unconscious mathematical transformations on the impinging stimuli that correct for the distance between the perceiver and the perceived object. Size constancy is very easy to demonstrate. A professor in front of a small class asks his students to estimate his height. The students in the front row obviously have a larger image of the professor on their retinas than students in the back row. Despite this difference, by a remarkable psychological transformation of the professor's image that takes the professor's distance into account, the professor is perceived—interpreted—as having the same size. There is some variability in both the front-row and the back-row estimates, but the average front-row and back-row estimates of the professor's height are virtually the same. (Actually, the back-row students will slightly over-correct for size and, on the average, perceive/interpret the professor's height as slightly—very slightly—larger than the estimate of front-row students.)

The critical point for dream science is that the interpretation of meanings, as with distance and size, presumably involves sophisticated, but mostly unconscious programs, that it is the business of scientists to unravel and make explicit. Research on depth-perception, which has been studied by psychologists for more than a century, has shown that depth perception is actually underpinned not by one but by a variety of "depth cues." Most of these cues reside in the stimulus (e.g., "interposition," "linear perspective," "relative size," and "continuity") but, in a few cases, internal cues (e.g., "retinal disparity," which results from the slight difference in the images subtended on the right and left eyes). The counterpart work on depth in the domain of dream science has hardly begun but, at least to some extent, is likely to yield overlapping principles. For example, most of the stimulus cues for depth—whether in perception or dream interpretation—involve context. This will be a crucial theme in our treatment of dreams, jokes, and other cognate phenomena. Also,

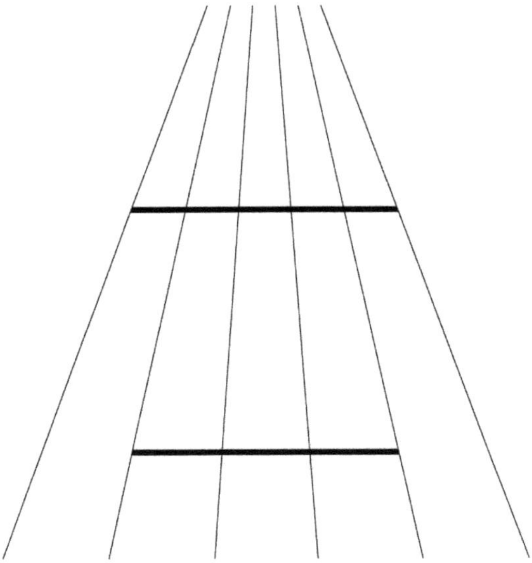

FIGURE 1.4 The Ponzo illusion.

in both the domains of perception and psychopathology (e.g., paranoia), misleading context can override objective reality and induce flagrant errors of interpretation.

Figure 1.4 depicts the *Ponzo Illusion,* which results from the perceptual system's overcorrection for the length of the top, horizontal line. The two horizontal lines are actually equal in length but the top line is seen as more distant because of the context (the linear perspective lines that embed the two horizontal lines). In the real world, a line at a distance would subtend a shorter image than an equivalent line at a shorter distance and, so, if the more distant line is objectively the same in length as the closer one, it must be (according to the perceptual interpreter) longer. This is a clever and highly adaptive heuristic—which happens to yield the wrong interpretation in this instance. Knowledge about standard illusions would help us to correct for them if we chose to recapture the objective magnitudes of the impinging stimuli.

Cognitive Psychology's Neglect of Dreams

Before we conclude this foreshadowing chapter, we might revisit the doleful claim made a few pages back (p. 13) that psychology has gone to sleep on dreams for some half a century.

It should not be surprising that behaviorists avoided dreams altogether since behaviorism, by design, excluded subjective phenomena (such as consciousness, "mental" processes, meanings, imagery, emotions, attitudes, personality traits, beauty, joy, and sadness) as falling outside the purview of science, to be relegated to a forbidden "black box" that was interposed between the objective stimulus and the objective response. But the "cognitive revolution" toward the end of the 1950s was supposed to have broken out of this straight-jacketing conception of psychology and, in effect, to have reformulated psychology as the science of the very topics that had been banished to behaviorism's black box. Yet, with the exception of seminal work on the biology of sleep and dreaming starting in the 1950s (to which we shall devote a chapter), dreams continued to be *terra incognita* to mainstream psychological science. We must contend with the fact that, in both the political and the conceptual arenas, "revolutions" are rarely complete—or completely real.

Over the last few decades several textbooks on "cognitive psychology" have appeared, focusing on topics such as conscious and unconscious processes, perception, imagery, memory, constructive processes, schemas, attention, biases, and distortions in cognition. And yet, the modal number of pages devoted to dreams in all these books on cognition is zero. The same results obtain in assays of the flagship journals of psychology—including *Psychological Review, Psychological Bulletin,* the *Journal of Experimental Psychology: General, Psychological Science, Perspectives in Psychological Science*, for which the modal number of pages devoted to dreams in each yearly volume over the last quarter-century is, again, zero. The good news is that there are signs of change. Some journals devoted to consciousness, unthinkable during the reign of behaviorism—for example, *Consciousness and Cognition*—have begun to publish important works on dreams and, crucially, the relatively new journal (actually, some 30-year-old by now), *Dreaming*, now provides a dedicated venue for the publication of research on dreaming.

Perhaps behaviorism should not take all the blame for psychology's neglect of dreams, just as Hobson should not take all the blame for the field's understanding—or misunderstanding—that dreams are essentially froth, random and meaningless effusions of the night. We must consider the likelihood that there is something deeply ingrained in the nature of academic psychology, both preceding and following the behaviorist era, that makes the field unreceptive to unwieldy phenomena of the real world. This recalcitrance of psychology probably arises from an excellent motive—the wish to safeguard the scientific bona fides of the fledgling discipline (officially no more than a century-and-a-half-old) and avoid its derailment by obscurantist impulses. Sweeping subject matters such as the meaning of dreams tend to inspire sweeping speculative leaps—as with Freud, Jung, and others—which inevitably yield sweeping errors alongside some of the sweeping insights. Academic psychology has chosen a far more cautious course, one which delimits the subject matter—and the stimuli studied. Yet, caution can be reckless too.

Memory and Dreams

One thematic example of excessive diffidence is experimental psychology's study of memory, which is critical for this project, since dreams may be regarded (as will be elaborated in Chapter 6) as noisy forms of remembering, or—by definition—forms of *implicit memory* (memory that is indicated indirectly, and of which the subject may actually be unconscious). The founder of the experimental study of memory,

Hermann Ebbinghaus (1885), introduced the ubiquitous *nonsense syllables* into the field on the grounds that nonsense syllables would not be contaminated by the superfluous associative contents that are inevitably attached to regular, meaningful stimuli, such as normal words. Now, this sounds like a commendable scientific caution—keep the stimulus pure and uncontaminated—and yet, on reflection, this scrubbing of the stimulus of meaning (never completely possible, by the way) can also be construed as an effort to keep psychology out of the stimulus. Why would we psychologists be interested in nonsense, and why should we be particularly interested in the common-sense and predictable yield of this program, highlighted in almost every introductory psychology textbooks, that memory (for nonsense) is forgotten over time (see the Ebbinghus curve of retention, plotted from his data, in Figure 1.5). In self-justification, Ebbinghaus noted that the mathematical fitting of his data yields a negative logarithmic function, which we did not appreciate until his work.

There are basic problems with the Ebbinghaus tradition that have implications for dream science. One of these is that by intentionally stripping the stimulus of associative context, Ebbinghaus concomitantly stripped stimuli of depth, which, as has already been much emphasized, depends on context. We thus get an (unintentional) methodological begging of the point: We need not worry about psychological depth because our experiments (which eliminate the contextual cues that are requisite for depth) do not yield depth.

Another basic problem is that, as Philip Boswood Ballard (1913) demonstrated in a seminal laboratory program, the course of memory over time depends on the stimuli being remembered. *Nonsense syllables* (in line with Ebbinghaus) are indeed amnesic but meaningful stimuli such as *poetry* are hypermnesic. More

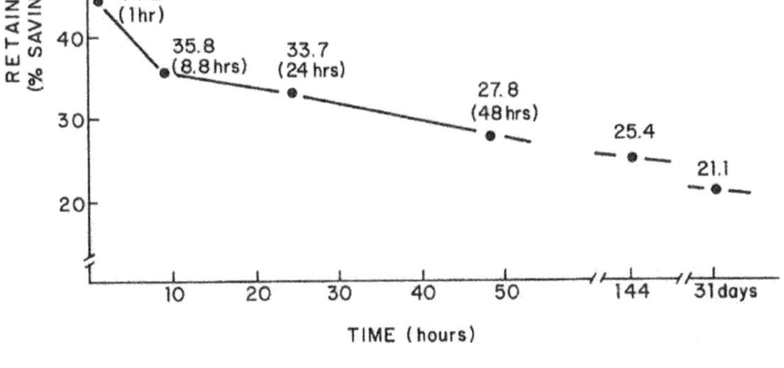

FIGURE 1.5 The course of memory over time according to Ebbinghaus (1885).

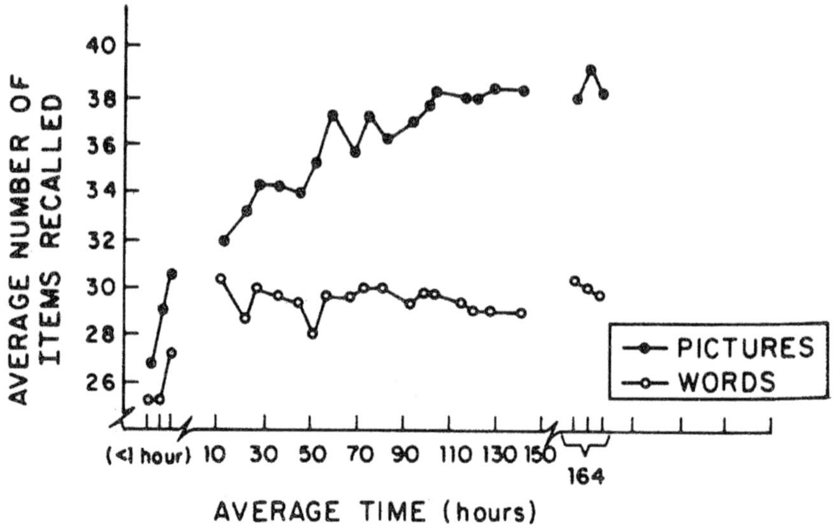

FIGURE 1.6 The course of memory over time for *pictures* and *words* (Erdelyi & Kleinbard, 1976).

recent laboratory work on memory for *pictures* and *words* has corroborated powerful stimulus effects (see Figure 1.6), with picture memory increasing over time but word memory remaining essentially unchanged (Erdelyi, 1996; Erdelyi & Kleinbard, 1978).

Perhaps Ballard's most seminal discovery (Erdelyi, 1996; 2010) was that memory over time is actually paradoxical (as dreams are), in that they *simultaneously* decrease *and* increase over time. For a group of subjects, there is, *invariably*, a loss of memory from a first recall test to a second recall test (this is hardly news; we call it "forgetting," Ballard called it *oblivescence*). What is surprising is that, just as invariably, there is also a recovery of memories from a first test to a later second test, which Ballard called, *reminiscence*. Thus, overall stimulus retention at any point in time is a *balance* between the two opposite tendencies of memory, oblivescence, and reminiscence. When reminiscence exceeds oblivescence on a particular trial, *hypermnesia* (improvement of overall memory) is obtained, which, notably, is the typical laboratory result with real-life stimuli such as pictures, poetry, jokes. We need not guess at the outcome with nonsense syllables since Ebbinghaus has already given us the answer: Memory is *amnesic* over time.

Can the reader intuit which stimulus laboratory psychologists overwhelmingly favored for most of the field's history? Yes, nonsense syllables, and lately, lists of unconnected words, which we may regard as close in spirit to nonsense-syllables. (In defense of Ebbinghaus's amnesia function, it must be noted that the experimental subject must engage in retrieval effort to obtain hypermnesia; without such retrieval effort, memory, regardless of the stimulus involved, is amnesic over a sufficiently long retention interval, although even here we can find exceptions, as in the case of traumatic stimuli, which can induce a pathological inability to forget, or, even, delayed hypermnesia.)

It is relevant for dream science that even after a long retention interval that results in decremental, or amnesic memory, it is the case that if the subject reinstitutes retrieval effort, amnesic memory will turn around and start to improve, becoming hypermnesic relative to its low point (see Erdelyi, 1996, Chapter 8). Thus, Freud's claim (1900, pp. 1–17; 589) that "dreams are hypermnesic" is compatible with the laboratory literature, and is actually to be expected if the subject/patient has begun to make repeated efforts to access long-lost memories which have become relevant (e.g., because of therapy). Also, the uncontested fact that dreams are typically rendered imagistically or as enactments ("dramatizations" [Freud, 1900, p. 50]), further favors their being hypermnesic, since it has been experimentally demonstrated that ineffective stimuli, such as strings of unrelated words, become hypermnesic if they are mentally recoded into images (for an integrative overview of the whole area, see Erdelyi (1996)).

Despite his brilliant research, Ballard ran away from the broader implications of his work, in line with experimental psychology's characteristic reluctance to grapple with murky real-life phenomena:

> When we leave the region of common experience and explore the realm of the abnormal we find evidence of reminiscence taking place on an abundant scale. We find instances of whole system of ideas passing for long periods quite beyond the possibility of recall. The study of hypnotism, trance-mediumship, double-personality, and the various kinds of amnesia arising from hysteria, epilepsy and insanity reveals abundant examples of this kind. But with none of these do I propose to deal here: I limit my enquiry to normal conditions.
>
> *(Ballard, 1913, p. 52)*

Ballard's findings actually point to grand unities, not only within psychology (experimental and clinical) but also between psychology and neuroscience, as the Ballard findings converge on the basic dualistic reality in neuroscience of both *excitatory* and *inhibitory* processes being at play. Memory, too, is dualistic, reflecting the dance of contradictory tendencies of memory (oblivescence and reminiscence) over time.

If overall retention is a balance between oblivescence and reminiscence, it follows that if we disregarded oblivescence and cumulated stimulus recoveries (reminiscences) over trials, we would get more markedly upward-trending memory functions. Figure 1.7 shows cumulative stimulus recoveries over time (disregarding forgetting in each trial) for lists of pictures or words. With cumulated recall over trials, we get upward-trending memory for *both* pictures and words.

Actually, research shows (see Erdelyi, 1996) that even for nonsense-syllables, cumulative recall increases over time. Obviously, and by now this is universally acknowledged in psychology, more is available in memory than accessible to consciousness (Breuer & Freud, 1895/1955; Erdelyi, 1996; Tulving & Pearlstone,

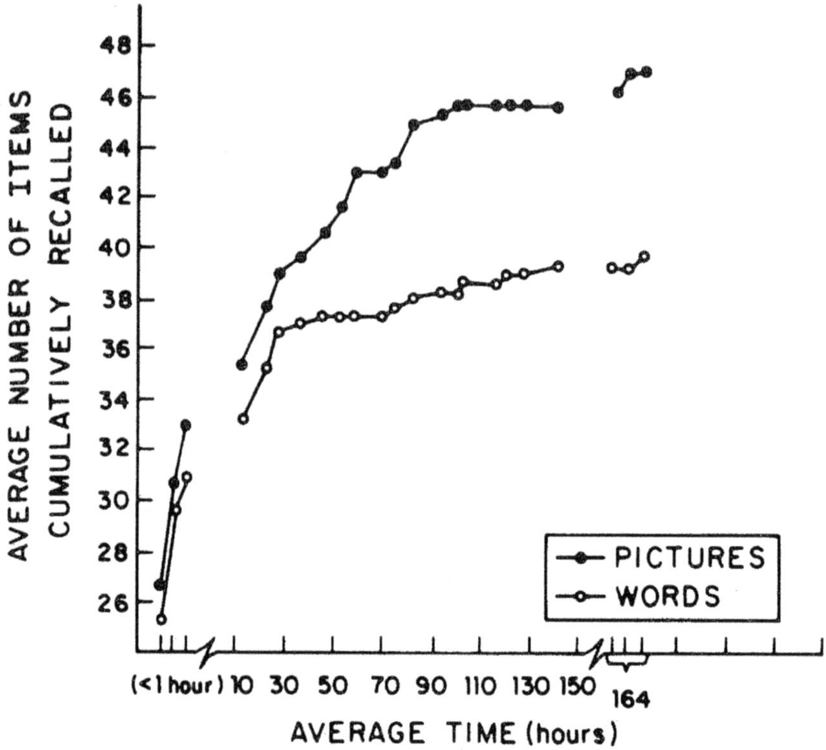

FIGURE 1.7 The course of cumulative recall over time for a list of pictures or words. (Data points represent recall trials.) (Erdelyi & Kleinbard, 1978, p. 283).

1967). If dreams were hypermnesic they would have much unconscious material to draw upon. In Chapter 6 (pp. 156–159), several real-life cases are given of dreams actually recovering materials inaccessible to waking consciousness (e.g., "The Watch Lost at the Beach and Found in a Dream" [p. 156]). Recent experimental work by Nicolas Dumay (2015) shows that, after a period of sleep, recall of recently learned materials significantly improves due (mostly) to increased access "to memory traces that had initially been too weak to be retrieved" (p. 6). It remains to be determined what role dreams might play in this "post-sleep boost in memory accessibility" (p. 6).

2

FREUD'S INTERPRETATION OF DREAMS AND HIS TREATMENT OF JOKES

Breakthroughs, Errors, Revisions

Freud's Transition from Neuroscience to Psychology

A deep understanding of Freud's approach to dreams and to other release phenomena of psychology—essentially the same, as will be seen—is much enhanced by our appreciation of his having begun his scientific career as a neuroscientist. He would have liked to remain so and continue his physiological work at the University of Vienna but was derailed from his path by a timeless problem in academia, the unavailability of regular long-term positions. He had become engaged to be married and was in need of some financial security and, so, he reluctantly left the University and opened a practice in medicine.

Given his background, Freud attracted patients suffering from a variety of illnesses resembling neurological disorders, sometimes called "neurosis" or "hysteria," which on close inspection turned out *not* to be neurological. These hysterical patients suffered from a range of symptoms, including paralyses, paresthesias (tingling sensations), memory problems such as amnesias, analgesias, and pain, which the world-renowned clinical neurologist, Pierre Charcot, of Paris, France, had shown could often be distinguished from the real thing. The paralyzed person, for example, might move his "paralyzed" leg in sleep or be temporarily cured by hypnosis, neither of which could happen with a true neurological paralysis. Charcot had also shown that the careful demarcation of the afflicted areas revealed correspondences to psychological reality (e.g., "hand") but not to neurological reality (there are no neural networks corresponding to "hand").

To advance his real-world medical expertise in the psychological domains in which he suddenly found himself and for which his academic training had not prepared him, Freud applied for and won a fellowship to spend some months in Charcot's clinic (the fabled "Salpêtrière" Clinic in Paris) and managed to get close to the much-in-demand Charcot by offering to translate some of his recent works

DOI: 10.4324/9781003300441-3

from French to German. From Charcot he was to learn a startling new fact about hysteria (a term derived from the Greek, *hystera,* meaning, womb) which, contrary to ancient tradition, turned out not to be an affliction caused by sexual frustration in females, as, for example, described by Plato in *The Timaeous*:

> In men the organ of generation—becoming rebellious and masterful, like an animal disobedient to reason, and maddened with the sting of lust—seeks to gain absolute sway; and the same is the case with the ... womb... of women; the animal within them is desirous of procreating children, and when remaining unfruitful long beyond its proper time, gets discontented and angry, and wandering in every direction through the body, closes up the passages of the breath, and obstructing respiration, drives them to extremity, causing all varieties of diseases
>
> (Plato, *The Timaeus, p. 514)*

The proof against the womb theory came from Charcot's observation of quite similar symptoms in a class of male patients. At the behest of an insurance company, he had concerned himself with the rehabilitation of railroad workers who had suffered "physical traumas" in their line of work. Despite the apparently complete healing of their physical wounds, symptoms resembling those of hysteria frequently persisted in these male patients, suggesting that hysteria was not, after all, an exclusively female disorder of the uterus.

Back in Vienna, Freud delivered a talk on the Paris breakthrough on "male hysteria" and got, not for the first time in his career, an acerbic reception from some of his colleagues. Today, of course, both male and female patients are known to develop "traumatic hysteria" or "traumatic neurosis," although the modern term for it (e.g., American Psychiatric Association, 2013) is "post-traumatic stress disorder" (PTSD).

Freud also made a brief visit to the world-famous, Hippolyte Bernheim, in Nancy, France, to get help with a patient (whom he brought along) and, also, to gain instruction in hypnotic suggestion therapy and *psychotherapeutics* (essentially, suggestive therapy without the formal induction of hypnosis). Soon, however, Freud began to learn from his own experiences with patients, and in 1895 published his first psychological book, coauthored with his friend and senior colleague, Josef Breuer, *Studies on hysteria* (Breuer & Freud, 1993-1895/1955). The book consists of five case-histories, the first one featuring Breuer's famous case of Anna O., and documents, over the course of the five cases, the rapid evolution of standard clinical techniques of the time—hypnotic suggestion, faradic treatment, massage, hot baths—into early versions of psychoanalysis. Many of the ideas in the *Studies on hysteria* anticipate *The interpretation of dreams*, published only a few years later. Hysterics, according to Freud (it is not clear if Breuer fully subscribed to this idea), "*suffer mainly from reminiscences*" (Breuer & Freud, 1993-1895/1955, p. 42). Thus, symptoms, like dreams, are forms of garbled memories. The notion of "remembering without awareness" (Jacoby & Witherspoon, 1982) is an idea that has only became mainstream in cognitive psychology and neuroscience since the

1980s. For Freud, symptoms (like dreams, later on), "have meaning" (Freud, 1917/1963, p.75) which the patients might not grasp consciously and which, at least in clinical work, required interpretation—with the help of free-associations. Freud viewed symptoms and dreams to be cut from the same cloth and sometimes explicitly suggested that "a dream is itself a neurotic symptom" (Freud, 1917/1963, p. 75) and that the task of the analyst was "the interpretation of the symptom" (Freud, 1917/1963, pp. 231, 236).

Dreams as Just One Dialect from a Family of Release-Phenomena

One of Freud's major contributions to dream psychology, actually, was the insight that dreams are only one class of phenomena in a family of phenomena—hysterical symptoms, daydreams and fantasy, art, jokes, psychotic delusions, *parapraxes* (Freudian slips)—that could be approached with essentially the same theoretical and practical tools. Almost immediately after the appearance of *The interpretation of dreams* (Freud, 1900/1953), Freud published one of his most popular books, *The psychopathology of everyday life* (1901b/1960), which dealt with the analysis and interpretation of everyday errors such as "slips of the tongue," "misreadings," "bungled actions," "memory malfunctions," and so on, collectively designated *parapraxes*, or, less formally, "Freudian slips." The crucial point for us is that these errors are not random but have meanings that can be interpreted—in the same way that dreams can be interpreted. Freud was explicit about the overlap between parapraxes and dreams: "The mechanism of parapraxes ... can be seen to correspond in its most essential points with the mechanism of dream formation which I have discussed in the chapter on the "dream-work" in my *Interpretation of Dreams* (Freud, 1901b/1960, p. 278).

Only a few years later, in 1905, Freud published his monograph, *Jokes and their relation to the unconscious*, which plays a crucial theoretical and methodological role in the present work. Freud showed the significant homologies existing between dreams and jokes, which feature the same distortions as those found in dreams termed the *dream-work* in dreams and the *joke-work* in jokes. Neither psychoanalysts nor academic psychologists have made much of jokes in their experimental and theoretical work—it is as if jokes lacked the gravitas to be taken seriously—even though it turns out that jokes are Goldilocks stimuli for psychology: They are not too simple like nonsense syllables or word strings, nor too complex like case histories or full-fledged dream samples; they are just right. In a later section, we shall examine how jokes help us understand dreams and solve some methodological and theoretical problems that are sometimes intractable in dreams.

In 1909 and 1911, Freud published two of his book-length case histories, respectively, "The Rat Man" and "The Psychotic Dr. Schreber" (as they are informally known), in which he shows the dream-like features of psychopathological disorders such as obsessive–compulsive disorders and paranoid delusions, and discusses virtually all the well-known defensive distortions, or defense-mechanisms, including *condensation, displacement, symbolism, repression/suppression (omissions, ellipses, hints, allusions), reversal, projection, concretistic representation, and representation by triviality*. These distortions are the same as those he had already identified and elaborated in his previous writings, including, *The interpretation of dreams.*

Before proceeding forward, we shall first step back to consider a critical, but unacknowledged member of this family of release phenomena, *aphasia*. Actually, we need to consider two of Freud's neuroscience works, the most important (but invisible), 1891 monograph, *On aphasia*, and the second, which Freud judged a failure and withheld from publication, *Psychology for neurologists* (completed in 1895), but which his followers published posthumously as *The project for a scientific psychology* (1895/1966).

Although *The project* provides a window into Freud's thinking at the time—it is much praised for its brilliant speculative theorizing (Pribram & Gill, 1976) but, also, lambasted for some of its mistaken notions (Hobson, 1988)—the work, after almost euphoric enthusiasm during its 9 months' gestation, was, on its completion, rejected by Freud, who was far from shy about publishing his works. Arguably, this misfired project caused much mischief for psychoanalysis. It led Freud to abandon neuroscience altogether and to pursue his ideas purely in the framework of psychology, with which Freud explicitly identified psychoanalysis. Recently, a small band of psychoanalytically oriented psychologists and neuroscientists, some of whom have played a prominent role in modern dream science (Kaplan-Solms & Solms, 2000; Panksepp,1998; Solms & Turnbull, 2002), have attempted to reverse Freud's decision by establishing the subfield of "neuropsychoanalysis" (and a correspondingly named journal).

It is now widely accepted in psychology that, as much as possible, the field should be anchored in, or at least coordinated with neuroscience. It is the case, however, that neuroscience at the time of Freud's death (in 1939) had not advanced sufficiently to make a big difference for psychoanalytic thinking or practice. The situation also applied to mainline psychology in the mid-20th century period, with behaviorists, Skinner for example, seeking to exclude physiology from the discipline altogether on the grounds that physiological factors were merely black-box variables that mediated the functional relation (in the mathematical sense) between observable responses and observable stimuli. All this, of course, has drastically changed and, if anything, has led to an overestimation of the role of physiology in psychology—and, even, to a pre-Wundtian counterrevolution of sorts that implicitly minimizes the legitimate scientific role of psychology.

Here we run the risk of being drawn into philosophic debates, especially regarding the much rejected notion (these days) of "psychophysical dualism." If the dualism is rejected, which it widely is, it is not the physical side that is discarded, leaving little scope for psychology. Thus, a crude materialism—ironically, often rejected in modern physics—pervades in which psychology can be seen as an atavistic distraction. The computer analogy (which Freud did not have at his disposal), and which is now widely embraced in psychology, yields the valuable distinction (a dualism?) between "hardware" and "software." Computer programs are, of course, implemented in some hardware medium but the material base of the program is not the interesting issue. Even if we do not formally accept psychophysical dualism, we may still embrace it as an informal heuristic stance to designate two important levels of analysis, which is what we have in regard to psychological and biological explanations.

Even within a purely biological framework that excludes psychology, we still have critical disjunctions among levels of analysis: One level of biological analysis cannot explain phenomena requiring another level of biological analysis. Thus, we might manage to master everything that can be known about the sensory systems in the eye-ball but have no clue about the biological foundations of depth perception, illusions, perceptual constancies, perception of motion, face recognition. The critical point in all this for dreams is that biological levels of analysis, similarly, cannot yield the necessary psychological levels of analysis required for dream interpretation. This is not a criticism of biology—the same could be said for chemistry or classical physics, for example—but a realistic acknowledgement that biology, at present, has no tools for mastering meanings in dreams, jokes, or poetry, just as it has no tools for mastering black holes or "spooky effects" in quantum physics. It will be suggested later on that Hobson's program, which has been identified (incorrectly, according to him) with the meaninglessness of dreams, arises from a foisting of a biological level of analysis beyond its legitimate domain (see Chapter 4, pp. 101–105).

Aphasia and Dreams

The pity—and the irony—is that aphasia, perhaps the most important neuroscience adumbration of the *The interpretation of dreams*, has been invisible in the dream literature. It is virtually absent in Hobson's work and it is absent in Freud's psychological works (presumably because of his abandonment of neuroscience). Aphasia, however, is an important key—a Rosetta-stone, in some ways—for understanding dream interpretation and distortion, which we now bring back into the foreground.

Perhaps the foremost historical figure in the study of aphasia (even if he did not give it its name) was the French clinical neurologist, Broca (1861)—though we might also add "Tan," the name of his first patient, who, as is often the case with famous neurological patients (such as "H.M.," in modern times), lead to scientific revolutions in the field that they themselves could not appreciate—or remember.

Originally, Tan was taken to the hospital in a confused state and could not answer questions about his name, address, or his family, answering all questions with the response, "tan," hence his assigned name. (It turned out later that Tan did retain a small class of words, namely, obscenities, a not unusual phenomenon in brain disorders.) After Tan's death, Broca carefully preserved his brain, a rendering of which is reproduced in Figure 2.1. It does not take deep neurological expertise to detect the catastrophic damage sustained by Tan's left frontal lobe from a stroke. (The location of the lesion was in "the third frontal convolution [Freud, 1891/1953, p. 21]). In the next several years Broca studied other patients with lesions in the general region of Tan's brain damage and found that such lesions produced severe problems of verbal production. Patients with this problem—now called *Broca's aphasia* or *non-fluent aphasia*—often have some spared language-production abilities but their speech is labored and extremely limited, often constituting a few telegraphic responses involving verbs and nouns (e.g., to the question, "What did you do today?," the patient answers, "Buy bread store" [Gray, 2011, p. 169]). Also, Broca was able to conclude that the brain infarct tended to be located in the *left-hemisphere*, although this lateralization was most reliably found in right-handed patients.

The next breakthrough in aphasia was produced by the German neuroscientist, Wernicke (1874), who found that a more posterior damage to the cortex (in the first temporal convolution [Freud, 1891/1953, p. 12]—see the circled area of Figure 2.1) produced another type of aphasia, *fluent aphasia*, or *Wernicke's aphasia*, which superficially seemed to be the opposite of Broca's aphasia. These patients lacked understanding of verbal communications but effortlessly—too effortlessly—spewed forth strings of incoherent verbalizations that included many neologisms. It has been noted by some researchers (e.g., S. Arieti, K. Goldstein, P. Schilder—see Brown, 1973, pp. 37–38, 55; also, American Psychiatric Association, 2013, p. 88) that the over-fluent verbalizations of Wernicke patients may correspond to the "word-salad" associated with highly regressed schizophrenics. The possibility cannot be excluded that the two conditions draw on the same "organic nucleus" (Schilder, in Brown, 1973, p. 38).

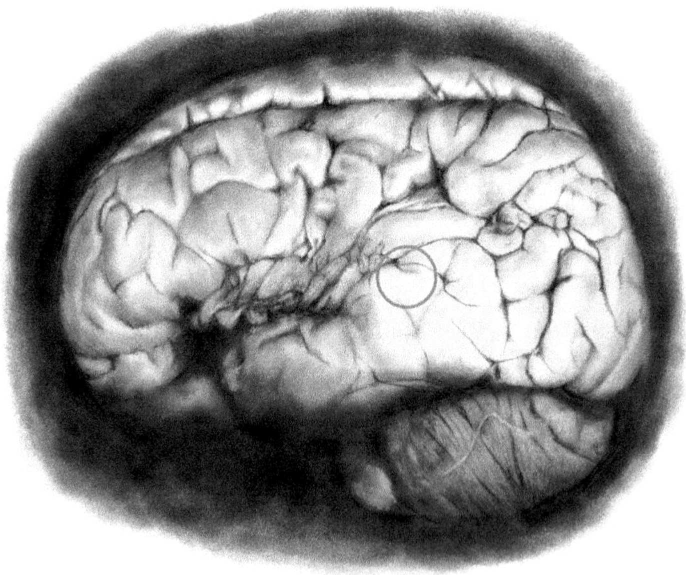

FIGURE 2.1 Frontal lobe lesion in Broca's patient, "Tan," and (indicated by the circle) the more posterior, temporal cortical region involved in Wernicke's aphasia. Ellie Lacourt, rendering artist.

The superficially clear brain loci for Broca's and Wernicke's aphasia led initially to the reasonable emphasis of the brain locales associated with the psychological dysfunctions. The problem with localization approaches, however, is that while they make sense initially, strict localization usually begins to unravel on further analysis. This became the situation in aphasia research. Neuroscientists in the late 19th century were struggling with how best to explain the variety of aphasic disorders that did not clearly correspond to the classic cases of Broca and Wernicke. The most typical approach, widely discussed by Freud (1891/1953) in his monograph, *On aphasia*, was to derive the heterogeneous variety of aphasic disorders from postulated "dissociations" among different nodal brain locales, with emphasis shifting from damaged brain centers to damaged brain circuits and loss of organization. Freud's final take on aphasic disorders followed the lead of Hughlings-Jackson in deemphasizing crisp localization and espousing a more holistic, or field-like positon (which anticipates Heinz Werner's emphasis of "spheres of meaning," discussed below) and concludes that "the apparatus of speech is "a continuous cortical area in the left hemisphere" (Freud, 1891/1953, p. 102). Freud also begins to move away from viewing aphasia as strictly a language disorder, broadening the problem to disturbances of *memory*, for example, rejecting the "differentiation ... between aphasias and amnesias" (p. 102) and introducing a term, still in use in modern neuroscience and psychology, *agnosia*, to designate "disturbances of the recognition of objects" (p. 78).

For our purposes, the most instructive part of this program were the psychological phenomena that were reported and analyzed by Freud and other aphasia scholars. Since Freud's 1891 monograph appeared early in the history of aphasia (Wernicke's classic publication had just been published in 1874), Freud's material will be supplemented by a number of other examples, especially those featured in Heinz Werner's (1956) brief article, "Microgenesis and Aphasia," which sought to demonstrate that the phenomena of subliminal perception, on which he was experimenting, found striking counterparts in the neurological phenomena of aphasia. Werner's project, curiously, provides an unwitting replication of a classic experimental literature in psychoanalysis, pioneered by Pötzl (1917/1960), a Viennese clinical neurologist of some note, who was also a long-standing member of the Vienna Psychoanalytic Society. (Werner may not have been aware of the work of Pötzl or Freud—at least, he does not cite them.)

Pötzl, who worked extensively with brain damaged patients, sought to demonstrate—in a reverse trajectory of Werner's later project—that the distortions and memory phenomena of aphasia that he observed in his neurological patients could be *experimentally* induced through subliminal presentations to *neurologically intact* patients. In one of the first subliminal perception experiments, Pötzl (1917/1960) showed that the fragmentary percepts produced by tachistoscopic presentations could develop, over time, into partial recoveries of the subliminal stimuli and—crucially—that these recoveries (invariably distorted) could occur in the subjects' dreams. It is this tradition that Charles Fisher, whom we have already encountered in Chapter 1, revived in the psychological literature during the high point of the "New Look" movement in experimental psychology (see Erdelyi, 1974). We shall return to some of Fisher's own work presently (in pp. 37-40).

Clinical Samples of Aphasia

In the early pages of his monograph on aphasia, Freud introduces phenomena that were to reappear in psychological guise in *The interpretation of dreams*. The issue of meaningful errors is broached early on. In aphasia, distortions are often designated as *paraphasias*, which Freud defines as distortions "in which the appropriate word is replaced by a less appropriate one, which however, still retains a certain relationship to the correct word" (Freud, 1891/1953, p. 22). For example, the aphasic patient might respond with "pen" when the correct response would be "pencil" or say "Potsdam" instead of "Berlin" (p. 22). Another example of paraphasia is when "two intended words are fused into one malformation," such as "Vutter" for "Vater" (father) and "Mutter" (mother). Such fusions were soon to be designated *condensation*, one of the principal distortions of the dream-work in *The interpretation of dreams*. Freud makes the important observation, which suggests the unity of release phenomena in psychology, that distortions in aphasic patients do not differ from the distortions produced by the "healthy person" under conditions of "fatigue or divided attention or under the influence of disturbing affects" (Freud, 1891/1946, p. 13).

Further on, Freud discusses a case of "mind blindness" (from C. C. Freund) in which the patient makes successive errors in attempting to name, *candlestick*: "spectacles"; "it is for putting on, a top hat"; "it is a stearin light" (Freud, 1891/1953, p. 80). The repeated responses are noisy but seem to converge on the recalcitrant target and, hence, are hypermnesic, as dreams are claimed to be in *The interpretation of dreams*. More recently, Weiskrantz (2002) found, to his surprise, that when one of his "blindsight" patients, on closing his eyes after the stimulus went off, reported a conscious after-image of the stimulus for which "he had reported absolutely no awareness ..." (p. 573). Late-developing consciousness for initially subliminal stimuli in, for example, hypnagogic imagery, is actually a classic phenomenon, going back to the works of Helmholtz, Purkinje, Johannes Müller, Urbantschitsch, among others, with the recovered materials undergoing "transformations, for example, condensations, fragmentations, displacements, rotations, and so forth, similar to those found in dreams" (Fisher, 1960, p. 3; see also Pötzl, 1917/1960, pp. 114–116).

Broca and Wernicke were certainly aware of the meaningfulness of paraphasias (see Goodglass, 1993, p. 78). In picture-naming tasks it is easy to discern (usually) the semantic relation of the intended response to the actual response. Interestingly, the patients are often aware of their errors, adding a "no" or "not" to their responses. Thus, Broca's Mr. W. produces the following distortions of intended target words (the target words are underlined and are followed by the patient's responses, in quotation marks):

stethoscope → "**telescope—not**";
asparagus → "**carrot—no**";
pinwheel → "**kite**";
nozzle → "**hose—no**."

Wernicke reports similar examples in the responses of a patient, Father L.:

stethoscope → "**octopus—no**";
seahorse → "**mandarin**";
globe → "**atlas**";
hourglass → **It's a weather**."

Sometimes the distortions, though meaningful, are more phonemic than semantic (Goodglass, 1993, p. 88), e.g.:

broom → "**broo** ... **croo ... broom**" (with the target word finally recovered);
scroll → "**scrip** ... **screwl** ... **script** ... **roll it up ... sholl ... scroll**" (again, a full recovery);
bench → "**fence** ... **park bence** ... **bench**" (full recovery, again).

An important emphasis in Werner's article on aphasia is the notion that distorted responses in aphasia fall within *spheres of meaning* (a term introduced in 1919 by Lotmar). The "sphere" often includes not just words but, also, behaviors. Thus, Werner cites a patient of Weisenburg and McBride (1935) who would sometimes be able to say "scissors" after he had wiggled two fingers back and forth as if cutting (in Werner, p. 349). Another patient of Weisenburg and McBride sometimes misread a word "which was nevertheless in the sphere of the correct one" (p. 350). The patient, for example, was presented with the word "son" but produced the response, "boy," but immediately after tried to correct himself: "no, it isn't ... boy ... no ... what my mother calls me ... (What is that?) ... 'Boy' ... no ... 'So ...' the ... no, son" (Weisenburg & McBride, 1935, p. 314 [in Werner, 1956, p. 350]). In this case the patient finally recovers the correct stimulus, but even if he had not, most of us could have easily extracted the correct response from the preceding associations. The interpretation of dreams through free-associations (which, as Freud emphasized, are never truly "free") involves the same processes.

Werner cites the paraphasic responses of a patient of Conrad (1948) which suggests that the patient was able to "apprehend the general, categorical nature of the word or sentence without grasping its specific content" (Werner, 1956, p. 351). The patient was trying to repeat words or phrases and was invariably wrong, but was also invariably right—right in that the incorrect responses fell in the target's correct sphere of meaning. This patient's effort to repeat the word Zunge (tongue) resulted in the response, "Something on the body, where and what I do not know." For the saying, *Eine flinke katze kriegt die Mäuse* (a quick cat gets the mice), the patient produced, "Fox and rabbit, or something; a proverb it was, I think; something to do with hunting."

Even without elaborative free-associations, efforts at interpretation would not yield random outcomes. It is obvious that in a multiple-choice test of interpretation, the interpreter would have no trouble correctly connecting the paraphasic responses with the target stimuli (a technique successfully used experimentally with cartoons in connecting punchlines with pictures [see Bergstein & Erdelyi, 2008; Erdelyi & Stein, 1981]). Similarly, "parphasic derailments"—e.g., reading "red" for green, or "peach" for "apple," or "Italy" for England; or, in attempting to give an example of a "preying animal," producing "Zebra" for (presumably) tiger (Conrad, 1949 1949 [in Werner, 1956, p. 352]); or uttering paraphasic statements such as, "He was to sail by train to the South" (Weisenburg & McBride, 1935, p. 253 [in Werner, 1956, p. 352]) or, "He spoke the violin" (Stengel, 1933, p. 266; in Werner, 1956, p. 352)—suggest that notwithstanding the mistakes in the surface contents (manifest contents), the underlying meanings (the latent contents) are substantially preserved.

The theoretical import of the "sphere of meaning" notion is that distortions are not just mistaken dictionary renderings of a target item but, more broadly, errors within an associative structure that includes behaviors, feeling tones, rhythms. Thus, "meaning" resides in associative structure. It is easy to see, then, that free-associations (which are not "free" because their contents are embedded in associative structures) may be key to interpretation: Free-associations map the meaning-sphere of the target content, providing necessary context for interpretation.

The "sphere of meaning" idea intersects with modern cognitive psychology's emphasis of the non-random "associative structure" of memory (Anderson, 1983; Anderson & Bower, 1983; Collins & Quillian, 1969; Collins & Loftus, 1975; Llewellyn, 2013; Rummerlhart, McClelland, & the PDP Research Group, 1986). Further, the "sphere of meaning" notion can be formalized mathematically (Andrews, Vigliocco, & Vinson, 2009; Landauer & Dumais, 1997) with mathematical procedures for defining and extracting "semantic representations" (meanings) from associative "neighborhood structures" (context, spheres) which succeed in simulating errors in which "one word mistakenly replaces the intended word" and exhibits "meaning resemblances to the intended word" (Anderson et al., 2009, p. 479; see also Freud's 1891 definition of paraphasia, quoted above, in p. 34). The emerging overlaps, not just in concepts but outright terminology, are striking, especially since the modern conceptualizations of cognitive psychology make no effort to contact the literatures on aphasia—or dreams.

Experimentally Induced Aphasia Through Subliminal Stimulation: The Pötzl Phenomenon

The aphasic samples discussed thus far were the result of brain damage that led to some insufficiency in the neural machinery for cognitive processing (of percepts, memories, language). Neural damage need not be the only cause, however. Freud, as already noted, suggested in his 1891 monograph on aphasia that such insufficiencies could result from fatigue, divided attention, or the disrupting effects of emotion (see pp. 37–38). Otto Pötzl (1917/1960; see p. 37) put the non-neurological aphasia idea to the experimental test, demonstrating, in neurologically intact patients, that subliminal stimuli led to impoverished perceptual responses that featured many of the errors, of both omission and commission, of aphasic patients. Pötzl further showed that some of the initially omitted stimulus content could be recovered with further effort and, also, in the content of dreams. As noted earlier, Pötzl's work drifted into obscurity, perhaps because the unfavorable behaviorist zeitgeist in experimental psychology and, also, because of his difficult writing style—according to Charles Fisher (1960), "Pötzl wrote in one of the must turgid and tormented styles ever to flow from the pen of man" (p. 1). Fisher revived and extended Pötzl's work a few decades later.

We will briefly consider in this section some of Fisher's striking examples of paraphasic perception and recovery which, according to both Pötzl and Fisher, instantiate similar phenomena in dreams. Like Pötzl, Fisher employed subliminal (inadequate, below the limen of consciousness) stimulation to get his aphasic effects, flashing his stimuli for 10 ms and then requiring his subjects (psychoanalytic patients) to produce a recall of the tachistoscopic stimulus, followed by free-associative fantasy of various sorts and, later, dreams from the ensuing night. For now, we will focus on the same-day data. Figure 2.2, which depicts two cats and a parakeet perched between them, was one of the stimuli used.

One subject, in reproducing the stimulus flash reported possibly seeing "two white and black animals which resembled dogs or pigs (Fisher, 1956, p. 22) (see Figure 2.3a). The recall is, of course, literally incorrect, as is typical in aphasic

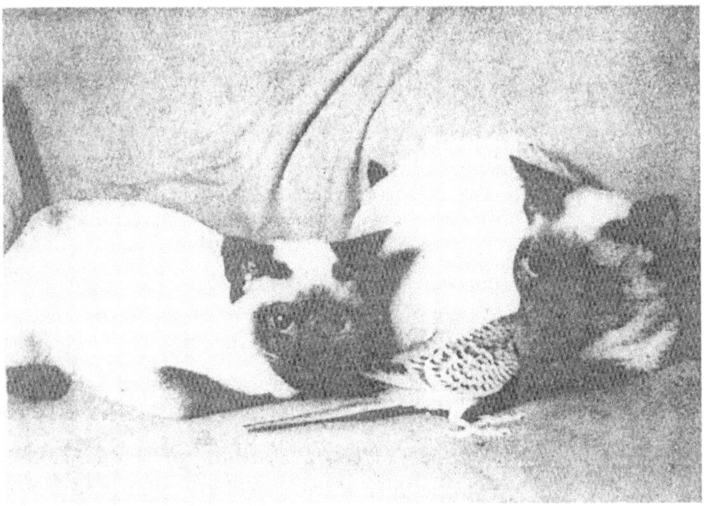

FIGURE 2.2 Fisher's (1956, p. 24) stimulus (flashed for 10 ms) of a parakeet perched between two cats.

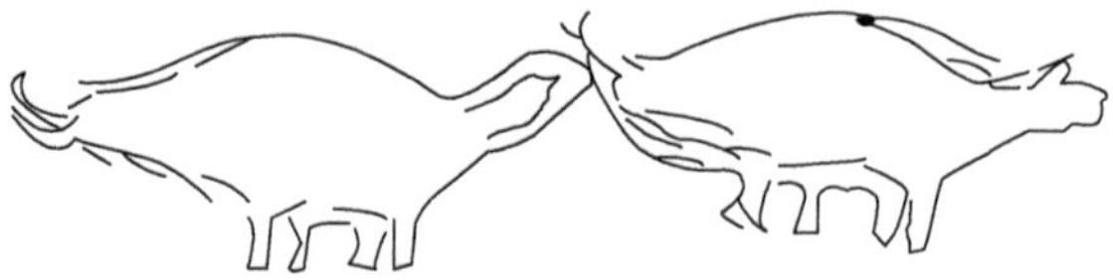

(a)

FIGURE 2.3a Subject's drawing of what she had seen from the tachistoscopic stimulus: "Two white and black animals which resembled dogs or pigs." (Fisher, 1956, p. 23.)

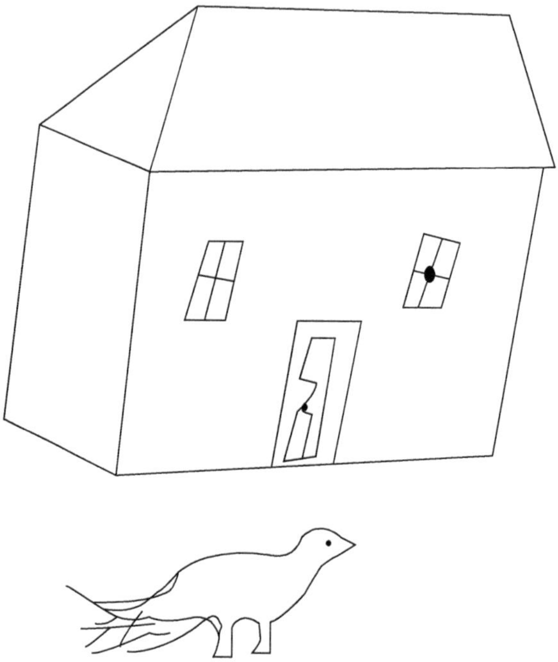

(b)

FIGURE 2.3b Subject's drawing of her free-associative image of a watchdog standing in front of the house (Fisher, 1956, p. 25.)

responses. Still, it is in the general sphere of meaning, featuring bird-like details, even though no bird was reported. In an association test, this same subject responded to the stimulus word, *dog*, with the word, *house*, elaborating that she had "imagined a watchdog standing in front of a house," which she drew (see Figure 2.3b). The "watchdog," as the subject noted, was strange. According to Fisher, she "became very confused, wanted to know what was wrong, could not understand why she continued to draw a bird, stating the she knew very well how to draw a dog, and had done so many times" (pp. 23–24).

In another study (Fisher, 1988), the compound stimulus shown in Figure 2.4 was presented for 10 ms to a handful of participants. None initially reported seeing

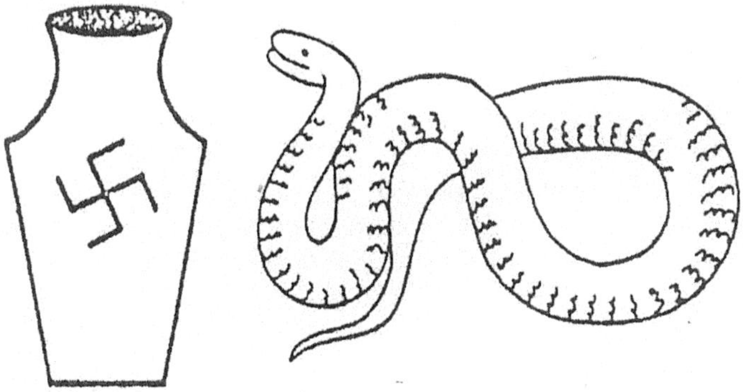

FIGURE 2.4 Compound stimulus of a vase-with-swastika and a snake, flashed for 10 ms (Fisher, 1988, p. 6).

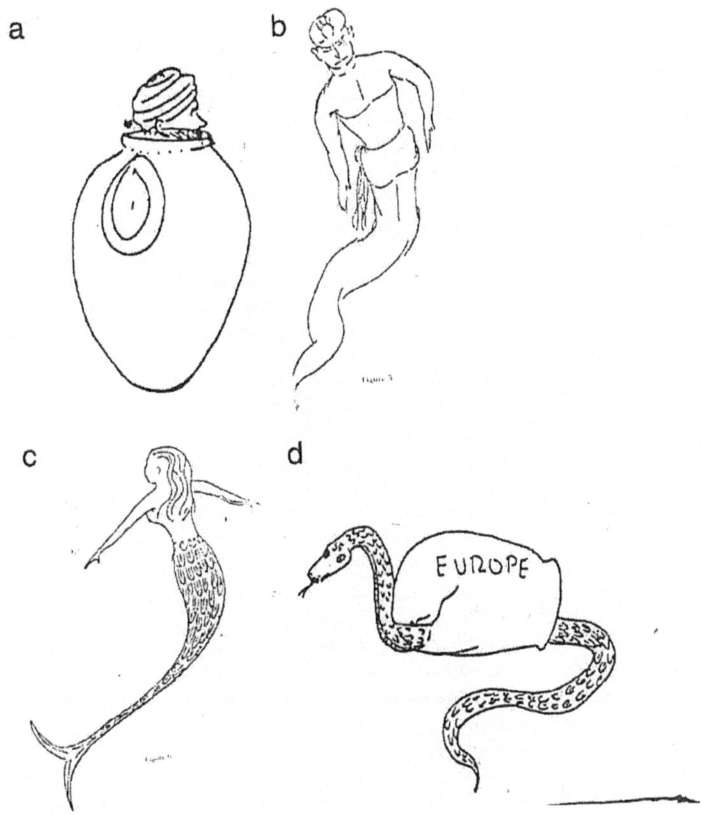

FIGURE 2.5 The subject's successive free-associative images drawn after the once-presented tachistoscopic stimulus in Figure 2.4 (Fisher, 1988, pp. 12, 13, 14, and 16, respectively): (a) "Ali Baba Hiding in a Jug"; (b) "A genie"; (c) "A mermaid," and (d) "The Rape of Europe by the Nazis."

the snake but the stimulus later emerged in dreams, daydreams, and fantasy imagery. In one case, a succession of free-associative images yielded the gradual recovery of the initially inaccessible snake (see Figure 2.5, a, b, c, and d) and, in the end, of the swastika (displaced onto the snake's forehead). These types of findings, as will be discussed in Chapter 5, have been corroborated with standard experimental controls and statistical procedures in studies of imagery and free-associative fantasy (Haber & Erdelyi, 1967; Shevrin & Luborsky, 1958; see Erdelyi, 1985, 1996, for overviews; and see Hartmann, 2011, pp. 31–42, 62–64, for a recent treatment of fantasy, daydreams, and dreams as largely overlapping forms of cognition on a "continuum of mental functioning," extending form focused waking thought to dreaming).

Dreams as the "Royal Road to the Knowledge of the Unconscious"

In *The interpretation of dreams* Freud asserts that "the interpretation of dreams is the royal road to a knowledge of the unconscious activities of the mind" (Freud, 1900/1953, p. 608).

This view, as noted in Chapter 1, recapitulates a classic tradition in dream theory, extending from Plato to modern neuroscience, which holds that because dreams are relatively disinhibited, ideas and emotions not normally allowed access to waking consciousness emerge in the content of dreams. It is for this reason that dreams are crucial for "dynamic therapies," which assume that intolerable ideas and emotions are defended against and normally excluded from consciousness.

Freud's quote, however, has a wider ambit, which becomes clearer with the evolution of Freud's conception of the "unconscious" (for a detailed exegesis, see Erdelyi, 1985, pp. 61–64). Beyond the *dynamic unconscious* (which, essentially, refers to materials that are unconscious because of repression), Freud began increasingly to emphasize (Freud, 1912/1958, 1915/1957, 1917/1963) a *Systemic Unconscious*, which he delineated (not with exemplary consistency) by capitalizing the first letter of the term (as above), or of its abbreviation (thus, "Ucs.").

The Systemic Unconscious, actually, does not so much refer to a level of consciousness, but to a primitive psychological system (the Ucs.) which is contrasted with a psychologically advanced system, the Systemic Conscious (or, Cs.). The polysemous use of terms led to category confusions—of the sort that would occur, absent necessary context, with the confusion of "intelligence" with "Intelligence" (as in "The Central Intelligence Agency") or of "justice" with "Justice" (as in the "Department of Justice"). As Freud and his colleagues began to trip over their own terminology, Freud (1923/1961) finally tried to simplify (perhaps too late) by renaming the Systemic Unconscious, the *id*, and the Systemic Conscious, the *ego* (and a later developing subsystem of the ego responsible for morality, the *superego*). This tripartite structuring of the mind is referred to as the *structural model* in psychoanalysis.

Freud's often repeated claim (with or without correct capitalization) that the laws of the unconscious differ from those of the conscious is to be understood as the difference between the "Ucs." and the "Cs."—or, between the id and the ego. In fact, the id and the ego are *defined* by two basic differences imputed to them in: (1) their respective *goals* as systems and (2) their *cognitive styles.*

The goal of the id (the Ucs.) is to have fun—and to have fun without delay. Freud's more formal rendering was that the id "obeys the Pleasure Principle," that is, it seeks to obtain immediate pleasure. (This is the "wish-fulfillment" that dreams purportedly provide.) The controlling objective of the ego (the Cs.), by contrast, is to be *realistic* ("it obeys the Reality Principle"). Although Freud does not actually say this, it would be in accord with his discussions to define the goal of the superego to be moral, whether being moral is or is not pleasurable or realistic. We might fill in for Freud by asserting that the superego "obeys the Morality Principle." As Freud noted, explaining the inherent difficulty of being a human being, it is very hard, perhaps impossible, "to serve three masters"—especially in this case, where the basic goals of the three systems are often at odds with each other, forcing us to resort, as happens in the political sphere, to a variety of shoddy tricks and self-deceptions. In Freud's theory the three systems are always in play, including during sleep, but—and this is significant for dreams—the balance of power among them shifts toward the id in dreams. Hence, dreams are "idish."

The second difference between the id and the ego is their contrary cognitive styles. The id's style of cognition is primitive, like the thinking of a young child. It is designated by Freud as *primary-process thinking*, which is characterized by a number of primitive features: It is not realistic; it does not abide by logic; it does not benefit from experience; time is not linear; distinctions do not hold, with one idea being easily confused with another similar idea; opposites coexist; and, importantly, representations are concretistic, typically involving imagistic or behavioral representations. In short, it is the cognitive style of many dreams—and of some psychotic thinking. The cognitive style of the ego is the opposite, a mature style, which is designated as *secondary-process* thinking: It is realistic; discriminating; it abides by linear time; it endures delays in gratification; contradictions are eschewed; there is learning from experience; and its mode of representation is abstract (e.g., words). The superego's cognitive style is an admixture of primary- and secondary-process thinking.

We see, then, that dreams (and cognate cognitive phenomena such as psychotic thinking, daydreams, jokes) are quintessential "release phenomena." Dreams, especially, are (relatively) released from inhibition and advanced cognitive control, hence their frequently bewildering nature—and their relative honesty.

The Manifest-Latent Content Distinction and the Dream-Work

A basic feature of psychoanalysis, which Freud regularly emphasized, was that psychoanalysis was a "depth psychology." Surface contents (which behaviorism treated as the sole legitimate data of behavioral science) were, according to Freud, only superficial slivers of the meaning of complex thoughts or acts. The specific formulation of this depth-psychology view in dreams was Freud's distinction between *manifest-* and *latent-content.* The manifest content is the surface content of a dream; it is the literal rendering of what can be recalled. The latent content, by contrast, is the deeper meaning, which can be accessed (easily or only with great effort, if at all) with interpretation. Examples will be provided below and in Chapter 3 for dreams as well as for other release phenomena.

Freud proposed that a complex of techniques is deployed by the dreamer to translate (mistranslate, really) the latent content into the manifest content. These techniques, which Freud collectively designated as the *dream-work*, comprise *censorship, condensation, displacement, concretistic (plastic) representation, symbolism*, and *secondary revision.* They were assumed by Freud to be techniques of disguise by which unacceptable psychological contents were defended against through distortion or outright exclusion from consciousness. An understanding of the dream-work techniques, which we may already intuitively grasp to some extent, as we do the cues for depth-perception, is critical for interpretation since, according to Freud, interpretation involves a reversal of the dream-work, a back-translation from manifest content to the latent content.

Censorship

Censorship is a term adapted to dreams from the social-political realm. (In his book, *Group psychology and the analysis of the ego,* Freud (1921/1955) suggests that "the contrast between individual psychology and social or group psychology ... loses a great deal of its sharpness when it is examined more closely" [p. 1]). Censorship, with which Freud was abundantly familiar as a denizen of the Austro-Hungarian Empire, involves various techniques for omitting or blunting troubling facts from being communicated. Censorship is the counterpart in dreams for repression, or suppression, in awake mental functioning. As is obvious from the political analogy, "censorship" is not necessarily the outright excision or redacting of some offending material but can involve softer, more subtle techniques of mitigation (as is the case with repression, or suppression (Erdelyi, 1985; 2006; Freud, 1917/1963)). One frequent variant of censorship is vagueness instead of direct, explicit communication, allowing only "hints and allusions" concerning the problematic material. Another technique is to misplace emphasis by the "displacement of accent" from the critical to the trivial. A creative example of this technique is exemplified by the Chinese press, which often employs dream-like techniques of censorship (as discussed in more detail in Erdelyi (1985), pp. 151–152). Thus, a highly problematic leader, Liu Shao Chi, the former head of state and a chief victim of the Cultural Revolution, and who had become a "non-person" (his name and references to him having altogether disappeared in the Chinese media), eventually died and the government sought to signal his death while minimizing references to him in public discourse. The displacement-of-accent techniques employed by the official Chinese press agency, Hsinhua, was to report that Wang Kuang-mei (the *widow* of Liu Shao Chi) had attended a Party celebration of the Chinese New Year.

Condensation

Condensation, as we have seen in our discussion of aphasia, is the fusing of two or more ideas into a composite idea. Thus, the fabled sphinx comprises the fusion of as many as four elements that make up the dangerous creature: human (the head), lion (the body), eagle (the wings), and serpent (the tail). Similarly, the *Minotaur* is part human and part bull. Condensation provides a crude juxta-positional logic for equating aspects of two or more ideas. The cover of our book features Pablo Picasso's (1932) painting, "The Dream," and makes use of condensation (mouth-penis) to suggest what the young woman might be dreaming about. The technique is quite common and will be illustrated by additional examples further below (e.g., "The Picture Dream of Dolores P.," in Chapter 3).

Displacement

Displacement is also a very common defensive distortion, occurring when we retarget feelings or thoughts from one problematic target to another less problematic one. Freud, for example, in his dream of "Frau E. L." (see, *On dreams* [1901a/1953], pp. 635–641) dreamt that Frau E. L. "was turning her whole attention to me and laid her hand on my knee in an intimate manner." This manifest content made no sense to Freud since he had never been friendly with Frau E. L., nor had wished to be—even in the dream, "he removed her hand unresponsively" (pp. 636–637). In an analysis of his dream, aided by free-associations, Freud came to realize that he had actually been "annoyed" not at Frau E. L., but at his wife, who had recently shown too much attention to a stranger. Before their marriage, Freud recalled, his wife-to-be had paid plenty of attention to him, and had even given him a caress under the table in acknowledgment of a letter he had sent her (Freud, 1901, p. 638). Here, the manifest content of this dream fragment involves Frau E. L.; the latent content, however, seems to be about Freud's wife.

Concretistic representation

Often translated as "*plastic representation*," concretistic representation refers to the concrete rendering of ideas in terms of visual images or behavioral enactments ("dramatizations"). It is a primitive form of representation, akin to a game of charade, in which abstractions or nuances are difficult to communicate. Concretistic representation and dramatization are exemplified by the verbalizations of two schizophrenic patients considered below who are trying to make a difficult discrimination between two very similarly colored disks, both beige or salmon colored, one of which is slightly redder. Despite the difficulty of the task, non-psychotic subjects managed the task easily enough:

Non-psychotic subject # 1: My God, this is hard. They are both about the same, except that this one might be a little redder.
Non-psychotic subject # 2: Both are salmon colored. This one, however, has more pink.

The schizophrenic patients, who had produced straightforward responses to an easily discriminated pair of disks (e.g., red vs. purple-blue) were clearly unsettled by the difficult discrimination task and responded with regressive, primary-process cognition that involved concretistic representation and dramatization:

Schizophrenic subject # 1: A fish swims. You call it a salmon. You cook it. You put it in a can. You open the can. You look at it in this color. Salmon fish.
Schizophrenic subject # 2: This is a stupid color of a shit ass bowl of salmon. Mix it with mayonnaise. Then it gets tasty. Leave it alone and puke all over the fuckin' place. Puke fish.

Cohen, Nachmani, & Rosenerg, 1974, p. 11

The disinhibition of obscene language is frequently observed in organic brain syndromes, including Tourette's syndrome and Phineas Gage syndrome. It might be noted that Ivan Petrovich Pavlov (1927/1960) also found, in his canine subjects, a regression of functioning when a discrimination task became too difficult. The dogs started barking and biting the equipment and when the task was made easier again, the dogs sill could not function, as they had done successfully before. Pavlov called this regressive phenomenon "experimental neurosis."

Symbolism

Freud was late in focusing on *symbolism* as a feature of the dream-work. Influenced by the work of K.A. Scherner, Wilhelm Stekel, and others, Freud substantially enlarged on the subject of symbolism in dreams in the third and fourth editions of the *The interpretation of dreams* (in 1911 and 1914). However, given the kinds of "symbols" Freud emphasized, the new departure was more terminological than conceptual. Freud himself notes that "symbolism" overlaps with substitutive representation and "even approaches closely to allusion" (Freud, 1917/1963, p. 137). The symbols Freud elaborated were analogous to the concretistic, or plastic representations he had discussed from the start in which objects or ideas are represented according to physical or functional resemblances. These "symbols" (as noted in Chapter 1, pp. 10–11) would be called in some cognitive and linguistic circles, "signs," and, thus, what has come to be known as "Freudian symbols" could be alternately referred to as "Freudian signs." The essential point is that representations in dreams are primitive ("primary-process" in character) and ideas are rendered as pictorial images or behavioral enactments. For this reason, Freudian symbols (which also operate in other release phenomena such as fairy tales, psychotic thinking, jokes) are easy to identify or memorize:

"long and stiff objects", **"revolvers,"** **"sabers,"** etc. ≈ **penis** or **phallus**
"cupboards," **"boxes,"** **"ovens,"** etc. ≈ **vagina** or **the uterus**
the number **"three," "the Fleur-de-Lis,"** a **"clover"** ≈ **the male sexual organ (penis and testicles)**

"King and Queen" ≈ **father and mother**
going up "steps," "ladders," "staircases" ≈ **sexual intercourse**
"water" ≈ **birth**
"little animals," "vermin," ≈ **children** or **siblings**
a **"journey"** ≈ **death**
uniforms" ≈ **nakedness** (involving representation by the opposite)

Freud toyed with the idea that symbols might provide a key to interpretation that bypasses the need for free-associations, wafting back and forth on the question, but, on balance, retained free-associations as the ultimate conduit to latent contents. Absent context, however, symbols may provide a first-blush estimate of meaning.

The whole area of symbolic representation in dreams has been neglected by modern experimental psychology and calls for a great deal of research. Could it be demonstrated (e.g., through developmental research) that Freudian symbols are "primitive"? To what extent are "universal symbols," universal? Here research, such as the work discussed in Chapter 1 on facial expressions and body language by Darwin and later scholars, should objectively determine what is more or less universal and what is mostly cultural or arbitrary. We might expect, as with facial expressions, that the answer will not be a crisp "yes or no," but a probabilistic "more or less," with some symbols being more universal than others. The question of *archetypes*, which is generalized here from Jung to designate innate tendencies (prepared cognitions) to represent certain ideas in certain ways, also needs to be followed up scientifically. It should be clear, however, even at this point, that the symbols proposed by Freud are more or less recognizable to humans. A matching test—the reader might informally check this on some untutored friends—in which the subject is obliged to match a scrambled list of the referents with the symbols listed above, should yield a significant rate of matches with the correspondences suggested by Freud.

Secondary Revision (or, Elaboration)

Freud proposes that after the multiplicity of distortions wrought by the dream-work, a final reworking of the material is undertaken to bring some coherence to the mangled manifest content. Freud is not so crisp on this final step, treating it only sometimes as part of the dream-work and, also, suggesting sometimes that this final reworking of the material occurs after awakening. In any event, secondary revision involves the types of reconstructions made famous by the research of Sir

Fredrick Bartlett (1932) a few decades later, which have become, after some resistance, widely accepted in modern psychology. In Chapter 6 (pp. 179–181) we shall explore the remarkable overlap of Freudian and Bartlettian reconstructions, which turn out, actually, to be identical but for motive (Erdelyi, 2006; 2014). For Bartlett, the reconstructions are largely cognitive and motivated by an effort at making sense of imperfect memories, while for Freud the reconstructions are largely defensive efforts at making emotionally acceptable sense of what is remembered. It will be suggested that both motives (cognitive, defensive) can be at play. Regardless of motive, however, the actual *distortions* are real and grounded on rock-solid empirical data.

It is also worth noting that we do not typically have on-line access to dreams during sleep and so whatever assertions we make about dreams are almost always based on the *memory of dreams*. Consequently, the "dream-work" operations that supposedly occur during sleep are inferences—backward extrapolations from the materials that are reported after awakening (next day, next week, or years later). It will be argued from modern research on the repeated recall of a dream-like story, "The War of the Ghosts," which Bartlett used in his classic experiments, that all we have for certain is "secondary elaboration" after sleep—which, however, might be redesignated, simply, as "elaboration," since the revisions are ongoing over time and change with each repeated recall effort.

The Dream-Work as Sub-work

Although it is not usually acknowledged (but see Anna Freud (1936/1946), p. 192), the "dream-work" as Freud usually presents it, involves an ambiguity, if not an outright self-contradiction. The problem is that the executive system—"reason," "the ego," part of the "prefrontal cortex"—is substantially debilitated during dreaming and yet Freud treats the dream-work as a special set of active operations of the executive dreaming mind. It is easy to appreciate, however, that censorship (which according to Freud is an operation of the ego, which is somnolescent during sleep) must be weaker in dreams than in awake consciousness. If one is on a job interview, a first date, or giving a professional talk, it can be expected that inappropriate or irrelevant thoughts or behaviors will be energetically inhibited. In intermediate states such as daydreams, exhausted or inebriated cognition, jokes, there is less inhibition compared to what would be found in sober, serious cognition. Distortions, also, may have nothing to do with defensive disguise. In aphasia we encountered standard "dream-work" distortions such as omissions, hints and allusions, condensations, displacements, dramatizations, which result not from any effort at defensive disguise but from cognitive debilitation caused by brain damage, which results in disorganized and disinhibited cognition.

What is being suggested is that the "dream-work" actually comprises not "work" but relative "non-work" (Erdelyi, 1985), or "sub-work" (Erdelyi, 2014) by the executive system. Dreams are revealing precisely because censorship is not operating at full strength; similarly, condensations or displacements are not distorting because they are imposed on latent contents but, rather, because the refinements of secondary-process thinking are not available to impose discipline on cognition; likewise, primitive symbols in dreams are used not necessarily for disguise but because this is all the debilitated mind can muster. Thus, *the dream-work distortions are real, but arise not from any extra "work" by the executive system (the ego) but from diminished cognitive work.*

From the standpoint of interpretation, nothing is lost by this reformulation; indeed, much is gained. Because associative structures are revealed in rawer form, with stitches and other imperfections showing more clearly, it is easier to discern, by this view, what ideas are associatively connected and, perhaps, disguised. Further, a reformulation of the dream-work as sub-work has liberating effects on Freud's dream psychology by bringing dream distortions into alignment with the distortions observed and empirically studied in other release-phenomena such as aphasia, subliminal perception, and long-distance memory.

Formalization of the Manifest-Latent Content Distinction

Manifest Content ≠ Manifest Content Interacting with Context

The "depth" metaphor is easy to understand and is frequently encountered in everyday language, as well as in psychology. We have noted Freud's treatment of psychoanalysis as a "depth psychology," in which contents can be superficial (manifest contents) or deep (latent contents). In modern psycholinguistics, "deep" and "surface" syntactic and semantic structures are posited. In memory research, "depth of processing" (Craik & Lockhart, 1972) has been a major research area (in which it has been shown that deeply processed stimuli are better remembered than more superficially processed stimuli). In everyday life, we regularly resort to deep-shallow descriptions of people or ideas. Thus, the young chess prodigy's gambit may be described as astonishingly deep; a college professor, despite his high IQ, may be deemed shallow. The metaphor of "depth" is certainly common, as well as useful, but, in the end, it is only a metaphor. As scientists we wish ultimately to move forward to explicit, even mathematical formulations of our concepts.

In Chapter 1 we already anticipated a formalization of the manifest-latent content distinction in terms of the inequality between the *manifest content* and the *manifest content interacting with some context*, i.e., *manifest content ≠ manifest content* × *context*. It might be noted that some of the context may be *external*, that is, events or details from the outside world, and some, *internal*, namely, knowledge and feelings we possess that can be brought to bear on the material to be interpreted. In statistical terms, the manifest content is a *main-effect* and the latent content, an *interaction*. Finally, it should be noted that *psychodynamic effects*, for example, defensive

TABLE 2.1 The semantic algebra game

The task is to solve for "x," which has the same meaning throughout the embedding statements. Starting at top and, proceeding line by line to the bottom, fill in your best estimate of *x*.

1. I broke my *x*. *x* = ____________
2. I told Mary that I broke my *x*. *x* = ____________
3. Mary did not seem to care that I had broken my *x*. *x* = ____________
4. I love *xball*. *x* = ____________
5. I broke my left *x*. *x* = ____________
6. I bought it at Bloomingdale's *x*wear department. *x* = ____________
7. American *xball* is different from European *xball*. *x* = ____________
8. What's a*x*? *x* = ____________

Source: Adapted from Erdelyi and Goldberg (1979).

distortions of cognition, can be understood in terms of the biased weightings of elements in the contextual ecology.

In most cases, the depth metaphor makes for ease of communication and we shall often revert to it, but for scientific purposes it is important to underscore unambiguously the role of context in the interpretation of meaning (which, actually, Freud himself often emphasizes (e.g., Freud. 1917/1963)) and show how context, in sufficient amounts, can yield crisp, incontrovertible meanings. Let us consider a "semantic algebra game" (Table 2.1) in which a semantic variable, *x*, is embedded in a succession of contextual statements, which at first yield little interpretative reliability but, with accumulating context, produce close to 100% concordance among independent judges. It will be seen that as the number of useful contextual elements increases, the number of "degrees of freedom" (*df*s) for correct solutions decreases.

From informal experimental probes, interjudge concordance in the forced interpretation of *x* in the first statement is low (not zero, in part because there is some constraint on possible solutions—for example, "the Milky Way," "oxygen," "infinity," do not fit). Statements #2 and #3 provide uninformative context; somehow we must manage to select the context that is helpful (the paranoid schizophrenic might be particularly weak at this task with respect to problem areas, producing false meanings, that is, delusions, because of the selection and emphasis of wrong contexts). Statement #4 is highly informative because it drastically whittles down degrees of freedom; the only legitimate options left for *x* are, "basket," "base," "foot," "hand," and "power."

Statement 5 delimits the remaining interpretative solutions to two possibilities, "*foot*" and "*hand*." Statement 6 pretty much cinches "*foot*" (unless Bloomingdale's introduced a "Hand-Wear Department"). By Statement #7, there are no degrees of freedom left; the only solution that works is "foot." Statement 8 provides "insurance," vetting our solution in Statement 7. Note that in this exercise we need not resort to the often convenient metaphor of "depth." There is potential meaning in the initially inscrutable *x*, but this meaning does not call for the notion of "depth."

The essential point of this exercise is that it demonstrates that interpretation, which at first can be chancy, can nevertheless develop to virtually perfect levels of reliability with sufficient context. Further on, the exercise will be generalized to the proposal that free-associations function as context generation and, for this reason, can be crucial for the interpretation of latent meanings.

Outright Errors in Freud's Dream Theory

Theories in science—from physics to biology to psychology—are invariably mottled, requiring corrections, revisions, qualifications, and, sometimes, outright rejection. Darwin's grand theory of evolution, for example, which had no mathematical underpinnings and lacked the necessary gene theory that was soon to become available, was beset with problems. His "blending" theory for the hereditary transmission of adaptive traits did not lead to evolution and was, arguably, not only wrong but impossible. Only with its turn-of-the-century synthesis with Mendelian genetics, leading to what is often called "the grand synthesis," was the revised theory able to achieve the exalted position it now occupies in biology (and psychology). Even today many aspects of Darwin's theory are in dispute—how, for example, to account for the evolution of altruistic and cooperative traits and the question of whether evolution can operate at the level of groups. Even Isaac Newton's theory of gravitational attraction, by which we can still fly to the moon, turns out to be wrong—once it transgresses into the realm of subatomic physics.

The challenge for scientists is how best to revise and improve a theory or, perhaps, decide at what point to discard it altogether. In this chapter we have examined problems in Freud's dream theory which required serious revisions. In the present section we briefly treat three notions which are sufficiently wrong as to require outright rejection. Of course, further research might overturn some of the problems, but the three theoretical notions discarded below have already run aground of much empirical evidence.

Dreams as Wish-Fulfillments

One of Freud's most obdurately held views, despite repeated criticisms, was the notion that dreams are wish-fulfillments (Freud, 1900/1953, 1917/1963, 1940/1964). Freud maintained that we try to satisfy in the hallucinatory world of dream fantasy what we cannot satisfy in reality, often pointing to daydreams as the waking analog of the process (Freud, 1917/1963). The problem with the wish-fulfillment conception of dreams is readily apparent: What is to be made of dreams which have nothing to do with pleasure or which, worse yet, are unpleasant. Freud tried a variety of explanations over the years.

Freud's most important defense of the wish-fulfillment hypothesis was to emphasize the distinction between the manifest and latent content of dreams. A dream which appears not to fulfill a wish at the manifest level may nevertheless be shown, through interpretation, to do so at the latent level. Unfortunately, this possibility is not always borne out by the evidence, and even Freud's examples often fail to support his claim (cf. Foulkes, 1978). Moreover, the meaning of a "wish" is soon stretched to include unpleasant events, with the justification that wishes may, after all, be masochistic; that is, the wish that is satisfied might be a guilt-induced wish to punish oneself (Freud, 1900/1953, 1917/1963).

What of anxiety dreams or nightmares? Freud here takes another tack. He suggests that because of the debilitated state of the ego during sleep, censorship may sometimes not be sufficient to the task and when threatened by primitive content breaking through into consciousness, experiences anxiety ("signal anxiety") which then awakens the dreamer from sleep. The awakened dreamer experiences the fright but remembers only a censored or reconstructed version of the wishful impulses that threatened to break through.

Freud's patchwork of explanations would appear to have introduced unlimited degrees of freedom into the theory, which is now a wish-fulfillment theory of dreams that is stretched to accommodate palpably hedonistic dreams, indifferent dreams, punishment dreams, and nightmares. A class of dreams, however, observed in tragic abundance during World War I, could no longer be explained away and finally undermined the wish-fulfillment hypothesis. These were the *repetition compulsion* dreams of war neurotics (traumatic neurotics, PTSD sufferers) which remorselessly reenacted, night after night (and in the daytime too) the traumatic events from their horrific combat experiences. These reenactments, as we have grown to expect from the reconstructive nature of memory, are often distorted, and may change over time (the type of changes having prognostic value). Freud finally had to yield ground, though he did so grudgingly. He came "to admit for the first time an exception to the proposition that dreams are fulfilments of wishes" (Freud, 1933/1964a, p. 29), substituting, at least for trauma dreams, a new principle, the "compulsion to repeat." Still, he tried to hold onto the general dream-fulfillment notion by suggesting that if dreams were not wish-fulfillments, they were at least *attempts* at wish-fulfillment (Freud, 1917/1963, p. 29). Perhaps Freud should have simply conceded that his hypothesis had been falsified.

In Chapter 4, which deals with the neuroscience of dreams, it will be seen that the disinhibition of more primitive systems, especially the subsystems of the limbic system, does release crucial emotions and drive states, notably, fear, aggression, sex, and general pleasure. Some of these released drive states do involve wish-fulfillment but, and this is the critical point, wish-fulfillment is only a subset of the released drive states.

Children's Dreams

According to Freud, the dreams of young children have a unique characteristic. Because of their psychological underdevelopment, children's dreams are relatively untrammelled by defensive distortions, and so the usual difference between manifest and latent content is not encountered, or at least not to its usual extent (Freud, 1900/1953, 1917/1963). For this reason Freud considered children's dreams to be particularly decisive for the wish-fulfillment hypothesis (which, as we have seen, does not stand). He gives examples of children's dreams which involve the satisfaction of some wish. For example, a 19-month-old girl—Anna Freud by name—who had been kept from food for a day because of a stomach problem, was heard to call out excitedly in her sleep: "Anna Fweud, stwawbewwies, wild seawbewwies, omblet, pudden!" (Freud, 1900/1953, p. 130).

From such examples, usually taken from dream reports of older children, Freud (1900) concludes that "the dreams of children are pure wish-fulfillments." Freud soon realized he was overstating the empirical evidence for his assertion and backpedaled by inserting, in later editions of the *Interpretation of dreams*, a "frequently" into his maximalist assertion. Thus, he modified his claim to: "the dreams of children are frequently pure wish wish-fulfillments" (see Footnote 1, p. 127, in Freud, 1900/1953). Even "frequently" is overstating the facts, which might be better rendered by "sometimes," as research shows that the majority of dreams are not manifestly wish-fulfilling (Foulkes, 1978). More recently, Foulkes (1999) has pushed the argument past wish-fulfillment and has suggested that, surprisingly, most children up to about 7 years of age do not have narrative dreams. A minority (perhaps 10%) do have such dreams but since verbal IQ does not correlate with dream frequency in the first 7 years of life (but imagery does) it is argued that the problem is not an inability to verbalize dream experiences. We shall return to these issues in Chapter 4, when we consider the relation between REM sleep and dreams—and the question of what mental activities of the sleeping person may be legitimately considered to be dreams.

Dreams as Guardians of Sleep

We turn now to one more hypothesis about dreams on which Freud was almost certainly in error. This was the notion that dreams are guardians rather than disturbers of sleep (Freud, 1900/1953, 1901a/1960, 1917/1963). The observation is more speculative than empirical. Freud argued (e.g., 1917/1963, pp. 115–116) that the sleeper is continuously assailed by stimuli, external and internal, which threaten to awaken the sleeper. In response to these disturbing stimuli, particularly unavoidable internal stimuli, the sleeper responds with a dream, in which the disturbing stimulus is dealt with and satisfied (through wish-fulfillment). By dealing with the mental stimulus in a dream, the dreamer can continue to sleep.

Experimental work on dreams casts serious doubts on the tenability of Freud's hypothesis (cf. Foulkes, 1978). First, one would expect that an experimenter-produced disturbance (such as a noise or a strong smell) would be incorporated into a dream so as to prolong sleep. Although there is some evidence for the occasional incorporation of external stimuli into dreams, this is hardly a regular occurrence and, actually, most external stimuli are not incorporated into dreams. Moreover, disturbing stimuli do not provoke dreams. Studies of REM sleep (see Chapter 4) suggest that stimulus incorporation of external stimuli, when it happens, occurs only when dreaming is already in progress (Foulkes, 1978, p. 95). The cyclic regularity of REM sleep (Dement, 1976; Foulkes, 1978; Van De Castle, 1971) further militates against any attempt to portray dreams as direct responses to external or internal disturbances threatening sleep (unless one wished to argue that such disturbances occur with precise regularity every 60–90 minutes, the typical interval between REM periods in adults).

Jokes

One of Freud's more original integrative efforts was the elucidation, in his 1905 book, *Jokes and their relationship to the unconscious*, of the underlying psychological overlaps between dreams and jokes. Freud's interest may have been spurred by his friend, Wilhelm Fliess, who complained, on reading the proofs of *The interpretation of dreams*, that the dreams in the book were too full of jokes (Freud, 1900/1953, pp. 297–298). Actually, some of the dream samples in Chapter 6 (e.g., the Ratatuille dream in pp. 156–158) also have a joking lilt to them. As we shall see, other release-phenomena, especially in the domains of abnormal psychology and art, are often perceived as funny.

As noted already, the book on jokes has been substantially neglected by both psychologists and psychoanalysts, perhaps because the subject matter is, by definition, not serious—and psychologists and psychoanalysts aspire to do research that is serious—and, further, because the content of jokes is often puerile and offensive and can invite disdain for a scholar involved with the material. Yet, actual research on jokes suggests that the more we work seriously with jokes the more serious value they yield as scientific instruments. Jokes, as has already been suggested, are Goldilocks stimuli: They are not too simple; they are not too complex; they are just right. Jokes provide an invaluable just-right model for the elucidation of more complex release-phenomena such as dreams.

The Interpretation of Jokes

There cannot be any question that jokes need to be interpreted. "Getting" a joke is interpreting the joke. Further, as will be seen, the "getting" of jokes involves the same processes as the "getting" of dreams, except that with jokes the processes are obvious instead of controversial. The operative context of jokes is often internal and we fail to get a joke usually because we do not have the requisite internal context—the relevant background knowledge—for interpreting them. Further, the very fact that jokes are not invariably gotten suggests that they are not necessarily "transparent" (as Hobson suggests for the more complex medium of dreams). Further still, research evidence suggests (Bergstein & Erdelyi, 2008; Erdelyi & Stein, 1981) that some "ungotten" jokes may be eventually "gotten" with further thinking, over time. The research evidence also shows (Bergstein & Erdelyi, 2008; Kozbelt & Nishioka, 2010) that, in line with common sense, some of us are more "sensitive" to the latent content of jokes than others and we may assume (although the research should be done) that individual differences also hold for sensitivity to the latent content of dreams and other deep stimuli.

The Joke-Work

Curiously, Freud does not use the terminology of "manifest- vs. latent-content" outside of dreams, even though the conceptual distinction between manifest- and latent-content clearly applies in jokes and other release-phenomena and is employed throughout our book to distinguish surface from deeper contents. With jokes, Freud distinguishes between the "outer-shell" (p. 55), or "the façade" (pp. 55, 106) of the joke, from its "hidden meaning" (pp. 106, 165). Moreover, Freud elaborates on "joke-techniques," which he terms "the joke-work," which are equivalent to the "dream-work" techniques for translating latent contents to manifest contents. In Freud's words, "the joke-work and the dream-work must, at least in some essential respect, be identical (p. 165); or, "the technique of jokes ... show[s] a very far-reaching agreement with the process of the 'dream-work'" (p. 159).

These joke-work techniques include omission/censorship, condensation, displacement, modification, allusion, representation by the opposite, and indirect representation. The only two dream-work techniques missing in the joke-work are symbolism and secondary-elaboration. The omission of symbolism in the 1905 book parallels Freud's treatment of dreams in this period, as symbolism (by name, at least) only became prominent in Freud's later editions of his dream book (the 3rd and 4th editions, published, respectively, in 1911 and 1914). Clearly, perhaps even more so than in dreams, primitive symbols are rife in jokes. Secondary-elaboration is also observed in jokes, with different versions of jokes often used by different jokers or, sometimes, the same joker. Obviously, the joke-work and the dream-work are the same processes. Since the dream-work, according to Freud, translates the latent content into the manifest content, it follows syllogistically (if $x = y$, and $y = z$, then, $x = z$) that the joke-work translates the joke's latent content (its "hidden meaning") into its manifest-content (its "façade, or "outer shell").

Jokes tend to cinch common-sense ideas that often are problematic in other realms of cognitive science. "Censorship," for example, which is the dream equivalent of the awake process of "repression," is still a controversial defensive operation to many contemporary cognitive psychologists (see the commentaries on the author's [2006] target article in *BBS*, "The Unified Theory of Repression."). It is perhaps not necessary to demonstrate experimentally, as it is too obvious, that we "censor" jokes—sometimes not enough. Virtually all the naughty ("tendentious") jokes reported in the pages that follow, tame as they are, have caused some offense or discomfort, with suggestions that they be excised.

Joke Samples, Tendentious and Innocent

We now turn to some concrete examples of jokes. The first of these (Figure 2.6) is a graffito that appeared many years ago on the bathroom wall of a now defunct

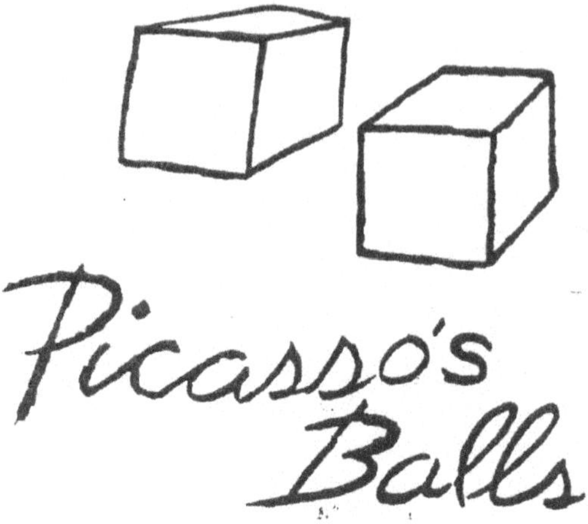

FIGURE 2.6 "Picasso's Balls."Visual joke (graffito from a defunct artist's café in Greenwich Village.

artist's café in Greenwich Village. It is slightly naughty—interpreted as the absurd assertion that a cubist like Picasso had cubes for testicles. Without knowledge about Picasso's cubism, the graffito would not make sense. The latent content requires this piece of internal context.

The second sample is a Groucho Marx joke brought into class by a student many years ago which some other students, though they laughed at it, criticized for not being a faithful rendition of the original (although they themselves had different recollections of the original). The different recollections of the joke do not affect our version and, if anything, suggests the obvious fact that jokes themselves are subject to "secondary-revision." According to the present rendition (used in Erdelyi, 1985, p. 93), Groucho Marx was interviewing a man on his TV show, "You Bet Your Life," and his risqué witticism scandalized too many viewers in this prudish era, resulting (if the report can be believed) in the cancellation of the program. Apparently, there was not enough censorship applied in this case.

****

Groucho: "How are you?"
Man: "Fine."
Groucho: "Well, tell me, are you married?"
Man: "Yes, I have been married for nine years."
Groucho: "Gee, that's swell! Do you have any kids?"
Man: "Yes, nine already and the tenth is on the way."
Groucho: "Wait a minute! Ten kids in nine years?!"
Man (sheepishly): "Well, I happen to love my wife very much."
Groucho: "Well, I love my cigar too, but I take it out of my mouth once in a while!"

****

Although, as Freud often notes, rendering primary-process thinking in secondary-process terms can be tedious (and not funny), it should be underscored for the sake of our conceptual analysis that the context in this joke, as in most other jokes, is crucial. "Cigar" and "mouth" may be transparent Freudian symbols (although one suspects Groucho Marx didn't learn this by studying Freud) but the context—the conversation preceding Grouch Marx's final retort—forces the extraction of deeper meanings ("penis" and "vagina") from the surface manifest contents ("cigar" and "mouth"). In the present case, context need not do that much work, as "cigar" and "mouth" (in contrast to *"x"* in the semantic algebra game) do seem to be effective universal symbols because of the physical or functional resemblances between symbols and referents (see pp. 10–11, 195-196).

Figure 2.7 has four panels, the two left panels constituting jokes and the two right panels, "pseudo-jokes" (cartoons with scrambled punchlines), which afford controls for the reactions to the true jokes in the left panels. The top left panel ("Your Strategic Withdrawal was a Failure, General!!") is correctly interpreted by most college students, although not all use the same terms to render their interpretation of the latent content (e.g., "*Coitus interruptus* failed."). The bottom left panel ("Ye Gods, Abdullah!!) is apparently more difficult, being missed by more than half of the students informally tested, who were puzzled by the interpretation, "A young woman is having the sexual experience of her life." We might note that the elephant trunk serves as a primitive symbol (of the penis); the threesome of trunk and two tusks correspond to the entire male sex organ (see pp. 44–46).

The three joke samples employed thus far all involved sexual or, at least, anatomical latent contents. It cannot be concluded that, therefore, most jokes are about sex, even if they often are. Serious sampling biases apply, which may have led to the omission of hostile or blasphemous religious contents which might cause deep offense—and even violence. In "safe" settings (where the joker is not likely to be condemned or assaulted), plenty of hostile and other offensive jokes can be encountered. Because of censorship—interestingly, not just a psychological but also a methodological issue here—we cannot easily estimate the percentage of jokes devoted to any particular theme by random selection.

Many jokes are not about taboo contents. Freud proposed for jokes—and it might have been a useful proposal for dreams also, which Freud did not make—that there are two kinds of jokes. The first, exemplified by the preceding samples, are *nasty or naughty jokes* (usually involving sex or aggression), which are termed *tendentious jokes* by Freud. The other type of jokes are *innocent jokes*, which are funny not because of the expression of taboo subject-matters but because of the prominence of primitive, primary-process features, for example, absurd logic, lack of realism, false equations, and so on, which, when playfully executed, can strike one as humorous. It seems that throwing-off the restricting control of secondary-process thinking can be experienced as pleasurable and, often, funny. Innocent jokes typically make us smile rather than laugh, although there are exceptions, as will be seen. Puns and other forms of word-play are standard examples.

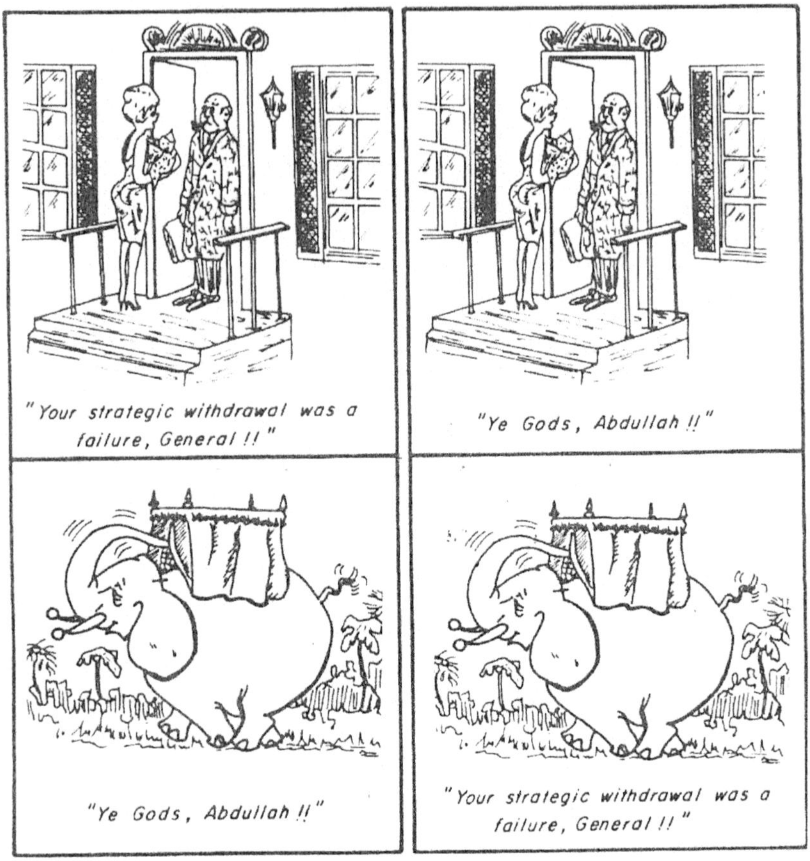

FIGURE 2.7 *Left panels*: Two cartoons (*Top:* "Your Strategic Withdrawal Was a Failure, General!!" and, *bottom,* "Ye Gods, Abdullah!!"). (From, Sex to Sexty # 2 [1971], SRI Publishing Co., Inc., John W. Newbern; Erdelyi, 1985, p. 172). *Right panels*: Corresponding pseuds-cartoons, with mismatched pictures and captions.

A somewhat cerebral example of an innocent joke (probably due to Abbott and Costello), depends on the derailment of secondary-process logic as a result of a confusion between two levels of meaning (the literal vs. the figurative meaning of "mother of"). The joke involves a trick question and answer:

Q. Why is a loaf of bread the mother of airplanes?
A. A loaf of bread is a necessity; airplanes are an invention; since necessity is the mother of invention, therefore, a loaf of bread is the mother of airplanes.

We have here a breakdown of logic, a faulty syllogism, which, nevertheless, succeeds in aping in everything but sense the lofty formalism of an algebraic proof:

a (bread) = *b* (necessity),
b (necessity) = mother of *c* (invention), and
d (airplanes) = *c* (invention).

Therefore, by substitution,

a = mother of *d*.
Q.E.D.

We conclude with an innocent joke routine that does produce full-throated laughter, Abbott and Costello's, "Who is on First?" The acting contributes importantly to the comical power of the piece and so the reader is urged to access the skit on the internet. The routine is based on the unlikely premise, which the actors manage to pull off, that some baseball players in recent times (the 1950s then) had been adopting highly unusual names. In this case, the player on first base is, "Who," the one on second base, "What," with other players, introduced gradually, with names like "Why," "Today," "Tomorrow," "Naturally." The extended joke is based on the polysemous names (e.g., "Who" and "What" are both proper names *and* pronouns). When Costello (the rotund one) asks Abbott, "Who is on First?" Abbott replies, "Yes, Who." Costello is annoyed: "Why are you asking *me*? Tell me, *I* am asking *you*," Costello responds, "Who." This leads to endless discombobulations and frustration (at some point poor Costello starts chewing on his necktie). Costello finally tries to approach the issue indirectly in the hopes of getting an answer in a roundabout way, for example, "At the end of the month, when he gets his salary, who gets paid?" but gets the mind-scrambling answer, "Yes." Still trying the indirect route, Costello asks, "If his wife gets it, who signs the receipt?" but again gets "Yes" for an answer.

Multiple Levels of Meaning and Content-Analysis

The Abbott and Costello routine is based on a theme that has become familiar to us, namely, that communications can involve more than one layer of meaning. The problem for the characters in this drawn-out joke is that each character is stuck in his own level of meaning and cannot make contact with the other level, hence the impossible communicative impasse. In Chapter 5, which deals mostly with content-analysis, it will be suggested that dream science has also been like two ships crossing in the night, with one committed only to latent contents (Freud) and the other to mostly surface contents (modern quantitative content-analysts). The dissociation between the two is completely unnecessary, as communications could be analyzed (quantitatively or qualitatively) at all levels.

Further, it should be noted that clever statistical techniques for producing more "sensitivity" or "power" for quantitative content-analysis will be unavailing if the content-analysis or interpretation is applied to the wrong semantic level, where target contents might not reside. Although quantitative content-analysis can yield extremely high *reliabilities* (the author and his students have not had difficulty in obtaining *r's* in the high .90s), the issue of *validity* (does the analysis measure what it is supposed to?) is often insufficiently addressed. Quantitative content-analysts have, as will be seen in Chapter 5, gathered crisp estimates of the frequencies of sexual, aggressive, negative, and other types of dreams, but these estimates are based on surface semantic levels and may be misleading (as it would be misleading, for example, in doing a "quantitative content-analysis" on the frequency of furnaces in New England houses to count only furnaces on the first floor of the houses while ignoring basements in our counts). It is clear from the tendentious jokes we have examined that nasty contents are relegated to the latent level and that we would not find them in the manifest content. This is obvious in jokes, representing a very general rule, and applies to dreams also, where the latent content is not only deep but also, often, unconscious.

The two cartoons in Figure 2.7 obviously have to do with sex, yet a literalistic quantitative content analysis would miss this. The first cartoon might get scores for "military strategy," or some such, and the second, some variant of "riding atop an elephant." The Groucho Marx joke, scored for surface content, would yield points on smoking of cigars. Yet, mechanical counts of surface contents, no matter how reliable, would miss the point, and it would be a methodological boondoggle if our best-effort measures of psychological content missed the point. Thus, jokes, which are in themselves not serious, incontestably demonstrate a serious methodological problem in content-analysis which, fortunately, can be effectively remedied. A simple rule of thumb may be proposed: If an interpretative or content-analytic scheme does not succeed in getting the deep content of jokes, the scheme is ineffective, or, at least, insufficient, being limited to surface contents. A full content-analysis needs to include all levels of meaning.

3

SAMPLES OF DREAMS AND OTHER RELEASE PHENOMENA, WITH INTERPRETATIONS AND COMMENTARIES

Freud's Standard Approach to Interpreting Dreams and Other Release Phenomena

Details aside, Freud's procedure entails the application of context to the material to be interpreted. The basic steps for dream interpretation are as follows:

1. *A dream report* is elicited.
2. A *preamble* is produced and inserted at the beginning (before #1) that explains some of the local details found in the dream. Thus, if the dream is about Irma, some facts are given about Irma and what role she plays in the dreamer's mental economy; the other characters and places are also expanded on to set the table for the dream analysis. The preamble provides some of the necessary context for the interpretation of the dream.
3. The dream is then segmented (by sentences, idea units, or some other reasonable scheme) and *free-associations* (more context) are produced to each of the segments. Free-association is the *basic rule* of psychoanalysis (e.g., Freud, 1917/1963, p. 154), requiring the subject to report *any* ideas that comes to mind. No idea is to be excluded, whether trivial, brutally upsetting, or seemingly irrelevant. One of the fundamental discoveries arising from Freud's technique is that the free-association task, which from a logical standpoint could not be easier—after all, any association goes and there are no wrong responses—turns out to be an impossible task. We simply cannot bear to communicate some of our innermost ideas to another person and invariably cheat on the basic rule. Freud soon came to realize that we cheat not only with other persons but we cheat also with ourselves. Apparently we cannot tolerate to be fully honest even with ourselves.

DOI: 10.4324/9781003300441-4

Free-associations, which to Freud constituted a "microscope of the mind," provide a conduit to defense processes, the myriad techniques we all use to deceive ourselves (although most experimental psychologists have not yet signed off on this—see Erdelyi, 2006a, 2006b). If we humans are computers, we are a very strange breed of computers who often, for the sake of emotional survival, compute incorrectly and come up with emotionally gentler but objectively wrong (conscious) answers.

As we free-associate to each segment of the dream, we gradually begin to see meaningful patterns emerge that may not have been obvious at the outset. As in the semantic algebra game examined in Chapter 2 (p. 48), the new patterns arising from successive free-associations begin to cohere into one or more interpretations demanded by the context.

4. The preliminary interpretations in #3 are organized into an overall interpretation of the dream, which reveals thoughts and feelings not evident in the manifest content. Since the overall interpretation tends to emerge toward the end of the free-association sequence in #3, the last two steps (#3 and #4) are often merged.

Freud's Interpretation of a Freudian Slip: The Fugitive "Aliquis"

As suggested in Chapter 2, one of Freud's important contributions to dream psychology was the insight that dreams belong to a family of release phenomena which are, essentially, dialects of each other and can be interpreted in the same fashion. It was also emphasized that simpler variants of release phenomena can serve as clarifying models for more complex ones like dreams. Taking advantage of this precept we begin not with a dream sample, several of which will follow later on, but with an analysis of a *parapraxis*, a Freudian slip, which Freud analyzed in exactly the same way he might have analyzed a dream. Unlike the analysis of his famous dream of Irma in *The interpretation of dreams* (Freud, 1900/1953, pp. 105–121), which is very long, comprising some 16 printed pages, and to which we turn in the next section, our first target text for interpretation is just one short line of poetry, six words in length—with one word missing. It might be wondered, and we shall return to this issue in Chapter 5, how modern quantitative content-analysis would handle the missing word and whether it would simply come up with nothing, as a missing word in itself carries zero explicit content.

The parapraxis was analyzed by Freud in his 1901 *Psychopathology of everyday life.* (A. A. Brill's 1938 translation is used in this section.) Since the target text consists of just a few words, it is incorporated into the preamble. Thus, we start with Steps 1 and 2 combined.

Preamble and Text

On a vacation, Freud met a young, much embittered academician, who was familiar with some of his works. Because of his Jewish background, the young academician felt consigned to almost certain failure, given the endemic anti-Semitism of the Austro-Hungarian Empire. To punctuate his outrage he quoted—or tried to quote—a line from Virgil's *Aeneid*, in which the wronged Dido prays for revenge:

> "*Exoriar aliquis nostris ex ossibus ultor.*"
> (Let someone arise from my bones as an avenger.)

The young academician, however, made a mistake, omitting the word *aliquis* (someone), producing:

> "*Exoriar ... ex nostris ossibus ultor.*"

He tried to correct himself but he just could not recover the fugitive word. Much embarrassed, he tried to turn the tables on Freud, and challenged him to prove his theory that such slips have meaning. Freud accepted the challenge on the condition that the young man commit himself to the basic rule of psychoanalysis, "to tell me frankly and without any criticism everything that occurs to your mind after you focus your attention, without any particular intention, on the forgotten word" (Freud, 1901b/1938, p. 10).

Free-Associations

The young academician's free-associations began with the "ridiculous" notion of dividing *aliquis* into *a* and *liquis.* From there followed, *reliquiem, liquidity, fluid.* Then followed a strange train of thought involving Simon of Trent, whose relics the young academician had seen two years before in a church in Trent and which brought to mind the old accusation of blood ritual sacrifice being brought again against the Jews. (The original event took place in the fifteenth century. Simon was a two-and-a-half-year-old child whom the Jews had been accused of killing for the purposes of blood ritual. As a result, Simon was declared a martyr and a saint. Only centuries later did the Catholic Church exonerate the Jews, since confessions of the crime had been extracted under torture.)

The young man's next association was that he had recently read an article in an Italian journal entitled, "What St. Augustine Said Concerning Women." Then, "I now think of something which surely has no connection with the theme." Freud interjected: "Oh, please abstain from all criticism..." (p. 10). "I am thinking of a fine old gentleman I met on my travels last week. He was a real *original,* with all the appearance of a huge bird of prey. His name was Benedict ..." (p. 10).

At this point, Freud broke into the young man's free-associations: "You give a grouping of saints and Church fathers: *St. Simon, St. Augustine, St. Benedict,* [and] the Church Father named Origenes" (p. 10). The next free-association was, "*St. Januarius* and his blood miracle" (p. 10).

Freud again interposed a comment: "Just stop a moment; both *St. Januarius* and *St. Augustine* have something to do with the calendar" (p. 11). Then Freud asked the young man to remind him of the blood miracle.

The young main explained that the blood of Saint. Januarius is preserved in a phial in a church in Naples, and on a certain holiday it miraculously liquefies. The people attach great significance to the miracle and become agitated if the miracle fails to occur, as happened once during a French occupation. The General then took the priest in charge aside, and pointing to the armed soldiers outside, expressed his hope that the miracle would take place very soon, which it did.

And then something interesting happened. The free-associations stopped and a look of consternation came over the face of the young academician. "Why do you hesitate?" asked Freud. The young man replied: "Something ... occurred to me ... but it is too intimate a matter to impart ... besides, I see no connection and no necessity for telling it" (p. 11).

The young man was trying to cheat on the basic rule. Freud said to him: "I will take care of the connection. Of course I can't compel you to reveal what is disagreeable to you, but then you should not have demanded that I tell you why you forgot the word '*aliquis*'" (p. 11). Finally, the young man continued: "I suddenly thought of a woman from whom I could easily get a message that would be very annoying to us both" (p. 11).

Interpretation

At this point, Freud delivered his interpretation in the form of a question: "That she missed her [period]?" The young man was startled. "How could you guess such a thing?" (p. 11). Freud replied:

> That was not very difficult. You prepared me for it long enough. Just think of the *saints of the* calendar, *the liquefying of the blood on a certain day, the excitement if the event does not take place, and the distinct threat that the miracle must take place....* .. Indeed, you have elaborated the miracle of St. Januarius into a clever allusion to the courses of the woman.
>
> *(p. 11)*

The young man's response was, "It was surely without my knowledge" (p. 11). Freud elaborated on his interpretation. The prefix *a* often means no; *liquis* means liquid. Thus, the young man was attempting to banish the frightening idea, "*a liquis*"—no liquid, that is, no menstruation—she is pregnant! From the sphere of meaning weaved by the free-associations, one may also surmise from the story of the martyred Simon that the young man was already thinking of an abortion as a solution to the problem.

The young man said, "Please stop. I hope you don't take these thoughts—if I really entertained them—seriously. I will, however, confess to you that he lady is Italian and that I visited Naples in her company. But may not all this be coincidental?" (p. 11)

The Irma Dream and Its Analysis (Sigmund Freud)

As already noted, this dream analysis of Freud's (1900/1953, pp. 105–121) is very long and requires some serious abridgment in its treatment here. Yet, it is of great interest because it is the first dream analyzed in detail by Freud and roughly follows the standard four-step procedure outlined at the beginning of our chapter. Also, the dream was regarded by Freud as a breakthrough in dream interpretation. In a letter to his friend, Wilhelm Fliess (Freud, 1900/1953, Footnote 1, p. 121), Freud shares a wishful fantasy about his feat:

Do you suppose that someday a marble tablet will be placed on the house ["Bellevue," where the Irma dream was dreamt] with these words?

In this House on July 24th, 1895
The Secret of Dreams was Revealed
To Dr. Sigm. Freud

The short-term reality was, actually, disheartening. *The interpretation of dreams* sold a meager 351 copies after the first six years of its publication and Freud fell into a depression over its failure to stir interest. Yet, interest eventually picked up and the book is still in print after more than a century since its publication. Throughout his life, Freud considered *The interpretation of dreams* to have been his most important work.

Preamble

In his preamble (pp. 106–107), Freud summarizes some of the essential facts touching on the Irma dream. First, he notes that during the summer of 1895 he had been giving psychoanalytic treatment to a young woman, Irma, who was on friendly terms with him and his family. (This would become, as Freud already sensed, an inappropriate situation for psychoanalytic therapy, which requires maximum openness and trust between patient and therapist and, therefore, complete separation from family and friends.) One day, Otto, a physician, who was a younger colleague of Freud and who was staying with Irma and her family, paid a visit to Freud who asked him how his patient was faring. Otto answered, "She is better, but not quite well." Freud was "annoyed" at Otto's remark, which he took as a reproof for promising Irma too much. She was less anxious but she continued to have her somatic symptoms. That same evening, Freud wrote out Irma's case history so he could send it to Dr. M., a senior member of Freud's circle, to "justify" himself (p. 106). That night or perhaps early next morning, Freud had his dream, which he set down immediately after awakening. The dream is reproduced below without any abridgements.

Dream of July 23rd–24th, 1895

A large hall—numerous guests, whom we were receiving. Among them was Irma. I at once took her on one side, as though to answer her letter and to reproach her for not having accepted my solution yet. I said to her: "If you still get pains, it's really only your fault." She replied: "If you only knew what pains I've got now in my throat and stomach and abdomen—it's choking me"—I was alarmed and looked at her. She looked pale and puffy. I thought to myself that after all I must be missing some organic trouble. I took her to the window and looked down her throat, and she showed signs of recalcitrance, like women with artificial dentures. I thought to myself that there was really no need for her to do that. She then opened her mouth properly and on the right I found a big white patch; at another place I saw extensive whitish grey scabs upon some remarkable curly structures which were evidently modeled on the turbinal bones of the nose. I at once called in Dr. M., and he repeated the examinations and confirmed it. . . . Dr. M. looked quite different from usual; he was very pale, he walked with a limp and his chin was clean-shaven. . . . My friend Otto was now standing beside her as well, and my friend Leopold was percussing her through her bodice and saying: "She has a dull area low down on the left." He also indicated that a portion of the skin on the left shoulder was infiltrated. (I noticed this, just as he did, in spite of her dress.) M. said: "There is no doubt it's an infection, but no matter; dysentery will supervene and the toxin will be eliminated." ... We were directly aware, too, of the origin of the infection. Not long before, when she was feeling unwell, my friend Otto had given her an injection of a preparation of propyl, propyls ... propionic acid ... trimethylamin (and I saw before me the formula for this printed in heavy type). . . . Injections of this sort ought not to be made so thoughtlessly ... and probably the syringe had not been clean. (Freud, 1900/1953, p. 107)

Free-Associations and Analysis

Freud divides the dream into 22 consecutive segments, to each of which he proceeds to produce free-associations and accompanying analyses (he calls this section, "Analysis"). Because of its excessive length, only a few segments are fully sampled here, with many segments jumped over altogether.

"A large hall--numerous guests, whom we were receiving." Freud and his family were spending the summer at "Bellevue," a house designed for entertainment, with a number of large reception rooms. It was here that Freud had his dream--a few days before his wife's birthday. On the previous day his wife told Freud that a number of friends, including Irma, would be visiting.

"[I] reproach her for not having accepted my solution yet. I said to her: "If you still get pains, it's really only your fault." The "solution" comprised an interpretation Freud had made to Irma about her case. It was Freud's view at this fledgling stage of psychoanalytic therapy that the acceptance of a correct interpretation would resolve the patient's symptoms. Although he insisted on it at the time, Freud notes (in 1900) that this early view was wrong. In his associations, Freud recognizes that he was trying to shift blame for the part-failure of the therapy (Irma was less anxious but continued to suffer from somatic symptoms). It could hardly be Freud's fault that Irma still had her pain if she had failed to accept Freud's "solution."

"If you only knew what pains I've got now in my throat and stomach and abdomen ... it's choking me." In his associations to this segment, Freud notes that pains in the stomach and abdomen were not Irma's most prominent symptoms; rather the chief symptoms were "feelings of nausea and disgust" (p. 109). Freud expresses perplexity over the dream's choice of symptoms.

"She looked pale and puffy." Irma, actually, had a rosy complexion, and Freud begins to suspect that reference was being made to another person. In later associations (p. 110), Freud notes that his wife was usually pale and once, although in good health, had looked "puffy." In a footnote, Freud adds that his wife had complained of pains in the abdomen. Thus, as Freud realizes, he is conflating Irma with his wife (as well as with a few other women). A sexual theme begins to intrude, although in a subtle, round-about way, in connection with the bolded "**Trimethylamin**" and "the turbinal bones of the nose," as explained further below.

"... a big white patch ... extensive whitish grey scabs upon some remarkably curly structures ... modeled on the turbinal bones of the nose." Freud here connects up some of these symptoms with various persons close to him--and, also, with himself. Freud had been concerned about his own state of health and had been making frequent use of cocaine to reduce some troublesome nasal swellings. (This account by Freud was a censored version of events, as in real life Freud was taking cocaine for its psychological effects and was recommending it to others, including his fiancé.) In his associations he notes that one of his women patients had "followed his example" (p. 111) but had developed extensive necrosis of the nasal mucous membrane. Freud then shifts to another case involving his recommendation of cocaine, which damaged his reputation in Vienna. He had a friend who was dangerously addicted to heroin and, worried for his life, Freud attempted to wean him from heroin by substituting cocaine for it, which produced some of the desirable psychological effects without, Freud thought, the dangers. This friend, however, overdosed on cocaine and died (p. 111). Only in later associations to the dream (to: **my friend Otto had given her an injection** [(p. 115]), does Freud return to this cocaine death, to emphasize that he had advised his friend to take the drug orally but his friend had at once given himself injections of cocaine. Presumably, then, Freud was not to be blamed for the death. Elsewhere, Freud turns to another case which resulted in the death of a female patient. He seems, again, to be trying to deflect blame by asserting that he had prescribed "what was at the time regarded as a harmless remedy (sulphonal)" (p. 111).

"I at Once Called in Dr. M., and He Repeated the Examination and Confirmed It." Dr. M. was a friend and a senior member of Freud's medical circle to whom Freud would turn for medical consultation. Freud notes that the patient who had succumbed to sulfonal had the same name as his eldest daughter. Several times in his analysis of the dream, Freud intimates that he had cheated on the basic rule. In a footnote to this section he remarks: "I had a feeling that the interpretation of this part of the dream was not carried far enough to make it possible to follow the whole of its concealed meaning" (p. 111).

"Dr. M. was pale, had a clean-shaven chin and walked with a limp." Dr. M., like the other characters in the dream, did not support Freud's treatment of Irma and Freud (as he admits) was taking his revenge on him, as on the others, in this case by noting his unhealthy appearance and inflicting a limp upon him. Also, he strikes out at Dr. M.'s masculinity by removing his beard, which in this time and culture was regarded as a manly feature. Also, Freud notes a connection between Dr. M. and his own elder brother, who lived abroad, was clean shaven, and had developed a limp.

"My friend Otto was now standing beside her as well, and my friend Leopold was percussing her through her bodice and saying: "She has a dull area low down on the left." Both Otto and Leopold were younger physicians who had been Freud's assistants while Freud was still in charge of the neurological out-patient unit at a children's hospital in Vienna. Otto, Freud notes, was quick but Leopold was slow but sure and remarks that he is drawing an unfavorable contrast between the facile Otto and the more prudent Leopold.

. . . . in spite of her dress." Children, in Freud's hospital, were examined undressed. In contrast, adult females in those days were examined through their clothes. At this point, Freud again intimates cheating on the basic rule. ("Frankly, I had no desire to penetrate more deeply at this point" [p. 113].)

"M. said: 'There is no doubt it's an infection, but no matter; dysentery will supervene and the toxin will be eliminated.'" This immediately struck Freud as "ridiculous" (p. 113), thus making the senior Dr. M., to whom Freud often turned for help with medical cases, something of a fool. Those who disagreed with Freud about Irma (as Dr. M. also did) were, apparently, subjected to the "vials of [his] wrath" (p. 119).

... when she was feeling unwell, my friend Otto had given her an injection. . . . Freud was, of course, connected to the injection of cocaine, which caused the death of his heroin-addicted friend. But poor Otto was once again saddled with blame and, also, the nasty accusation of having used an unclean syringe. Freud emphasizes that he himself is extremely conscientious in making sure that his syringes are clean.

"Trimethylamin."

The issue of sex begins to insinuate itself toward the end but it is virtually subliminal. Trimethylamin had been linked by Freud's eccentric friend, Wilhelm Fliess, with the chemistry of sex (p. 116) and Fliess had also proposed a relation between the turbinal bones of the nose and the female sexual organ. Freud more explicitly raises "the immensely powerful factor of sexuality" (p. 117) by noting (pp. 117, 119) that Irma was a young widow.

In the conclusion of his dream analysis, Freud more than once notes his self-censorship in his analysis of the Irma dream, for example, "it will be understood that I have not reported everything that occurred to me during the process of interpretation" (p. 118). He defends himself with a challenge: "If anyone should feel tempted to express hasty condemnation of my reticence, I would advise him to make the experiment of being franker that I am" (p. 121).

In this first major dream analysis, as already noted, Freud does not neatly demarcate his free-associations from the analysis of the dream. He produces interpretations to the associations as the interpretations occur to him. He does have a concluding few pages in which he draws together some of the local interpretations. The overall "meaning" of the dream, according to Freud, is that: He is not responsible for the persistence of Irma's pains (the various reasons having already been given); he is angry at his friends for disagreeing with him (especially, Otto and Dr. M.); he is taking revenge on the doubters; and he is a scrupulous and conscientious physician (notwithstanding some of the evidence to the contrary).

The dream, then, was a dream of exculpation and revenge. There might have been additional layers of meaning in the dream, of which Freud may or may not have been conscious, but he chose not to go there in this public venue.

The Picture Dream of Dolores P. (Matthew Erdelyi)

Unlike the Irma dream, which is complex and long, the ensuing dream of Dolores P. is a study in contrasts, being short, crisp, and probably transparent to most of us—even if it was not to Dolores P.

The dreamer, Dolores P., was a student in the author's "Introduction to Psychoanalysis" course at Brooklyn College, some 30 years ago. The picture-dream (Figure 3.1) is reproduced from very long-term memory of the original dream drawing. Dolores P. was an excellent student who seemed to be quite involved in

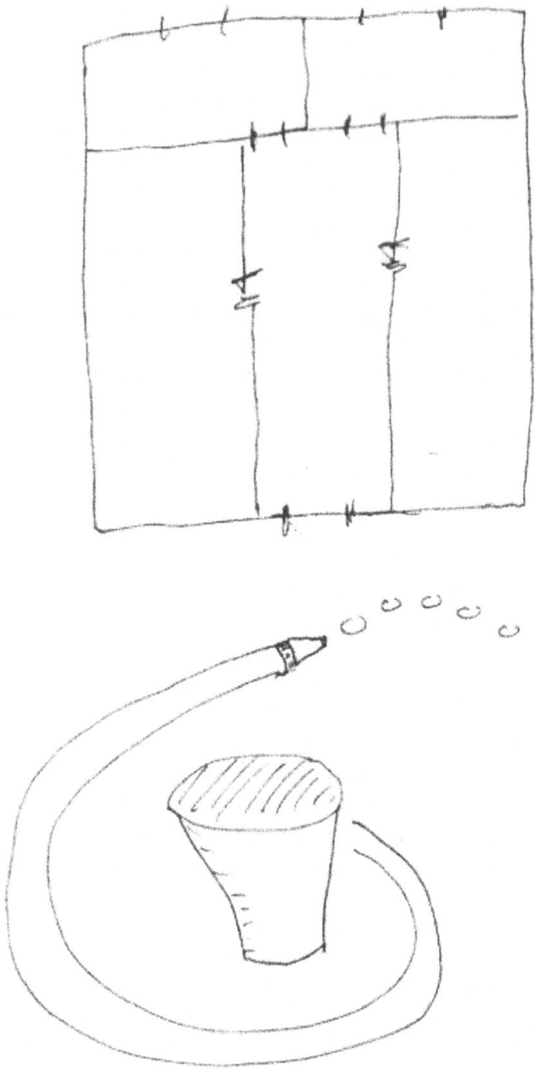

FIGURE 3.1 The Picture Dream of Dolores P.

the course—twice before, she had visited her professor during office hours to go over some finer points in the readings and lectures. Her third visit, which occurred toward the end of the semester and a week after a class lecture on sexual symbols in Freud's theory, was presumably to take advantage of a standing offer to all students in the class to go over a dream of their own that they had analyzed according to Freud's technique.

We can easily agree that there are three basic elements in the manifest content of the dream report: a spouting hose; a bucket; and something of a mystery, a rectangle containing other rectangles. The dreamer's free-associations would likely have identified the mystery element but the dreamer never produced free-associations. Fortunately, the author can provide the information: It is a diagram of *Room 4307, William James Hall, at Brooklyn College*—the author's *former office complex*, with various subdivisions, including offices and laboratory rooms.

Dolores P. arrived for her appointment in a visibly agitated mood—she actually looked angry. She gruffly sat down next to her professor's desk and (inappropriately) slammed her drawing of the picture-dream on the desk and asked, "What does it mean?!" She indistinctly muttered something (presumably related to the bucket and the hose) about having had to wash her car recently. Then, still apparently angry, she again demanded "What does it mean?!" adding that she had asked her boyfriend, a psychiatrist, but "he didn't want to touch it!."

In looking at the "dream" on the desk, the author had three immediate, unvoiced questions:

1. Is this really a dream-report, and if so, what is the problem? Dolores P. was a top student and should have had no difficulty with Freudian symbols (whether she believed in them or not)—or with the juxtapositional logic of *condensation*.
2. Is this, perhaps, not a dream but a joke?
3. Or, is this, possibly, an untoward proposal?

The interesting theoretical point is that the latent content would be the same, regardless.

The author asked Dolors P. if she had typed her preamble and free-associations (a requirement). She had not. (Students almost invariably fail to bring in their free-associations and thus lose a chance of going over their dream interpretations with their professor.) And so, the author was able to dodge dealing with an awkward latent content. Dolores P. never came back for another office visit. She did get a high A in the course.

The Elephant Dream of Alice V. (John Nemiah)

Preamble

Alice was a 25-year-old married woman who already had five children. She had fraught relations with her father (who, she said, "was poison" to her) and avoided him as much as possible. Even so, her father had recently gone out of his way to help her out of a financial jam.

Alice reacted strangely to his generosity: She developed obsessions which involved irruptions into consciousness of unbearable "obscene" images of herself and her naked father having sex. She would "desperately try to push the images out of her mind by shaking her head or thinking of other things" (Nemiah, 1984, p. 55), but to no avail. She became increasingly anxious and depressed and was finally hospitalized.

The dream presaged Alice's breakdown. The very morning after the dream, Alice experienced the first episode of the frightening imagery of sexual activity with her father.

In therapy sessions in the hospital, Alice recovered a memory of having had a similar transitory obsession some 15 years earlier (when she was 11 years old), which she claimed to have forgotten. She also reported that until she was five she had slept in a crib in her parents' bedroom.

The Dream

> She was ... at a zoo. It was nighttime, and she heard strange noises in the darkness. She asked an animal keeper standing next to her what these noises were. "Oh," he replied casually, "that's only the animals mating." She then noticed a large gray elephant lying on its right side in the grass in front of her. As she watched, she saw the creature moving its left hind leg up and down as if it were trying to get up onto its feet. At that point she awoke with a sense of terror (Nemiah, 1984, p. 56).

Associations to the Dream

In associating to the dream, Alice recovered a long-forgotten event going back to when she was 4 or 5 years old. She had awoken one night in her crib and saw her parents naked, having sex. Suddenly aware that Alice was watching them, the parents sprang apart and tried to hide their nudity: Alice's mother covered herself in the bedclothes, her father rolled over onto his back. Alice noticed her father's erection, which he tried to hide by lifting up his left leg. He then sat up and screamed at Alice to go back to sleep.

Comments

The dream by itself—excluding preamble and free-associations—is a reasonably coherent, if puzzling story, which does not obviously mirror Alice's wakeful life. A standard content-analysis would pick up sexual content ("animals mating") but would not link the elephant to Alice's father, who, the later information reveals, found himself in an analogous situation in Alice's childhood.

The dream recapitulates the traumatic event from Alice's childhood, with the "elephant" corresponding to her father, who had been "mating" with Alice's mother. The dream depicts the primal scene, so unbearably upsetting to Alice in real life, in an emotionally muted way—the animal keeper at the zoo responds casually, in an assuaging fashion: Animals mating, no big deal. Alice's father, regardless of how generous he might have been, was, actually, "poison" to Alice because he cued the traumatic memory which Alice was trying to avoid.

The contextual background of the dream—the preamble and the free-associations—interacts with the officially demarcated dream. Only with the context can the "elephant" in the dream be reasonably considered a stand-in for Alice's father.

Allan Hobson's "Mozart at the Museum" Dream

The next dream we take up is a dream reported and analyzed by Allan Hobson in 1988 in his book, *The dreaming brain*. Clearly, Hobson sees some meaning in his dream but, it should be noted, he does not produce free-associations to the dream elements and manages to extract only surface contents.

The dream, obviously, is substantially meaningful. It mirrors many events in the dreamer's life, including emotions and personality characteristics. Thus, from the dream we can surmise that Hobson is a Mozart aficionado; that he is quite knowledgeable about music; that he has been married, and for over 20 years; that his wife's name is Joan; that Joan has a responsible position at the museum. There are some puzzles in the dream, however, which limit its semantic "transparency." What, for example, is the meaning of Mozart's having become overweight?

The Dream

> *My wife, Joan, and I are at the Museum of Fine Arts in Boston to attend a concert in the larger Remus auditorium. It is someone (perhaps John Gibbons) playing a Mozart piano (concerto?) on a large Steinway (no orchestra, but image vague anyway). [The piano is reminiscent of the large Steinway grand in the great hall of the Phillips Collection in Washington, which I visited the previous Saturday.] As is usual on such "museum" occasions, I am restive, feeling like the third wheel on Joan's bicycle, and hence inattentive.*
>
> *I decide to explore and go down to the smaller, older theater (near the Egyptian sarcophagi). This theater is now limited to small lectures but was, twenty years ago, the place where, as young members, Joan and I attended museum programs of the type that are now in Remus, and now under Joan's direction.*
>
> *I hear music and the faint bustle of excitement. Opening the door a crack, I am amazed to realize that Mozart himself is on stage, playing the same concerto (again without orchestra) on an antique harpsichord from the museum collection (not the Mozart pianoforte). Although the door is open only for an instant, I notice Mozart's rich red brocaded frock coat (the curlicues are gold-embossed) and his white powdered wig. He has a beatific smile, and the arpeggios stream through the door into my ear. I also notice that Mozart has gotten a bit overweight, and wonder why.*
>
> *I close the door with a shhh!, and try to figure out how to tell Joan of my discovery.*
>
> Hobson, 1988, pp. 221–222

Preamble and Associations

As already noted, Hobson doesn't provide a preamble or free-associations to the dream. He does, however, supplement his dream with some commentary, which may be treated as the missing preamble and associations:

> The music I 'heard' in the dream is quite familiar to me. I often listen to Mozart piano concertos while driving. The scenes (in the museum) are also familiar. I go there often with my wife, who is a program director. I have just been at the Phillips Gallery.
>
> *p. 221*

> Mozart is Mozart. I have seen the film (*Amadeus*) at a special museum showing ... [an incongruous plot feature is that] *my* belly has begun to bulge!
>
> *p. 221*

> I am faintly distressed by the incongruities; no orchestra, wrong instrument; Mozart's corpulence.
>
> *p. 221*

> What does the Mozart dream mean? . . . . Transparent: I would love to see Mozart, to have my wife "score" by attracting him to the museum, and to discover him there so that I could report her coup to others.
>
> *p. 222*

Hobson concludes:

> At a deeper level I am prepared to admit that this dream might have a psychoanalytic 'meaning'; I *am* ambitious, I *do* admire Mozart. I *would*, consciously, like to be as brilliant as Mozart. Some of my most devoted friends have even called me 'Mozart' . . . . But ... Mozart is Mozart. . . . I also enjoyed telling my wife this story. From a social point of view, my dream was a belated wedding present!
>
> *p. 222*

Hobson's discussion of his dream is itself dream-like. There are puzzles of meaning and idiom choice (e.g., "from a social view" the dream is "a belated wedding present!" ... "I would love to see Mozart, to have my wife 'score'... "). Hobson is "prepared to admit that, after all, "this dream might have a psychoanalytic 'meaning'" but the deeper meanings supplied are not particularly psychoanalytic. Perhaps there is a hint of undeveloped latent content that is Freudian, revolving around the observation by Hobson that some of his most devoted friends call him 'Mozart'. Twice he declares that "Mozart is Mozart," but, at the same time, Hobson virtually invites another equation: Hobson = Mozart. Hobson notes that he saw the film *Amadeus*, in which the central conflict swirls around the warfare between the genius, Mozart, and the more savvy (and often masked) wannabe, Salieri. Salieri never appears explicitly in Hobson's dream text or his discussion but is nevertheless implicitly in the background for anyone, such as Hobson, who saw the film *Amadeus.* In *Amadeus,* as in Hobson's dream, a wife plays an important role. Free-associations to successive elements of the dream might have shed light, for example, on the specific concerns of a long-married, aging (pot-bellied?) man, and the theme's continuation. (The author surmised from the dream that Hobson's marriage was unraveling, a latent content that was subsequently confirmed publicly by Hobson (2005; 2011)). From a methodological viewpoint, it is noteworthy that Hobson insists on the transparency of his dream without engaging in the free-associative elaborations thought by Freud to be essential for uncovering deeper meanings

Hobson's assertion, "Mozart is Mozart," lies at the heart of the question of dream interpretation. If there is only manifest content, then, self-evidently, any item must be equal to itself (Mozart = Mozart). If, however, latent contents exist, then an item may have multiple meanings. In this case, the context suggests some of the alternate meanings (e.g., the wishful equation, Hobson = Mozart, or the aggressive one, Hobson = Salieri). To deny in principle the possibility of polysemy would be to retrogress back to a discredited radical behaviorism of decades past that insisted on the reality of only surface phenomena.

"Worst Case Scenario" Dream of Zelda (With Biographical Notes on the Dreamer)

It will become evident that Zelda had fraught relations with her parents, both of whom have since died. (The "Worst-Case Scenario" dream, written out in August 2013, occurred after the death of her mother but before the death of her father.)

More than once Zelda expressed the half-serious suspicion that "the stork had dropped her down the wrong chimney." Even though Zelda would be the first college graduate in her family, her parents opposed college for her and wanted her to focus on getting married and, until that happened, to get a job and contribute to the household expenses. They refused to pay for Zelda's one college application.

Zelda found college to be dishearteningly unchallenging. She was fascinated by psychology but could not abide the behaviorist views of her psychology department. She did manage to gain the sponsorship of one of her professors to do an internship at a famous dream laboratory in Brooklyn, where they assigned her to the "red-eye" contingent responsible for observing and testing laboratory subjects throughout the night. Zelda was also tasked with recording and scoring the sleeping subjects' EEG waves for later analysis. Thus, while still a college student, Zelda gained concrete, first-hand experience with dream research. She was to grouse later on that many dream scholars, including a world famous dream scientist, obviously did not dream (technically, did not remember their dreams). Zelda is quite familiar with Freud and his approach to dreams but found his segment-by-segment free-association procedure to be excessively linear and plodding (she tried it for one of her dream samples but rapidly abandoned it and produced associations, or "commentaries" to each dream as a whole).

After college, Zelda won a full-tuition fellowship to a doctoral program in Europe but life got in the way and Zelda only took up her graduate studies many years later in the United States. She managed, despite a full-time job, to complete her PhD studies in the evening in an exacting doctoral program in experimental psychology and is conversant, as any well-trained experimental psychologist can be expected to be, with methodology, statistics, psychophysics, neuroscience, and basic content areas in psychology. Her parents never developed any enthusiasm for their daughter's academic accomplishments and Zelda complained after her PhD graduation that they did not know the difference between a PhD and HTC.

Preamble

(The preamble, the dream, and her associations were typed out by Zelda.)

> I had an appointment with the dentist the following week which would involve a wisdom tooth that needed work. My dentist said that he would try to save the tooth (by filling the deep cavity), but warned me that he might have to extract it if it looked as though that wouldn't work. He wouldn't know the outcome until he started filling the tooth and evaluated the situation. I've always been terrified of going to the dentist but I was trying to be brave about this upcoming appointment and was trying not to catastrophize the situation.

Zelda's Dream

> *I was at a dentist's office for my appointment (it wasn't the office of my usual dentist, but somewhere else). I was immediately perplexed because there were two dentists waiting to see me, and I didn't understand why I needed both of them for this appointment. I was told that there was going to be a lot of preparation before they got started, and that I was to come back after lunch. Again, I couldn't understand what sort of preparation they would need: after all, it was to be a pretty routine visit. I was getting very anxious in my dream.*
>
> *After a while, I returned (presumably after lunch), and found that I needed to cross through the lobby, which was, by this time, filled with evangelical people praying and chanting. I was encouraged to join in, but declined. I was told that it would be in my best interest to join in the prayer group because it might help me with my "procedure." By now I was getting very upset and kept asking why everyone was making such a big deal about this – after all, it was just going to be a simple filling – or,* in the worst case scenario, *an extraction. I was getting agitated and started yelling at people, asking that they stop pumping this up into something monumental.*

Associations

About five years ago, I was called to Florida to take care of my father while my mother was going into the hospital to have an urgent operation: her heart valve needed to be replaced. I was panicked about the prospect of having to take care of my father back then, especially if anything happened to my mother (the "healthy one") as a result of her surgery. (Even back then, my father was already very frail and had dementia; he needed to have everything done for him and required constant care, which my mother provided.) I had asked my parents several years before to move back North so we could be closer to each other but they chose to stay in Florida. To deal with this health emergency I spent most of the summer in Florida. Before her scheduled surgery I tried to get my mother to make arrangements to take care of things while she recuperated, as well as to develop a plan for the long term care for my father "just in case," in the worst case scenario, something went wrong with her operation. This involved my getting access to their accounts, having information about bills, learning about the management of the house, having contact information regarding doctors and lawyers, instructions regarding my father's many medications, etc. She insisted that she'd only be in the hospital a few days and would be able to resume her normal life without any major interruptions. My mother was refusing to make any provisions, saying that "we'll cross that bridge when we get to it," and that I was making too much of it. I kept insisting that we were "at the bridge" and that I would be the one saddled with all of the problems and responsibilities in her absence, regardless of how long that would be. I kept telling her, "Mom, you're not just going to the dentist! It's not as if you're having root canal, or having your tooth pulled! You're going in for heart surgery – we need to make plans – just in case your recovery isn't what we expect" (and even, I thought, in the worst case scenario, if she didn't survive). She didn't want to hear this, naturally, and we fought about making any plans or arrangements—it was like "pulling teeth." Now, five years later, with the death of my mom, the worst case scenario has actually come to pass.

Of note, I started writing this dream one evening, and then returned to the text the following morning. I was quite surprised to see that my dream wasn't necessarily a dream about my fears of the dentist. Although on one level it appears to be a very elegant reversal of reactions—my mother not reacting strongly enough to her serious heart surgery and people in my dream reacting too strongly to my routine dental visit—I see that I've actually been writing quite a bit about my father and the current situation that I find myself in. I am overwhelmed with caring for my father, which brings up all sorts of past resentments. My experience this last year has been one of being depressed and angry about it, and I've found myself very short-tempered and agitated most of the time. . . . [Zelda censored some of her associations at this juncture.]

On the morning of her surgery (five years ago), my father and I were with my mother and her surgeon as she was about to be wheeled in to the operating room. To my surprise, her surgeon asked that we all hold hands while he said a prayer for divine guidance and spiritual support. This is definitely not the kind of thing that sits well with me, but I saw that my parents were eager to participate, so I went along with it silently. Actually, not only am I not religious, but I've become quite anti-religious in recent years, and this is precisely the kind of thing that irritates me. My mother survived the surgery and was in rehab (in a local nursing home in Florida). I had my father admitted there in respite care so that he would be taken care of while she was recuperating. However, as soon as I flew back to New York, my mother immediately undid all of my work and preparations for her recovery, and even moved my father into her rehab bedroom, where she was constantly fussing over him all day and night, and thereby not fully allowing herself to recover properly. At my complaints, she told me to "mind my own business."

Also: About a year ago, my daughter had a dental emergency in California. One of her wisdom teeth had become seriously infected and she was in excruciating pain. She saw the dentist on an empty stomach, anticipating that she might need to have anesthesia. When the dentist saw her, she told her to go and have something to eat and to try to relax. She gave her a tranquilizer and told her to come back after lunch. During the procedure, however, things got even more serious: the dentist needed to work deeply on her jaw, and the Novocain was just not doing the trick (worst case scenario). She decided that my daughter would require general anesthesia, and called an anesthesiologist in at the last moment. However, because my daughter had just finished eating lunch, and had taken a tranquilizer, they needed to wait several more hours before the general anesthesia could be safely administered. They were long hours of torture for my daughter.

Postscript: I did have to have the tooth extracted, but it turned out not to be that horrible. As a young child, I used to have a terrible time at the dentist. I had many cavities, and they did not use Novocain in those days. Additionally, my parents would punish me whenever I had a cavity, blaming me for not taking care of my teeth properly. I actually had two extractions as a teenager, and both times was severely punished by my parents for being so irresponsible and costing them so much money in dental bills. I have always felt anxious and ashamed whenever I went to the dentist and guilty if I needed to have work done. My brother, on the other hand, had orthodontia done, which was prohibitively expensive for them at the time. He also had his front teeth broken in a school yard accident, but my parents were always very supportive about his having a good set of teeth—sparing no expense or sympathy. Ironically, a woman at the nursing home where my father had been living complimented me on having beautiful teeth and a nice mouth. My brother, at this point in time, has seriously neglected his teeth and has lost almost all of them, without having yet replaced them with dentures.

Author's Postscript (Matthew Erdelyi)

Although not always obvious from the surface content, there is a whirl of negative affect coursing through the dream—fear, rage, resentment, guilt. Zelda, however, is aware of this. She complains outside of the dreaming context that she is too honest with her negative emotions and cannot hide from them, as most people do. Zelda agrees that the latent structure of the dream is exceedingly complex, with associative structures incorporating a diversity of events and emotions spanning decades. There is some prodigious version of *unconscious inference* operating which somehow manages to incorporate extremely disparate events into appropriate associative structures. The unconscious structuring obviously holds for other release-phenomena and is much in evidence in the *parapraxis* involving the missing *aliquis*, discussed in the early pages of this chapter (pp. 61–64). This unconscious, automatic structuring of materials appears to be a fundamental feature of both sleep and awake cognition. It is striking how Zelda manages in her dream—with no conscious cognitive effort—to interweave three separate dramas in her life (her dreaded visit to the dentist, her mother's heart operation, and her daughter's dental crisis) into one dream story.

Freud Dreams Chinese Poetry

弗梦汉诗 *(Fú Mèng Hàn Shī)*

(by Diane M. Zizak)

Interpreting a dream is, in many ways, much like interpreting a Classical Chinese poem. At first blush, there appears to be a kaleidoscope of images, but then we are drawn to look deeper. With cloaked allusions, metaphors and symbols, it is on the shoulders of the beholders to uncover the camouflaged meanings.

While it is certainly the case that all poetry, by design, invites a degree of interpretation, Classical Chinese poetry, in particular, requires the creative participation of the reader. In part, this is because the Chinese language simultaneously expresses thoughts and symbols both semantically and graphically. Both Freud (1900/1953) and the anti-Freudian neuroscientist, Allan Hobson (1988, 2002, 2011) emphasize the imagistic nature of dream representations. Thus, the highly visual nature of the Chinese language makes it a natural parallel to the dream world. Each written word—or character—is itself a piece of poetry. Complete thoughts are illuminated with the strokes of a brush. "Poetic thought works by suggestion, crowding maximum meaning into the single phrase pregnant, charged, and luminous from within. In Chinese character[s] each word accumulated this sort of energy in itself" (Fenollosa & Pound, 1936, p. 28).

The Chinese writing system is unique. It is highly visual—and artistic—in ways that alphabetic languages cannot be. There is no alphabet. Instead, each of the characters is pronounced as a single syllable and represents a discrete concept. Multiple characters are clustered to form new words and ideas, which are then arranged to design sentences and verse.

Unlike English (but very much like a dream), many of the components that are used to create a traditional Chinese character contribute to their unique story. And, as in dreams, it is the constellation of the fragments, along with their historical referents that give rise to their particular meanings. Although a derivational analysis of an English word could help to illuminate its earlier meaning, such an analysis of a word in English only goes so far; we do not dig down to the level of the individual alphabetic letter in the word's spelling in order to reconstruct its meaning. "There is little to nothing in a phonetic word to exhibit the embryonic stages of its growth. It does not bear its metaphor on its face" (Fenollosa & Pound, 1936, p. 25). However, Chinese characters are, in a sense, metaphorical representations, and by reading them we have access to the roots of the Chinese language—and culture.

In the mid-20th century, approximately one third of the most frequently used Chinese characters used in Mainland China became abbreviated versions of the more traditional characters that had been around for millennia. Many of the strokes and components in these simplified characters are lost to history in the name of efficiency. Only hints and allusions remain to suggest what they once referenced, and, just as the manifest content of a dream often misses—or masks—what the dream might actually be revealing, a modern version of a character does not always reveal its latent content so easily.

Like most dreams, Chinese is a quintessentially visual experience. Chinese characters have been modified over their 3,000-year history, starting with the earliest etchings of oracle bones, and on up through today's modernized and simplified forms. In any event, the Chinese language was, and basically remains ideographic. Even today it is possible to visualize what some of the characters are signifying, for example, three (三), mountain (山), and person (人). Since each character is, in a sense, a visible metaphor or a concrete representation of a concept or idea, the reading of Chinese poetry is a unique experience. The closest we come to this in English is with "concrete poetry" in which the actual shape and morphology of the printed words add substance to the meaning of the poem (e.g., Lewis Carroll's (1865; 1871) "The Mouse's Tale" from Alice in Wonderland).

Moreover, many of the poets were also artists and calligraphers, which adds further to their rich visual and dreamlike creations. Their calligraphic styles were expressions and extensions of the poet's thoughts in a way that we just do not see with alphabetic languages. In Western writing, penmanship is irrelevant. Whereas, for example, the great poet and artist, Ni Zan, is appreciated just as much for his calligraphy and art as for his verse, we seldom (if ever!) conjure up Shakespeare's handwriting when we are reading one of his sonnets. These artistic expressions add to the dream-like quality of Chinese poetry.

Interpreting a Classical Chinese poem is, in many ways, much like interpreting a dream. In both cases, we see aspects of primary process thinking (see pp. 41, 101TS: 104). And, as with dreams, Classical Chinese poetry often creates a surreal world with loose ties to reality, complete with instances of displacement, condensation, and substitute formation (see pp. 30, 34, 41TS: 46, 168). Chinese poets typically used elements of nature and the natural world (e.g., waterfalls, birds, and mountains) as indirect metaphors for the human condition. In addition to the rich use of metaphors and symbolism in poetry, the same may also be said about each of the individual Chinese characters. In some cases, the symbolic, or concrete representations are obvious; in others, they are more difficult to parse. However, both in dreams and in poetry, the metaphors become more decipherable when we trace their origins. In speaking of dreams, Freud has said, "Things that are symbolically connected today were probably united in prehistoric times by conceptual and linguistic identity" (Freud, 1900/1953, p. 352). This conceptual and linguistic inquiry rings especially true with Chinese.

Classical Chinese poetry is as concise as it is elegant. Many genres of Classical Chinese poetry prescribed strict rules regarding the number of characters (syllables) permitted per line, parallel syntax, rhyme schemes and tonal inflections. These guidelines created exacting challenges to the poets, and each character in a line of verse was selected with much deliberation.

The conciseness of Classical Chinese poetry is realized by having many of the critical elements we would expect in Western works left to the reader's imagination. Dreams, too, often contain examples of such "omissions." The results are often cryptic. In Classical Chinese poetry, it is most notably the personal pronouns, or agents that are left to the imagination. The result is an ambiguous stream of thought that is in neither the first nor third person point of view. In this dreamlike swirl, there exist multiple perspectives, sometimes simultaneously. This uncommitted structure and "mobile point of view" results in an elusive ego presence (Yip, 1997, p. 12). Are the actions being committed by the poet? Or are they being observed by the reader? Perhaps, even, it is a story being told from the point of view of an other-worldly being. As in the dream realm, these revolving perspectives give the poems their shimmering, almost holographic quality, and creates an aura of timelessness. With the absènce of a definitive subject, or point of view, the verse seems to drift in the air, waiting to be claimed by the reader. This dreamy sense of non-linearity and primary process elements create a magical realm wherein much of the structured logic of the waking world is suspended. Freud found in the Chinese language many analogies to the types of indefiniteness exhibited in dreams (Freud, 1917/1920, p. 206). Much of Classical Chinese poetry certainly exhibits this dreamy sense of indefiniteness. It has even been suggested that Freud may have used the Chinese language as a model for his own interpretive strategies (Zhang, 1992, p. 9).

As we read a line of Chinese text, we are able to visualize the unfolding of a scene in its natural order. "In reading Chinese we do not seem to be juggling mental counters, but to be watching *things* work out their own fate." (Fenollosa & Pound, 1936, p. 9).The cinematic representations, or dramatization of ideas, are reminiscent of how Freud describes dream narratives. Chinese grammar is quite different from Western languages, especially in classical times. Syntax is flexible. Punctuation is absent. Any given character may function in a variety of ways without having to adapt to case endings, tense, gender, plurals, or even time, and so the reader must rely on the context to make sense of the verse (Yip, 1997, p. 2). The result is an emotional engagement with the poem on a primary level, and, as Ben Wang, a well-known authority on Chinese Classical poetry, has said, "Chinese may be a unique language eminently suited for poetry, for in poetry this visceral quality would ultimately join the cerebral in expressing art, beauty, and all things related to heaven, earth and how they relate to the humans in between." (Wang, 2018, p. vii).

Every sound in the Chinese language could have multiple meanings (even when accounting for the tones), and so we need to rely on conversational contexts to disambiguate what the speaker is saying. However, the homophones are not written alike (much like in English, e.g., "piece" and "peace"). Puns and jokes often work because of their play on words, relying on just this type of ambiguity to make their point. The graphic nature of Chinese is poised for such word play. For example, it is not uncommon to see a picture of a bat hanging upside down used as a decoration. That is because the Chinese word for "bat" sounds just like the word for "fortune"—"*fu,*" and the word for "upside down" sounds just like the word for "arrive"—"*dao.*" So, when you see a picture of a bat upside down, you would say "*fu dao le*" (the bat is upside down, 蝠倒了), which *sounds* exactly like the phrase for "fortune arrives" 富到了). Sometimes, instead of a bat, just the character for fortune, 富, is hung upside down—a wish for good luck that is pouring out and arriving at your home! An upside down bat (or the character, *fu*) is a visual pun that, when spoken, is actually a hail of good fortune. Some people with a superstitious streak believe that by making these references indirect, you are keeping away the evil eye!

Symbols, puns and metaphors are similarly an indirect way of expressing latent content in dreams, perhaps as a way to soften their impact on the dreamer. Without the aid of contextual references, unraveling a dream could be a nightmare. There are some words in Chinese that may contain their opposite meanings, (e.g., *jie* 借 (borrow/lend)), and so we need to rely on the context to disambiguate their meaning. We see these examples of "reversal" or "reaction-formation" in dreams, too, in that a manifest element could have very different, even opposite, latent contents. "...since in the dreamwork opposites coincide, it is in every instance uncertain whether a specific dream-element is to be understood in a positive or a negative sense...". (Freud, 1917/20, p. 204).

The many indirect references, subtle word play, and potential antonyms often result in multiple interpretations. Just as a simple content analysis of a dream may miss the nuanced associations and contextual cues that a deeper analysis could yield (e.g., pp. 57–58), likewise merely skimming across the surface of a verse would not do justice to the poem's deep meanings. "Discretion is the first part of Chinese poetry; it is like a riddle" (Ben Wang, lecture, 2022). Freud has likewise likened the interpretation of a dream to the solving of a riddle where the displaced latent meanings of the manifest symbols need to be deciphered in order to be fully understood. He even went so far as to say that "...dream-symbols...frequently have more than one or even several meanings, and, as with Chinese script, the correct interpretation can only be arrived at on each occasion from the context." (Freud, 1900/1953, p. 353).

Whereas it is inconceivable that anyone would say that poems are meaningless, there are those who nonetheless consider etymological and historical analyses to be a misguided route to understanding Classical Chinese poetry. They claim that it amounts to little more than fool's gold because, in their opinion, "no more than three percent of characters are historically pictorial or properly ideographic" (Tsu, 2022, p. xvii). This point is debatable.

Critics have also argued that the classical poets were unaware of the etymology of their characters, and therefore to pursue such a deep analysis is little more than the reader's conceit. But this hardly rings true. A classical education in those days would certainly have included the study of the language in depth. The etymological stories that the characters tell reveal the culture and history of the Chinese people, and the poets selected each word and wrote each character with meticulous deliberation. This skeptical line of argument mirrors much of what has been criticized about dream analysis and interpretation.

Just as some contemporary scholars have taken issue with etymological analyses of Chinese characters and poems, we have seen the tendency of 20th century behaviorist psychologists to criticize what they considered to be archeological digs into the deeper meaning of dreams; they cautioned not to look for meanings that were never there. Many dream scientists today still adhere to this line of reasoning. Freud noted this criticism when he said, "Dream interpretations have been accused of being strained, specious, dragged in" (Freud, 1917/20, p. 208). Freud could just as well have been referring to the deeper etymological reading of Classical Chinese poetry.

And, in a similar claim that poets were not cognizant of etymology, critics of dream interpretation have challenged whether a dreamer is ever aware, on any level, of the camouflaged imagery, metaphors, and puns when they produce their dreams. Perhaps it is the interpreter who is inserting and projecting analyses of their own. Is the "true meaning" in the hands of the poet/dreamer, or in the eyes of the beholder? I would argue that the answer is "both." To be engaged with a dream, or relishing a poem, the dynamic experience is at once personal and subtle.

In summary, what Wang Laoshi has said about Chinese poetry also rings true for dreams: "What you see is not all there is to see – There is so much more underlying the surface luster – But once you find the inner meaning, it becomes all the more profound!" (Ben Wang, lecture, 2021).

The following sample poem is by the Tang poet, Meng Hao Ran, as taught by Ben Wang, aka "Wang Laoshi" (respected teacher Wang). The words beneath the characters are the literal word-for-word definitions, and what follows are samples of their etymology. If we were to examine the earliest versions of these characters (which appeared as oracle writing), the symbolic representations would certainly be more evident. However, when reading these traditional characters (and even more so with simplified characters), we sometimes need to stretch our imaginations a bit in order to "see" their earliest images. In addition to getting a glimpse into the etymology of the characters, this sample demonstrates the concise nature of the verse, with personal pronouns, tenses, etc. omitted. When reading the lines of verse (from left to right), we can see how the cinematic trajectory of the characters tell their story. However, as in quantitative content-analysis, a straightforward reading of the words do not tell the full story. The references to the natural world are but metaphors for the realm of human experiences—left to your imagination to interpret. I have included a straightforward rendering of each line of verse, then provided my full translation of the poem.

A Tang poem written by Mèng Hào Rán 孟浩然 (689–740 AD)

春曉
spring dawn

春眠不覺曉
spring sleep not sense dawn

處處聞啼鳥
place place hear cry bird

夜來風雨聲
night come wind rain sound

花落知多少
blossom fall know how-many/much

The title: 春曉

春 This is an image of the plants emerging with the sun (日), meaning "springtime."

曉 The sun is on the left. On the upper right side are three pictures of soil (土), sitting atop a stove. The making of morning preparations, meaning "dawn." By itself, the right side means "to dawn on me," "to suddenly know." It is also the name of a mythological king.

Does this title suggest spring is dawning, or awakening? Or is it the dawn during springtime? Can it be that something is dawning on someone, somewhere?

1st Line: 春 眠 不 覺 曉

spring sleep not sense dawn

春 An image of the plants emerging with the sun (日), meaning "springtime."

眠 The left side is the symbol for "eye" The right side is the component that signifies "working people." They are tired, this means "sleep."

不 This glyph is an aerial view of a bird flying away. In other words, "there is no more." This character signifies negation, or "not."

覺 The upper portion depicts two hands folded on a desk. The lower portion indicates a sensation. Taken together, they represent the feelings typically experienced by a student at his desk, feeling the pain of intense instruction, meaning, 'to sense', 'to feel', to know'. This character is often connected with discussions of Buddhist writings.

This first line elicits images of springtime, still slumbering, with no sense of the new day.

Second Line: 處 處 聞 啼 鳥

place place hear cry bird

處 This signifies "places." It is repeated for emphasis, meaning "all around."

聞 There is a symbol of an ear between the doors of a gate; in other words, meaning "listening" or "hearing."

啼 There is a mouth on the left side, and the element for king, or emperor, on the right, meaning "to cry out," "to wail," "to weep."

鳥 This is a stylized depiction of a bird, complete with head, tail and feathers. It means "bird."

The second line conveys that everywhere, birds can be heard crying.

Third Line: 夜 來 風 雨 聲

night come wind rain sound

夜 Under a roof, a person sits with the moon, meaning "evening," "night time."

來 The character shows 2 persons (从) behind a tree (木), meaning "comes" or "arrives."

風 The inner part signifies insects; they are all around, meaning "the wind."

雨 There are droplets falling from under the clouds and sky, meaning "rain."

聲 The upper portion represents hands striking a mallet with stones, creating chimes. The lower portion is a symbol for the ear. Taken together, they mean "sound."

This third line, taken as a whole, paints a vivid image. We can visualize the scene: a person, sitting inside the house, waiting, as the night returns. The squall of the wind engulfs him. The rain drips down, making its distinct sound.

These five characters create an entire scene, complete with setting, mood, and sound.

Fourth Line: 花 落 知 多 少

blossom fall know how many

花 The top indicates foliage. This character means "flowers" or "blossoms."

落 Again, the top is foliage. There is water on the left side. On the right, there is a hand above a mouth. This character means "to fall," or "the fallen."

知 On the left, is an arrow or a dart against a person. On the right is a mouth, implying a knowledge that allows a person to give an opinion with precision, like a bull's-eye. This means "to know."

多 This depicts two moons—that's too many; it means "many" or "much."

少 These are few grains of sand, or something small or insignificant. This phrase is comprised of its opposites: 多少 "many/few." Taken together, they mean "how many?" Or "How much?"

This last line shows that blossoms have fallen; we know there are many or few.

Put all together, we have the following translation:

Spring Dawn

Spring sleeps, oblivious to the dawn
All the while, birds are crying far and wide
Throughout the night, the wail of wind and rain persists
Heedless to the countless blossoms perishing

Now, back to the title of this section:

Freud Dreams Chinese Poetry
弗梦汉诗

(The character "弗" is being used to represent Freud's full name "弗洛伊德" in order to keep with the Chinese tradition of using just four characters to convey an expression or proverb.)
So, what is this title saying?
Could it be an enumeration of items that are being discussed (Freud, Dreams, Chinese, Poetry)?
Or, are we talking about Freudian dreams and Chinese poetry?
Perhaps it is Freud, himself, dreaming of Chinese poetry?
As with dreams, it's open to interpretation.

Problem-Solving Dreams (Deirdre Barrett)

In this section we turn to creative variants of enhanced consciousness in dreams in which problems that stump awake consciousness are solved in dream consciousness. The current editor of the journal *Dreaming*, Deirdre Barrett, has organized and expanded on a variety of creative tasks that seem to be (sometimes) facilitated in dreaming—from musical composition, to literature, to science and math, to engineering, to medicine, to brain-teasers, among others.

For example, the 19-year-old, Mary Wallstoncraft Shelley, pregnant with Shelley's child, was trying to make good on Byron's challenge to his group of brilliant bohemian friends to write a horror story. She had a dream about "a pale student of unhallowed arts kneeling beside the thing he had put together ... (Barrett, 2001, pp. 40–41). On awakening she knew she had found her story, which was to become the immortal classic, *Frankenstein*. Stephen King, a modern giant of the horror genre, readily attributes some of his inspirations to materials in his dreams. He claimed, "I've always used dreams the way you'd use mirrors to look at something you couldn't see head-on" (in Barrett, 2001, p. 46).

Original musical composition is also often ascribed to dream creation. Paul McCartney, at the age of 22, heard a classic string ensemble playing in a dream and woke from the dream with "a lovely tune in my head" (Barrett, 2001, p. 66). Because he heard the tune in a dream he could not believe it was his own music. "It took me little while to allow myself to claim it, but then, like a prospector, I finally staked my claim. . . . Okay, it's mine! It had no words" (pp. 66–67). The lyrics provisionally used went, "Scrambled eggs, oh, my baby, how I love your legs" (p. 67). Eventually, it became the hugely popular song, "Yesterday." Similar dream-inspired music is to be found in the classical music genre. Richard Wagner claimed that his complex opera, *Tristan and Isolde*, was the creation of a dream. He wrote a friend, "For once you are going to hear a dream. I dreamed all this: never could my poor head have invented such a thing purposely!" (p. 73).

Science and math creations also sometimes draw upon dreams for inspiration and execution. A proponent of dreaming with a scientific purpose was the great chemist, August Kekulé. In a keynote speech delivered in 1890 to the German Chemical Society, he adjured his audience, "Let us learn to dream, gentlemen, then perhaps we shall find the truth" (p. 84). One of his two greatest contributions to organic chemistry, the "Structural Theory," had its origin in a waking reverie (*Traumerei*). Later, he was to achieve a breakthrough in the sleeping state, which yielded the problematic structure of benzene. He saw "atoms ... gamboling before my eyes ... all twining and twisting in snake-like motion. But look! What is that? One of the snakes had seized hold of its own tail, and the form whirled mockingly before my eyes. As if by a flash of lightning I awoke" (p. 86). He spent the rest of the night working out the hint in the dream: The benzene molecule was a ring, not a straight chain. Carl Gustav Jung, no doubt, would have noted the connection between the circled snake and the *mandala* (*magical* wheel) archetype for *individuation* (a universal drive, according to Jung, prominent in middle age, to achieve integration and wholeness in the heretofore dissociated mind).

A Nobel Prize winning idea, laying the foundation for the operation of *neurotransmitters* in neural communication, came to Otto Loewi in successive dreams. He hurriedly jotted down some of the essential ideas from a first dream but was not subsequently able to decipher his scribbles. But the next night, the idea returned in a dream which pointed to a design for proving the chemical underpinnings of neural transmission. This time, Loewi took no chances with his handwriting and headed straight to the laboratory to carry out the experiment on a frog's heart that led to his Nobel Prize in 1936.

Mathematical discoveries have also been imputed to dreams. The Indian mathematical genius, Srinivasa Ramanujan, claimed that all his mathematical discoveries came from the Hindu goddess, Namagiri, who conveyed to him the mathematical insights in dreams. The Muse, apparently, is a universal goddess—one who does not restrict herself only to poetry.

Barrett discusses some more down-to-earth puzzles that dreams can solve for the flummoxed awake mind. In her Chapter 9 ("What Word Starts and Ends with 'He?' Sleep on a Brainteaser and Wake Up with a Headache"), she poses a problem used by her friend, the psychiatrist, Morton Schatzman, a physician fascinated by the nocturnal solution of brainteasers—and also the author of an influential work on "The Psychotic Dr. Schreber," to be discussed briefly in our next section. The brainteaser posed in Barrett's Chapter 9 was given by Schatzman to a young colleague, a fellow physician, with the hint that the problem had two solutions. The young physician had a very long dream that night which included a lot of silly laughter ("hee ... hee ... hee ...") by the characters in the dream. In the dream, the young physician has a heart attack but the doctor treating him refuses to discharge him until the young doctor can tell him, in plain language, what his problem was. The answer, "I have had a coronary," is rejected as being mere jargon. The hospital doctor keeps laughing at the young physician ("hee ... hee ... hee ..."), who is furious, having expected sympathy, not laughter. He declares, "You could call it anything, even heartache" (p. 162). The laughter stops. The hospital physician in the dream now gives the young physician permission to go home even though some nonspecific pain persists, but urges the young physician to see "another doctor, a word specialist." Now Morton Schatzman appears in the dream and tells the young physician, "You must juggle words and pains" (p. 162). The young physician responds, "Riddles give me headaches" (p. 163). Suddenly, the pain disappears completely and the dreamer awakes with the solution to the riddle: HEartacHE and HEeadacHE (p. 163).

The famous Stanford dream researcher, William Dement, did his own studies of brainteasers on over a thousand college students. Here is one of the brainteasers used: "The letters, O, T, T, F, F ... form the beginnings of an infinite sequence. . . . According to your rule, what would be the next two letters in the sequence?"

(Barrett, pp. 163–164). Of 1148 students tested, seven students solved one of the brainteasers in their dreams. One student, in a dream, started counting paintings at an art gallery—one, two, three, four, five—but the sixth and seventh paintings had been ripped out from their frames. The dreaming student suddenly realized that he had solved the puzzle, the solution being, O, T, T, F, F, **S, S** . . . . (**O**ne, **T**wo, **T**hree, **F**our, **F**ive, **S**ix, **S**even, . . .)

It is clear that significant individual differences exist in solving brainteasers—or realizing that one's dream has actually provided the solution. Deirdre Barrett and her friend Morton Schatzman are very good at it; Barrett's friend, Nancy Parsifal, has a hard time with brainteasers. (On the other hand, facing a real life-or-death conundrum, Parsifal managed to save the life of her newborn baby by heeding a dream over the objection of two physicians and her husband [Barrett, pp. 131–134].) Here is a brainteaser that Parsifal appears to have solved in a dream without realizing she had solved it:

"What phrase does the following represent?" (pp. 177–178)

****

B.A.B.S.

0

****

Parsifal dreamt that she was in a frigid room. She finds the thermostat, which reads, 0. She then tries to raise the temperature but can only manage to get a couple of degrees higher. Parsifal had solved the problem in her dream without realizing it, the solution being, "Two degrees above zero."

Many examples of dream solutions to problems are given by Barrett for other domains. Clearly they abound. The challenge (as Barrett agrees [personal communication, 2015]) is to find experimental methodologies that would extend the findings from striking anecdotes to significant effects with statistical samples of subjects, along with controls for non-dreaming solutions.

Dream-Like Cognition in Schizophrenia

Around the turn of the 19th century, Carl Gustav Jung was a young psychiatrist who, in a few short years, had risen to second in command at the world-famous psychiatric institute in Switzerland, the Bürgholzli, headed by Eugen Bleuler. Bleuler is known for introducing the nosological entity, *schizophrenia*, which replaced the earlier *dementia praecox*. The Bürgholzli staff had periodic meetings to discuss new developments in psychiatry. The group was quite fascinated by a recent book, published by an obscure physician, Sigmund Freud, with the title,

The interpretation of dreams. What especially intrigued the group were the many similarities to be found between schizophrenic thinking and dreams. Jung wrote Freud and proposed a meeting between them, which turned out to be exciting for both. For over a decade, until their falling out, Jung was a leading figure in the psychoanalytic movement. Dreams and schizophrenia, it became clear to Jung and Freud, shared many cognitive features, especially the prominence of primary-process thinking, dream-work distortions, and disinhibition. Here are two clinical examples illustrating some of the overlaps:

The Case of N. (Matthew Erdelyi)

This patient, a former engineering student in his late twenties, continually rails against homosexuals, whom he detests with a violent passion. After a brief, unsuccessful marriage, followed by impotence, he began to experience delusions of persecution, according to which the CIA and the FBI were continually observing him with the ultimate purpose of getting him to submit to the sexual advances of Richard Nixon. He gave up all attempts at heterosexual sex because he would "not make love in public," that is, in front of the lurking agents. He soon came to understand also that his impotence had been imposed on him, via laser rays, by Nixon's agents. Satellites specifically sent up for the purpose began to bombard him with homosexual messages. Finally, he constructed a special protective metal hat, fitted with a complex jamming device. He wore this hat continually, at home and in public places, including restaurants and work. Even so, the messages that he should submit to Nixon increase in intensity and began to "penetrate" at times. Around this period he took all his jackets to a tailor and had the tailor sew up the slits (or flaps) in the back of the jackets. He implores his male acquaintances to do likewise, lest they be taken for "slot-jacket ass panderers." He deplored tight dungarees because they revealed buttocks too openly and therefore constituted a disgraceful invitation to sodomy. He complained that the CIA was spreading rumors that he was a homosexual; indeed, they had contrived to find "doubles" for himself and a friend and photographed them—the doubles—in "disgusting" homosexual acts, all for the purpose of blackmail, so that he might submit to the homosexual importunings of the "anarcho-communist sodomite" Gerald Ford, the new President, who, as he now came to realize, was really "behind" the conspiracy. (Nixon, it turned out, was just a "front."). N. consciously hated homosexuals; indeed the extent of his hatred was worrisome, for he began to mutter darkly about destroying them, seeing himself as an innocent heterosexual victim of homosexual persecution. (Adapted and elaborated from Erdelyi and Goldberg (1979, p. 372)).

There are many dream-like features in the Case of N. Almost all students (even the skeptical ones) tend to perceive the latent homosexuality of N. Presumably N. denies the obvious because he finds the obvious intolerable. A major reason for suspecting N.'s underlying homoeroticism is that he does not let go of the issue and some of his claims are preposterous. He sees homoeroticism everywhere, talks about it incessantly; only, he attributes it to others, who tend to persecute him. Almost all of the dream-work operations—censorship, displacement, condensation, symbolism, concretistic representation—are in ample evidence, along with a substantial breakdown of reality-testing. N. concretistically represents his efforts at defense by constructing a black-colored defense helmet—which looked like a painted Nazi helmet (he claimed to have been tortured by the Nazis in his home country), which he stuffed with a variety of electronic devices to jam the laser rays being directed at him by Nixon's satellites. Additionally, the black helmet had several holes drilled into it, from which antennae protruded, to defeat Nixon's laser rays. The black helmet worn by N. made for a disturbing sight.

Despite his efforts, N.'s defenses are not holding (he seems to be saying symbolically) when he asserts that the homosexual messages (from President Nixon) had increased in intensity and began to "penetrate" at times. An astonishing piece of defensive symbolism is illustrated by his having all the slits or flaps in the back of his jackets sewn together (lest others take him for a "slot-jacket ass panderer"). It is as if N. were saying in some behavioral code: "I am closed there; you may not penetrate."

It may be worth noting in conclusion a poetic quality to some of N's communications. Terms like "penetrate," "behind," "front," "softening up," along with the act of sewing up of flaps or slits, belong to this poetic mode. Freud noted such artistic features in his patients' symptoms—as we have in the preceding section—and connected up some of his ideas about insanity and defense with art.

The Psychotic Dr. Schreber (Sigmund Freud)

The Case of the Psychotic Dr. Schreber (Freud, 1911/1958) bears many similarities to the brief Case of N. of the preceding section. Dr. Schreber, like N., is consumed with homosexual (and also, in his case, sexual-identity) preoccupations which are formulated in bizarre delusional notions that are both persecutory and megalomaniacal.

Freud never treated or, even, met Dr. Schreber but, rather, wrote his case history on the basis of an autobiographical work, *Memoirs of my nervous illness*, published in 1903 by Dr. (of jurisprudence) Daniel Paul Schreber. Dr. Schreber was an important German jurist whose career was destroyed by mental illness. He managed to recover from his first breakdown (in 1885) after spending six months in the clinic of Geheimrat Professor Dr. Flechsig, who was to become a central figure in Schreber's subsequent delusional system. At first, Professor Flechsig was gratefully given credit for Schreber's initial recovery—his wife, according to Dr. Schreber (caveat emptor, here) "revered Professor Flechsig as the man who restored her husband to her, and hence it was that for years she kept his portrait standing upon her writing table" (Freud, 1911/1958, p. 108). His recovery lasted some eight years but then Dr. Schreber began to have dreams, which turned out to be premonitory, that his mental illness was returning. Around this time he awoke from sleep one morning with the thought "that after all it must be very nice to be a woman submitting to the act of copulation" (p. 108). This episode was followed in short order by fulminations of the most extravagant hypochondriacal delusions: his brain was softening; he was dead; his body was decomposing; his body was being handled in all kinds of revolting ways.

Now his former savior, Dr. Flechsig, was seen to be his "soul murderer" (p. 108). At first, Schreber sees God as an ally against his enemy, Dr. Fleichsig, but comes soon to realize that "God himself had played the part of accomplice if not instigator in the plot whereby my soul was to be mutilated and my body used like a strumpet" (p. 115). Eventually, Fleichsig and God are condensed into "God Fleichsig" (p. 149). Schreber complains that,

> Rays of God not infrequently thought themselves entitled to mock me, calling me Miss Schreber, in allusion to the emasculation which, it was alleged, I was about to undergo. . . . Or they would say: "So *this* sets out to have been a Senatpräsident, this person who lets himself be "f____d." ... Don't you feel ashamed in front of your wife?
>
> *(p. 116)*

These nightmarish delusions are eventually parlayed into the megalomaniacal idea that all this suffering, including his emasculation, had the higher purpose of leading to his "impregnation by divine rays to the end that a new race of men might be created" (p. 117). Even the act of defecation, which preoccupies Schreber a great deal, is invested with special status, e.g., "the call to sh___" is always accompanied by the generation of exceedingly strong feelings of spiritual voluptuousness" (p. 123).

Concretistic representations abound in Schreber's delusions. Through a technique Schreber calls "drawing," he conjures up visual images of his body being fixed with female breasts, buttocks, and genitalia (p. 130). He ascribes his "cultivation of femaleness" (p. 131) to the demands of God, who requires that he be a woman "luxuriating in voluptuous sensations" (p. 131).

The entire paranoid case can be seen as a vast, unending nightmare. More generally, Freud asserts that "it is legitimate to judge paranoia on the model of a far more familiar mental phenomenon--the dream" (p 137).

In this case-history, Freud elaborates on several specific techniques of defensive distortion, including, *reaction formation* (p. 165), *projection* (pp. 166, 171), *displacement* (p. 161), *denial* (p. 267), and *repression* (pp. 170–171). In his theoretical summing up, Freud claims that the "dominant element in Schreber's case ... is the father complex" (p. 161). Presumably, Fleichsig and God are symbolic representations of Schreber's own father, a physician, who was himself a famous and formidable figure in his time. Freud only passingly deals with Schreber's father, Dr. Daniel

Gottlieb Moritz Schreber, who introduced palpably sadistic techniques, by our standards, for the proper upbringing of children through "therapeutic gymnastics" (p. 151).

It is here where Morton Schatzman (1973)—and also W. G. Niederland (1959)—make major contributions to the case the Psychotic Dr. Schreber by showing, through scholarly analyses of the program of Schreber's father, of the substantial extent to which many of Schreber's (the son's) experiences are hyperemnesic, constituting unwitting recoveries, in distorted form, of some of the "educational techniques" imposed on him by his father which Schreber (the son) often conceptualizes as "miracles." Schatzman surmises that the adult Schreber was re-experiencing the pains that he had experienced as a child being subjected to his father's techniques. Thus, the various symptoms (or "miracles") which torture Dr. Schreber are "reminiscences" of the dreadful experiences the father imposed upon his young son (Schatzman, 1973, pp. 44–52). In a sorrowful plaint, Schreber declares, "God [presumably, his father] is inseparably tied to my person through my nerves' power of attraction which for some time past has been inescapable; there is no possibility of God freeing Himself from my nerves for the rest of my life" (*ibid,* p. 209).

Theoretical Cautions on the Overlaps between Dreams and Schizophrenia

It is clear that there are many commonalities between dreams and schizophrenia, which include neurological links (see Gottesman & Hanson, 2005; Solms & Turnbull, 2002). Both are characterized by an excess of primary-process thinking—breakdowns of logic and reality-testing, concretistic representation, cognitive distortions, outlandish symbolism, disinhibition, and other perversions of secondary-process thinking. Notwithstanding the overlaps, the two domains are not equivalent. Certainly, none of the psychiatric cases sampled would be confused for a dream.

Nevertheless, the overlaps are important to note because they point to future theoretical developments that may yield a unified framework for release phenomena in general. At present, however, we must reckon not only with limitations of the extant research but, also, of our basic constructs. "Schizophrenia" is not a stable concept. It keeps being recast with each edition of DSM (the *Diagnostic Statistical Manual* of the American Psychiatric Association). The latest edition (DSM-V, American Psychiatric Association, 2013) significantly differs in its treatment of schizophrenia from previous conceptualizations (e.g., in DSM-IV). Schizophrenia may not even survive in subsequent DSM iterations, just as "neurosis" has not survived. Similar problems, as will be seen in our next chapter, bedevil conceptualizations of what a "dream" entails. The simple identification of dreams with REM turns out to be oversimple. There is a modern trend for treating dreams with maximum generality as all conscious experiences occurring in sleep" (Hobson, 2002, p. 7; Malinowski, 2021, p. 5), and not just REM-sleep, with distinctions being made among various kinds of mental activities that are more or less dream-like, which are associated with different phases of sleep.

If both schizophrenia and dreams are no longer held to be stable constructs, analogizing becomes chancy. To propose that $x = y$, or even that $x \approx y$, loses conceptual crispness if it is not clear what "x" and "y" entail.

4

NEUROSCIENCE FOUNDATIONS OF DREAMING

REM Sleep: REM's, Short-Wave EEG's, Motor Inhibition, Genital Arousal—and Dreams

In the early 1950s, Eugene Aserinsky, working in the laboratory of the internationally famous sleep scientist, Nathaniel Kleitman, at the University of Chicago, was interested in doing research on attention in children. He was frustrated by a practical problem: Young children's attention tends to flag after a short while and they often drift off into sleep. Aserinsky decided to place electrodes near to the children's eyes to have an objective recording of eye closings. His first subject was his 7-year-old son, Armand, who produced an unexpected but highly reliable finding: As the young child drifted off to sleep, the eyes became active behind the eyelids, darting back and forth and up and down. This unexpected movement of the eyes in sleep, soon found to be associated with dreaming, has come to be known as *Rapid Eye Movements*, or, *REM's*, for short. (As Hobson noted, Aserinsky was a lucky researcher since only in children do REM'S appear soon after sleep onset and not, as in adults, in later phases of sleep.)

It turned out, as Aserinsky, Kleitman, and another member of the group, William Dement, soon discovered, REM's were only one component of a complex pattern of psychophysiological activities regularly ebbing and flowing in sleep over the course of the night in humans, cats, and, as later documented, in virtually all mammals (Aserinsky & Kleitman, 1953; Dement, 1976; Dement & Kleitman, 1955, 1957; Hobson, 2002; Jouvet, 1999; Solms & Turnbull, 2002). The complex pattern of correlated activities—including, REM's, short-wave EEG's, genital arousal, inhibition of motor activity—has come to be known as *REM Sleep, or, the REM State*. Humans, who can, unlike animals, report their psychological experiences when awakened from REM sleep, are highly likely to report a rich dream ("rich"

DOI: 10.4324/9781003300441-5

because such dreams involve hallucinatory, complex, story-like narratives) and so *REM's* have come to be considered (at least until recently; the complications will be discussed presently) as objective indicators of dreaming. In adult humans, these complex of events occur for approximately 10-20 minutes about four to five times a night, at intervals of approximately 90 minutes.

EEG's and Dreams

Let us consider the objective gauging of brain waves in humans, a simple yet epochal contribution of the German psychiatrist, Adolf Berger (1929), whose work was initially met with derisive skepticism in Germany but which, after the confirmation of his findings by British researchers and others, gradually gained international recognition.

The brain has an enormous number of neurons—the number is currently estimated as 100 billion—which at any time fire or are quiescent, depending on varied circumstances. The firing of a nerve cell (i.e., a neuron) constitutes an electrochemical event, subject to standard electrical recording. Berger concerned himself with voltage differences between different regions of the surface of the brain, the cortex, measured from recordings on the scalp. He placed electrodes on different places on the scalp and measured voltage differences between brain areas over time. This type or recording—fluctuating voltage differences over time—is known, after Berger, as the *electroencephalogram* (*EEG*, for short)

The critical finding was that voltage differences (usually measured in microvolts, μV) vary coherently over time and indicate different brain states—and, as it turns out, different states of consciousness. Figure 4.1 depicts several EEG patterns, each associated with a specific brain state. Pattern *a* reflects a very special kind of brain state: It is the EEG of a dead person. Pattern *b* is associated with wakefulness; pattern c with non-REM (NREM) sleep; and pattern *d* with deep, short-wave sleep (SWS). Finally, pattern *e*, which is easy to confuse with *b*, is the EEG associated with REM's—and with rich dreaming. When the person is asleep and producing REM's, the person seems also to be in a state resembling wakeful activation and is engaged in complex conscious activity. Mental reports can also be obtained from NREM awakenings but these are usually simpler, less rich narratively, and shorter, though it turns out that the picture is more complicated than originally thought, since dream reports from *late-sleep* NREM periods are often indistinguishable from those obtained from REM awakenings (Cicogna & Occhionero, 2013; Domhoff, 2018; Hobson, 2002; Solms & Turnbull, 2002). Also, reports of mental activity in the transition from wakefulness to sleep and from sleep to wakefulness often yield *hypnagogic imagery* that is also visually rich but less dynamic narratively. (Hypnagogic imagery obtained from awakenings in the transition from sleep to wakefulness is sometimes called *hypnopompic imagery* to distinguish it from the imagery obtained in the reverse transition from wakefulness to sleep.)

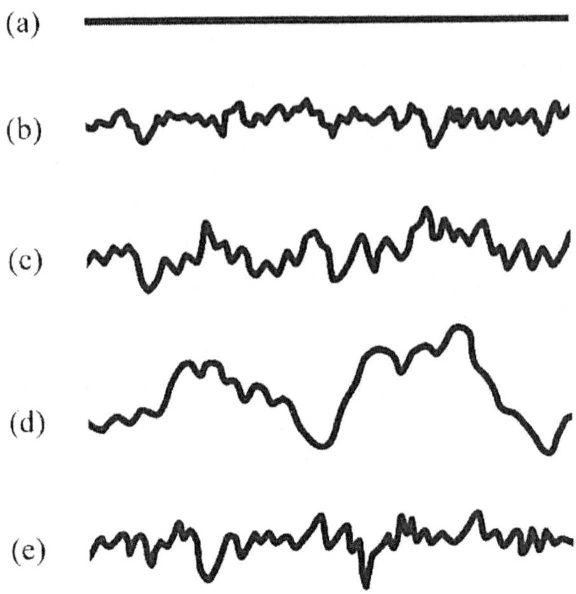

FIGURE 4.1 Several EEG patterns: (a) Brain-dead; (b) awake (mostly beta [β] waves [18–25 Hz], low amplitude, 5–20 microvolts [μV]), and some alpha [α] waves [8–13 Hz]); (c) NREM Stage 2 (4–15 Hz; 50–150 μV); (d) deep, short-wave sleep (SWS), rich in delta [Δ] waves (0.5–4 Hz; 100–200 μV); (e) REM (15–30 Hz, <50 μV).

Motor Inhibition in the REM State

We now turn to something of a paradoxical feature of dreaming—presently we shall more generally define dreaming as a paradoxical state, elaborating on Michael Jouvet's treatment of dreaming as "paradoxical sleep." In the REM state, the dreamer typically is involved in complex, dramatic activities, like running, fighting, flying, which involve energetic motor activities on the part of the dreamer, and yet the dreamer fails to enact the activities behaviorally. This inhibition of behavioral enactment of dream activity is adaptive since behavioral expression of the dream would be dangerous for the dreamer—or for the partner of the dreamer. Actually, in some cases, usually found in older persons, who may progress to neurocognitive disorders such as Parkinson's disease, this behavioral inhibition during the REM state breaks down, a condition recently recognized in DSM-V (Diagnostic Statistical Manual, 5th edition, *American Psychiatric Association,* 2013, pp. 407–410) as "Rapid Eye Movement Sleep Behavior Disorder." Of course, not all motor activities are suppressed, REM's themselves constituting an exception that is harmless to the dreamer.

Genital Arousal During REM Sleep

As noted earlier (p. 94), another striking correlate of dreaming is the occurrence of genital arousal. This was first noted for penile erections (Fisher, Gross, & Zuch, 1965; Ohlmeyer, Brilmeyer, & Hüllstrung, 1944) and later established for females, who evidence clitoral engorgement and vaginal lubrication during the REM state (Fisher, Cohen, Schiavi, et al., 1983). Awakenings from REM sleep during these episodes of genital arousal do not, however, yield reports of corresponding sexual arousal, and so REM sleep cannot be unambiguously identified with sexual arousal. This is a perplexing but not unusual problem in physiological research. Hobson's (2015) plausible explanation for this case is that only incomplete, early components of sexual arousal are being indicated by REM.

The Unraveling of the REM = Dreaming Consensus

"The story was too good to be true"

Coenen, 2003, p. 133

For several decades psychologists and neuroscientists enthusiastically believed that they had discovered an objective indicator of the subjective state of dreaming. Thus, it was assumed that the *REM state* = the *dream state*. From the start this equations was known not to be perfect since REM's were not perfectly correlated with dream reports and non-REM (NREM) reports also, if less frequently, yielded dream reports. The data were actually quite variable, depending on the criterion of what constituted a "dream report" and the manner in which awakened subjects were questioned (Foulkes, 1962; Snyder, 1967). Different researchers published different percentage of dream reports associated with REM and NREM sleep (see Snyder, 1967, p. 24: e.g., 74%–7% (Aserinsky & Kleitman, 1955); 88%–0% (Dement, 1955); 79%–7% (Dement & Kleitman, 1957); 82%–54% (Foulkes, 1962); 86%–23% (Rechtschaffen, Verdone, & Wheaton, 1963)). More recently, a concordance of 95% between REM and dreaming was reported by Hobson (2002), p.11. Although there clearly is a relationship between dreaming and the REM state, the relationship is statistical (the median difference for the entire Snyder data set is 83% versus 13%, for REM and NREM awakenings, respectively. The picture becomes murkier with the recent realization that the REM-NREM differences tend to disappear when the dream report samples are elicited in the later phases of sleep (see p. 95).

The breakdown of the REM = dreaming equation was theoretically inconvenient, especially for Hobson, who claimed to have discovered a biological clock in the brain-stem structure, the *pons*, which turned REM sleep on and off with the required periodicities and, when on, sent out impulses to many sites in the brain, including the frontal cortex. This pontine activation led to the famous *analysis-by-synthesis* hypothesis of dreaming of Hobson and McCarley (1977) which explained dream experience as resulting from the partial inhibition during REM sleep of the prefrontal cortex (which is associated with advanced cognitive processing) having to analyze and make sense of the chaotic impulses it was receiving from the activating pons. It was from this picture that the impression was widely drawn that dreams were basically chaotic, random neural phenomena.

Even if the model had not required revision by Hobson to accommodate further neurological findings, especially from the neuropsychoanalyst Mark Solms and his associates (Solms, 2003; Solms & Turnbull, 2002), the inference by many in the field that dreams were meaningless was illogical. Just because the (pontine) stimulus was random or chaotic, it did not follow that the subject's interpretation of the resulting experience was itself random or chaotic. The remote control of our TV does not contain any interesting, meaningful stories, such as we expect to see on TV, but merely contains the requisite information to trigger the TV channels which give us our meaningful stories. The analysis-by-synthesis model is, actually, a projective-test model: The stimulus is impoverished and the question is how the subject draws on his or her own internal psychological structures and biases to make sense of the experiences generated by the chaotic stimulus.

Double-Dissociation between the REM State and Dreaming (Mark Solms)

A fatal blow to the classic REM-dream connection was delivered by the neuropsychonalyst, Mark Solms (1997, 2003), who demonstrated, by aligning dreaming phenomena with brain pathology, that dreams and REM's could be "doubly dissociated": REM's could occur without accompanying dreaming, and dreaming could occur without accompanying REM's. Solms concluded that dreams and REM's were controlled by different brain mechanisms, with dreaming controlled not by the brain-stem pons but by two more phylogenetically advanced "anatomical groups" (see Figure 4.2), *the ventro-medial quadrant of the frontal lobe* and *the parietal-temporal-occipital junction* (or, the *PTO junction*, around Brodman Area 40). The phylogenetically more advanced instigating mechanisms (relative to the pons) suggested that dreams were not, after all, passive responses to the chaotic effusions of the pontine brain-stem but active creations of the cognitively advanced frontal systems.

The problematic REM-dream connection was revisited by a large number of dream scientists in a December 2000 special issue of *BBS*—the prestigious journal, *Behavioral and Brain Sciences*—which featured five major theoretical papers (including one by Hobson and his associates and one by Solms) and the commentaries of some 100 dream/sleep scientists. The special issue was soon republished as a book, with a new introduction and conclusion section (Pace-Schott, Solms, Blagrove, & Harnad, 2003). Although the statistical connection between REM's and dreaming was undeniable and, from a practical standpoint, determinative—a researcher wanting to get a dream report would be well advised to awaken the

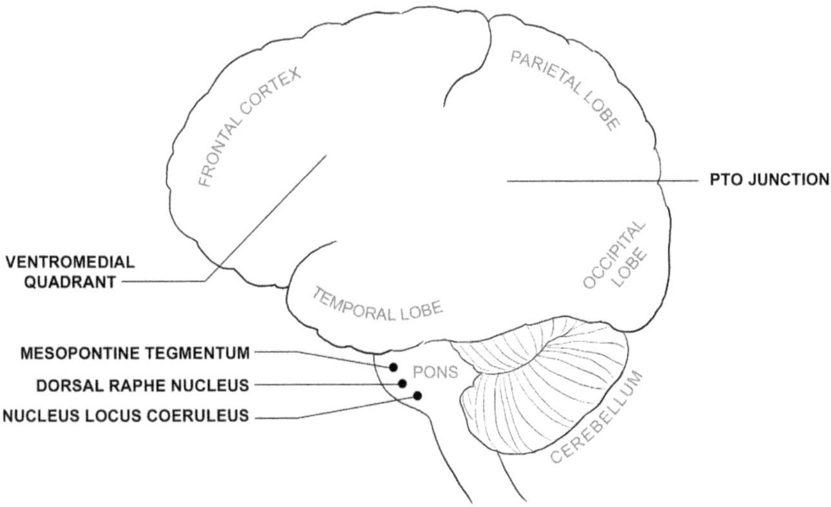

FIGURE 4.2 Schematic diagram of the brain and the brain stem, with the two regions identified by Solms as necessary for dreaming, *the ventro-medial quadrant of the frontal lobe* and the *PTO junction* (around Brodman Area 40). Included in the figure are the three brain stem regions that had been emphasized by Jouvet and Hobson as instigators (or inhibitors) of REM's, *the mesopontine tegmentum*, the *dorsal raphe nucleus*, and *nucleus locus coeruleus*. (It appears that REM's are actually biochemical release phenomena [Hobson, 2005, p. 29]: The REM-activating *mesopontine tegmentum*, a cholinergic system, is released by the cessation of firing of two aminergic systems, the *dorsal raphe nucleus* (rich in serotonin).

subject during a REM period—a growing contingent of scholars were moving in the direction of theoretically decoupling REM sleep from dreaming.

Hobson's Revision of the Activation-Synthesis Hypothesis: The "AIM" Model

Hobson proceeded to revise his classic analysis-by-synthesis hypothesis with a new, three-dimensional formulation, the "AIM" model, where A = *activation*, I = input mode, and M = chemical modulation (Hobson, 2011; Hobson, Pace-Schott, & Stickgold, 2000). The common denominator between the previous model and the new one was *activation*. REM's presumably are correlated with dreaming because REM's are high-activation states that are often sufficient to engender dreaming. Other sources of high-activation could, however, also produce dreaming. The AIM status of the subject is in continuous flux and so Hobson (2011, p. 248) suggested that a fourth-dimension, *t* (time), might be incorporated into his model, although he did not rename it, AIMT, and continued to treat it—as we shall—as a three-dimensional scheme (in which the values of the *X*-, *Y*-, and *Z*-axes happen to vary over time).

The "I" dimension of the model refers to input and output gating. During dreams, both the perception of the external world as well as the reactions to it are substantially shut down, rendering dreams a compelling form of virtual reality—much happens in the dream, but the rich environment of subjective perception and action is largely disconnected from the external world of perception and actual behavior.

The "M" (chemical modulation) component of the AIM Model became very important for Hobson because it provided an explanation for the strange cognitive style, or "form," of dreams, which no longer needed to be tied to the defensive distortions ("censorship") of Freud's dream-work. The strangeness of dreams was ascribed to mental activity taking place under the control of a different chemical environment than in waking cognition. Dreaming, according to Hobson's (original) view, is *cholinergic* (under the control of the neuromodulator, *acetylcholine*) whereas wakeful cognition is under *aminergic* control (notably, two amino acids, *serotonin* and *dopamine*). The chemical modulation of dreaming has, however, fallen into dispute (for an overview, see Domhoff, 2018, pp. 207–210), with the cholinergic hypothesis being challenged by a *glutamatergic* (glutamate) or a glutamatergic *plus GABAergic* (gamma aminobutyric acid) control view (Domhoff, 2018; Hobson, 2007; Jones, 1986; Luppi, Clement, and Fort, 2013). Or, still, all three neuromodulators may be involved, with dreams being glutamatergic, GABAergic, and cholinergic (Boucetta, Cissé, Mainville, Morales, & Jones, 2014). It may even be the case that REM activation is somewhat different in humans than in animals (Edlow, Takahashi, Wu, Benner, Dai, Bu, et al., 2012, p. 531). Obviously, the M dimension is an unfinished story.

The "Hot Zone" of Dreaming (Giulio Tononi, Francesca Siclari, et al.)

Recently, an international group of researchers, prominently including Giulio Tononi, head of the University of Wisconsin Center for Sleep and Consciousness and Francesca Siclari, now at University Hospital of Lausanne, Switzerland, appear to have discovered a more basic indicator of dreaming than REM, a "hot zone" in the posterior cortex (comprising the occipital lobe, the precuneus, and the posterior cingulate gyrus) which, when active, accurately predicts (though not perfectly, e.g., 87% of the time) the occurrence of dreaming, whether reports are elicited from REM *or* NREM sleep (Siclari, 2019; Siclari, Baird, Perogamvros, et al., 2017; Siclari, Bernardi, Cataldi, & Tononi, 2018). The work has been done with "high-density EEG" recordings collected from a net of electrodes covering the subject's head and face, which yields more simultaneous recordings (e.g., 256) than the usual two-dozen or so recordings of traditional assays. The high-density EEG's show that dream contents, for example, running, speaking, hearing, recruit the standard brain centers that would be active in corresponding awake activities, suggesting that dreams are ongoing activities in consciousness, and not spontaneous creations concocted upon awakening (see Chapter 6, pp. 163–164). Unwittingly recapitulating the classic *continuity principle* from psychology (see our next chapter, pp. 200–301),

Siclari concluded from the neurological data that "maybe the dreaming brain and the waking brain are much more similar than one imagined" (Siclari, 2019).

Form vs. Content: Hobson's "Formalistic" Theory and the Question of Dream Meaning

The Formalistic Approach

From his earliest book, *The dreaming brain* (1988), to his late work, *Dream life* (2011), Hobson emphasized a set of universal features that are characteristic of dreams (and of psychotic cognition also). Not all dreams evidence these characteristics but many do and even a small sample of dreams (such as are included in our Chapter 3) are bound to include them.

Before we consider these "formal" features, we might note a surprising fact about them that is not spelled out by Hobson: The proposed universal dream forms overlap substantially with Freud's *primary process*, discussed in Chapter 2 (p. 41). (For Freud's own exposition of the primary process, see his *The interpretation of dreams,* 1900/1953, pp. 597–609; *On dreams,* 1901a/1953, pp. 676–677; his article, "The Unconscious" (1915/1957, pp. 186–187); and his monograph, *Beyond the pleasure principle* (1920/1955, pp. 34, 62–63).) The labels used by Freud and Hobson are not always identical and there are some differences in details and emphases, but Hobson's and Freud's primitive dream characteristics are sufficiently overlapping to be considered the same basic set of features.

Another point that should be made before we proceed to Hobson's universal dream forms is that Hobson unaccountably treats *dream form* and *dream content* as antagonistic scientific issues, crowning form as the true scientific approach to the nature of dreams and demoting the interpretation of personal content to a failed venture that verges on "superstition" (Hobson, 2011, p. 161). It is for this reason that, to be faithful to Hobson's treatment, our subject heading is "Form vs. Content," when the heading should be "Form *and* Content."

Here, then, are the basic "formal" features that, according to Hobson, are characteristic of dreams in general (see Hobson, 1988, pp. 210–214; 2002, pp. 5–7; 2011, p. 129).

1. *Dreams are hallucinatory.* We see, hear, and feel things that are not objectively impinging on us. Freud's corresponding formulation is that dream representations are concretistic, or "plastic," comprising visual depictions and behavioral enactments ("dramatizations"). We have encountered numerous examples in our Chapter 3. Hobson's Mozart Dream has Hobson actually see Mozart and hear some of Mozart's music—played on the wrong instrument and without an orchestra. He perceives that Mozart has gotten a little overweight. He sees Mozart's rich red brocade frock coat and his gold-embossed curlicues and white powder wig. He sees Mozart's beatific smile and hears the arpeggios stream through the door (p. 72).

In Freud's Irma Dream, Freud examines the recalcitrant Irma, who looks pale and "puffy" and, looking down her throat, sees a big "white patch" and, at another place, "extensive white scabs upon some remarkably curly structures modelled on the turbinal bones of the nose" (p. 65). He sees that Dr. M. is very pale, walks with a limp, and has a shaven chin, and hears him make a ridiculous medical pronouncement. Dolores P. does not even try to render her visual dream in words but proceeds directly to providing a drawing of her dream. Alice V. is engrossed in witnessing the struggle of a gray elephant trying to right itself.

It is the case that the brain region associated with imagery, the PTO junction (but not the primary visual center in the back of the occipital lobe involved in veridical perception), is activated during dreaming, representing a "brain-mind isomorphism" (Hobson, 2002, p. 33), but this imagistic aspect of dreams is cinched by phenomenal experience and, not surprisingly, has been widely noted by scholars before the advent of modern neuroscience.

2. *Dreams are delusional.* Dreams are constructed from numerous false beliefs and memories. In Freud's language, dreams do not abide by the "Reality Principle" and readily violate logic and experience. In the Irma Dream, Freud is surprised that Leopold can determine, notwithstanding Irma's bodice, that portions of her skin on the left shoulder are infiltrated. It is not realistic, and, therefore, delusional, that Hobson should have an encounter with the long-dead Mozart. Again, a biological account can be given, namely the deactivation of frontal regions responsible for abstract reasoning and reality testing but, again, this feature of dreams has been grasped long ago.
3. *Distortions abound with regard to time, place, and persons* (Hobson, 1988, p. 212). Zelda has a peaceful conversation about *ratatouille* with her friend Jean who has, actually, been dead for some 15 years (pp. 156–158). Zelda is struggling with her mother's heart operation but soon transposes the "procedure" to her own dental extraction and, also, to her daughter's traumatic experience with a dental procedure gone wrong (pp. 74–77). The dream, moreover, surprises Zelda by being more about her father than the nominal problem in the dream, her mother. For Freud, *displacement*, *condensation*, and the *abrogation of linear time*, are distinguishing features of primary-process cognition (Freud, 1915/1957, pp. 186–187),
4. Dreams are *hyperassociative*, featuring "looseness of associations" (Hobson, 2002, p. 6). This, of course, is standard fare in Freud, who seeks to elaborate dream associations through the free-association technique. In highly regressed schizophrenic states, associations can be so loose as to constitute "word salad." In less extreme cases, the associations can be abnormally loose and yet make sense—very good sense sometimes, and be humorous to boot. Here are the loose verbalizations of a schizophrenic woman which feature both nonsense and wisdom, laced with, perhaps, unintended humor (note, Freud, Jung, Hobson, and Solms are committed to the virtual equation of dreams and psychopathological cognition):

> I am a doctor, you know. . . . I don't have a diploma, but I'm a doctor. I am glad to be a mental patient, because it taught me how to be humble. . . . When I was a little girl, I used to sit and tell stories to myself. When I was older, I turned off the sound on the TV set and made up dialogue to go with the shows I watched. . . . I am a week pregnant. I have schizophrenia--cancer of the nerves. My body is overcrowded with nerves. This is going to win me the Nobel Prize for medicine. I don't consider myself a schizophrenic anymore. There is no such thing as schizophrenia, there is only mental telepathy. I once had a friend named Camilla Costello. She was Abbot and Costello's daughter. . . . I'm in the Pentecostal Church, but I am thinking of changing my religion. I have a dog at home. I love instant oatmeal. When you have Jesus, you don't need a diet. . . . California's the most beautiful state in the Union. I have been there once, by television. . . . (Quoted in S. Sheehan, 1982, pp. 72–73) [In Bootzin, R. R., Acocella, J. R., & Alloy, C. B. (6th Ed., 1993), p. 367]).

5. *Dreams are amnesic.* Unless we write down our dreams on awakening we forget most or all of what we have just dreamt. Hobson's explanation is that "During REM sleep, the aminergic neurons do not send their 'remember' instructions to the forebrain, which, if not instructed to remember, will forget" (Hobsons, 1988, p. 214). Freud's almost surely incorrect explanation of the phenomenon (just as with infantile amnesia) is censorship, or repression, an issue that we shall revisit.
6. Finally, according to Hobson, dreams are *hyperemotional*. Here it is Hobson who is almost surely incorrect, or at least overstating the case, especially if one sticks only to the manifest content of dreams, which Hobson decidedly does ("the manifest dream is the dream, is the dream, is the dream" (Hobson, 2002, p. 161). Although it deals with an explosive issue for her, Alice's Elephant Dream at the manifest level is strikingly peaceful; the noises heard by Alice are explained reassuringly by the zoo keeper as, "it's just the animals mating" (p. 71). Alice does awake "with a sense of terror" but does not locate this terror in her dream. There is not much surface emotion in Freud's Irma Dream or in the Dolores P.'s Picture Dream. Hobson's Mozart Dream does express some amazement but the dream would not be considered by most to be particularly "emotional." Zelda's dream toward the end does break out in anger, so, obviously, dreams *can* be emotional but, and this is the point, they are not characteristically emotional, at least not at the surface level. Freud, of course, was an exponent of the view that dreams are about primal emotions and drives, notably *sex* and *aggression*, accompanied sometimes by *fear* ("signal anxiety"), but the sexual and aggressive material is largely confined to the latent content.

A perplexing feature of Hobson's approach is his either-or stance on form and content. Perhaps carried away by his enthusiasm for brain imaging and brain chemistry explaining the formal aspects of dreams, he states at one point: "The story keeps getting better and better. We might even wonder what is left for a psychology of dream content to do" (Hobson, 2002, p. 113).

The distinction between form and content is useful—both Freud and Hobson make it—but there is no reason why *both* form and content should not be concerns of dream science. The fact that neurology cannot provide us with a science of personal dream contents—or of the meaning of jokes, or of poetry, or of paraphasias—does not mean that personal content is not a legitimate scientific issue.

Misunderstandings About the Meaninglessness of Dream Content

From Hobson's frequent deprecations of personal dream content, it would be reasonable to assume that Hobson did not hold much hope for a science of personal dream meanings and has often given the impression of outright denying the existence of personal meanings in dreams. The Hobson-McCarley (1977) activation-synthesis model led, actually, to the widespread impression in academic psychology that dreams constitute random neural events lacking meaning. Of late, however, Hobson has claimed that he has been "misunderstood" ("I have been misunderstood by many colleagues who attribute to me a nonsense theory of meaning" (Hobson, 2011, p. 239)). It is true that from the beginning (Hobson & McCarley, 1977), Hobson asserted that dreams have meaning and actually gave some interpretations of personal meanings in his Mozart Dream, as he does for many other of his published dreams. Yet, he often seems to take back what he seems to be giving.

A close reading suggests that Hobson's position is hard *not* to misunderstand. In Hobson's "experimental memoir," *Dream life*" (2011), he "raises questions about our assumption that dreaming as a psychological experience is, in and of itself, terribly important" and concludes that "dreams themselves are not only illusory but may be dispensable" (p. 176). Yet, in the conclusion to this same book, he declares: "Dreaming is a glorious mental state worthy of our respect, interest and enjoyment. A life without dreaming would not be life" (p. 280).

In a frontal attack on the problem of dream meaning, Hobson and Kahn (2007) make a case against "the hypothesized individuality of dream content" in favor of "generic" meanings (p. 850) based on the "formal properties of dreams" (p. 855)—for example, pictorial representation, incongruities, discontinuities, delusions, amnesia, and so on. But what specifically is being proposed? Are we to understand, for example, that there are no personal meaning differences between Freud's Irma Dream and Hobson's own Mozart Dream (see Chapter 3)? Hobson and Kahn actually suggest that we are likely to fail to connect dreams to the dreamers if we removed "specific identifiers" such as proper names, places, relationships, and so on. The experimentally inclined reader could probably show easily that the prediction fails with the Irma vs. Mozart dreams, even with the excision of personal identifiers. These unwelcome identifiers, by the way, undermine a strict formalistic position, since truly generic dream contents would not yield specific names of characters and places in a dream.

In a rebuttal of Hobson and Kahn, Domhoff and Schneider (2008) review some of the quantitative content-analytic literature (see our next chapter) showing the pervasive correlations existing between the dream contents of individuals and their awake concerns, feelings, and emotional biases.

The denial of personal meanings in dreams can be understood to result from a procrustean impulse to impose a neurological solution on the psychological problem of meaning. Perhaps one day this venture will bear fruit, but its premature foisting has tended to derail dream science.

Another notion calling for reconsideration is Hobson's regular assertion that, to the extent that dreams are meaningful, their meaning is transparently obvious. This, however, is not our experience with dreams, such as the dreams sampled in Chapter 3. Laboratory research on the simpler modality of jokes shows not only that there are individual difference in sensitivity to latent contents, but also that sensitivity to latent contents can increase with effort over time (Bergstein & Erdelyi, 2008). Thus, the deeper meaning of cartoons (some of which are not transparent because we do not always "get" them) can be made more transparent. Jokes too have primary-process or formal features (the same ones as dreams (see pp. 53–57)) but this fact is in no way inconsistent with jokes having individual meanings. One joke is not equivalent to another joke, even if both rely on the same primary-process ("joke-work") techniques. There is no conflict between primary-process/formal-features and meaningful individual contents.

Dreams as Paradoxical States of Simultaneous Activation and Deactivation

The notion that dreams comprise "paradoxical sleep" was, as has already been noted, advanced by Michael Jouvet (1993/1999) to indicate that during dreaming the subject gives the appearance of being *both* asleep and awake. Specifically, Jouvet demonstrated that dreaming subjects (usually cats) show an activated brain state, as indicated by lively REM activity and also high-activation EEG patterns but, contrarily, the same subjects show postural *atonia* (e.g., the drooping of the cat's head during REM periods) and the inhibition of gross motor activity. Further research has shown that many objective brain and body indicators act in similar contradictory fashion during REM periods.

The simple picture—over-simple, as we will see—is that the frontal cortex, responsible for advance executive functions, is substantially deactivated (some authors refer to this condition as "hypofrontality" (Pace-Schott, 2007)) while, simultaneously, more primitive systems deeper in the brain, the *limbic system*, associated with emotions and drives are, contrarily, highly activated.

The usually anti-Freudian Hobson provides a bridge between the modern neuroscience view and Freud's clinically derived conception of a century earlier: "[T]he ego/super-ego equivalents are the dorsolateral prefrontal cortex" [which is deactivated].... [D]ream consciousness owes its often primitive character to 'release' of these brain programmes from the inhibition that holds them in check during waking" (Hobson, 2002, p. 145). In line with Freud's emphasis of the continuous tug and pull between the ego and the id, Hobson asserts, "The frontal lobes and the limbic brain are in a constant battle for control of the mind" (Hobson, 2005, p. 41).

Neuroscience research over several decades has led to a growing list of regions in the central nervous system that are either activated or deactivated during REM sleep (Braun, Balicin, Wesenten, Carson, et al., 1997; Braun, Balicin, Wesenten, Gwadry, et al., 1998; Dang-Vu, Desseilles, Albouy, Darsaud, et al., 2005; Hobson, 2002; 2011; Jouvet, 1962; 1999; Maquet, Péters, Aerts, Delfiore, et al., 1996; Maquet, Schwartz, Albouy, Dang-Vu, et al., 2004; Nir & Tononi, 2010; Nofsinger, Mintum, Wiseman, Kupfer, & Moore, 1997; Schwartz & Maquet, 2002; Solms, 1997; 2003). The *activated* areas include: reticular brain stem regions (e.g., the pons); thalamic nuclei; limbic-paralimbic areas (e.g., the amygdala; the hippocampus, the insula); motor and premotor cortices; the temporal-parietal-occipital (TPC) junction (around Brodmann's Area 40). The d*eactivated* sectors include the dorsolateral prefrontal cortex (the DLPFC), the right inferior parietal cortex, the posterior cingulate cortex, and spinal motor neurons.

Figure 4.3 provides a sketch of many of the CNS structures listed earlier.

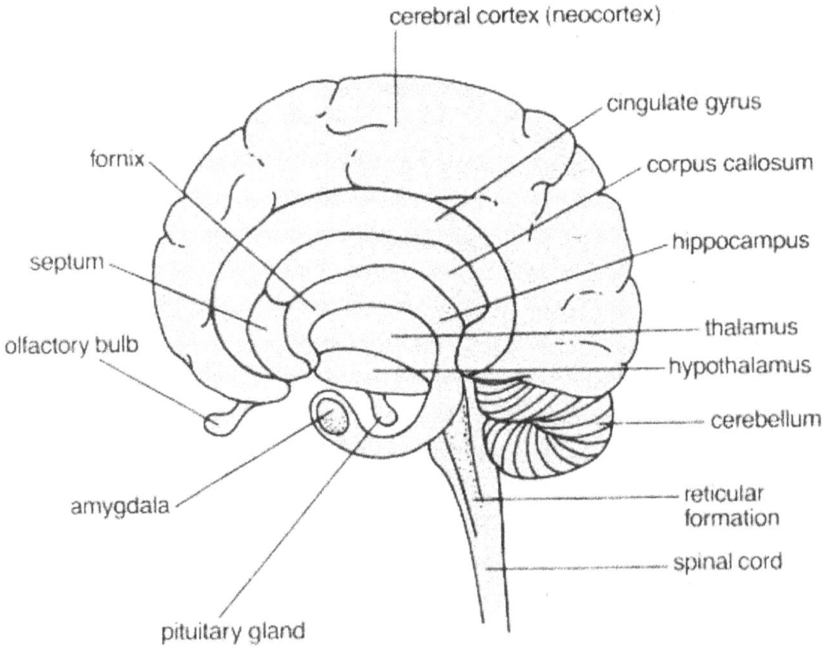

FIGURE 4.3 Some internal brain structures, including components of the *limbic system* (the *amygdala, septum*, the *hippocampus*, the *cingulate gyrus*), the *pituitary* (master) gland, and regions of the *brain stem* (e.g., the *pons* and the *medulla*). The *septum* is a limbic structure that tends to have a calming effect, lies to the front of the hypothalamus; not shown is the *insula*, a "paralimbic" structure (lying inside the temporal lobe of the neocortex), is major pleasure-center.

Note that the pons is activated during REM. Also, areas of the limbic system (the amygdala, hippocampus, and septum) and para-limbic structures (e.g., the insula) are activated, along with the cortical region associated with *imagery* (the PTO junction; (see Figure 4.2). Thus, activation of these parts yields emotional/drive activations which are experienced as emotions or drives. Also, the activation of the imagery center yields the imagistic representations of dream contents emphasized by Freud (1900/1953) and universally appreciated in the modern literature. The *insula*, tucked in the folds of the temporal lobe of the neocortex, is a major pleasure-center, which when electrically stimulated yields the experience of euphoric pleasure.

The deactivated regions associated with executive functions include not only the dorsolateral prefrontal cortex (the DLPFC) but also the right inferior parietal cortex and the posterior cingulate gyrus. We might note that the large structures in the brain, including the cingulate gyrus, have a semi-circular shape, roughly resembling an inverted letter "C," and so "frontal" and "posterior" loci tend to draw closer at their extreme ends.

Many of the constituents of the limbic system (e.g., the amygdala) have effects on the hypothalamus (which, actually, some neuroscientists do not recognize as a part of the limbic system). However we conceptualize the hypothalamus—or the limbic system—the hypothalamus gives us a notion of the kinds of drives and emotions supported by the brain, as the hypothalamus is prominently involved with basic drives such as fear, aggression, sex, hunger, thirst—and general pleasure.

Complications with the "Frontality" Notion

We shall restrict ourselves to noting two salient points. First, some of the *deactivated* systems associated with REM sleep are not in the front-most part of the frontal cortex (the prefrontal cortex) but also include the *right inferior parietal cortex*, the *posterior cingulate cortex*, and *spinal motor neurons.* Further, the "frontality" notion is itself too general, as its constituents do not necessarily go the same way. The *dorsolateral prefrontal cortex* (the DLPFC) is markedly deactivated during REM sleep but the *medial prefrontal cortex* (the MPFC) may, contrarily, show marked activation (see the discussion of the "default network" at the end of this chapter). Thus, we get only partial hypofrontality during dreaming. The tempting but ultimately too facile equation of Freud's "ego" with the prefrontal cortex—or the limbic system with the "id"—does not really hold on close inspection (see also Erdelyi, 1985, pp. 128–144).

Complications with the "Limbic System" (Does It Even Exist?—Joseph LeDoux)

The simplistic view of the limbic system is that it is the emotional brain. Paul Broca introduced the term (*le grand lobe limbique)*, which was extended by enterprising later neuroscientists, especially Paul MacLean, and recast variously as the *rhinecephalon* (the smell brain), the *visceral brain*, and the *paleomammailan brain.* There are many complications with the concept, however it is called and popular as it is (see LeDoux, 1997, 2016). Solms and Turnbull's (2002) comments on the subject are very helpful:

> The limbic system ... is really a *theoretical concept* about a group of structures that many neuroscientists feel are linked together in a functionally significant way ... different neuroscientists include different structures under the term.... It is therefore a rather vague definitional entity (the very usefulness of which some neuroscientists question).
>
> *pp. 16–17*

Thus, the limbic system is really an *interpretation*. The constituents—the brain stuff—are real enough, but how (and whether) they are organized as a "system" is an interpretation. The world authority on the limbic system, LeDoux (1997; 2016), has gradually moved to the position that the system does not really exist.

Fortunately, we need not resolve here the problems of the limbic system construct. Rather, we shall examine several of the structures usually associated with the limbic system and focus on some of the very interesting features that have implications for dreams.

The Hippocampus and Memory

The hippocampus ("horse's tail" in Latin—see Figure 4.3) is a traditional constituent of the limbic system and yet it is not commonly known for its contributions to drives and emotional life (though rabies, which selectively destroys the hippocampus, produces terror and rage in the afflicted animal). Instead, the hippocampus occupies a prominent position in cognitive science for its pivotal role in the encoding and storage of recently acquired memories. Destruction of the hippocampus results in *anterograde amnesia,* the inability to remember newly acquired memories (beyond a few seconds).

Anterograde amnesia was recognized more than a century ago as a key feature of *Korsakoff psychosis* (after Seregei Korsokoff, the Russian neuropsychiatrist who discovered the syndrome), which results indirectly from chronic alcoholism (as a result of the disruption of thiamine, or Vitamin B_1 metabolism, which leads to damage of the hippocampus). A classic clinical example, long ignored in the literature but now cited frequently, is the brief article by Edouard Claparède (1911). The patient, a 47-year-old woman who had been institutionalized for several years in a Swiss hospital, was incapable of learning new information, including her whereabouts and the names of her physicians and other attendants. Claparède sought to examine the patient and was formally introduced to her, shaking hands with her. He eventually left and returned later. Not surprisingly, on his return, Claparède found that she was unable to remember him and continued not to remember him even after several visits. Claparède decided to play a trick on her. He hid a pin in his hand which, on shaking hands again, caused her to suffer an unpleasant pinprick.

Would the patient remember Claparède better after this nasty experience? The answer was, yes and no.

As before, the patient could not remember Claparède on his return but, unlike before, she refused to shake hands with him. Claparède asked her why she would not shake hands. She replied, "This is a free country; one is not obliged to shake hands." But why, Claparède asked, would she not do him the honor of shaking his hands? Her answer was, "People sometimes hide things between their fingers." "What brings you to think of such a strange possibility?" he asked her. The patient replied, in dream-like fashion, "An image of such an event came to my mind." Even fastidious experimental psychologists tend not to cavil at the interpretation that her disinclination to shake hands had to do with a partial or unconscious memory of the unpleasant hand shake with Claparède. Sigmund Freud's conceptualization of such strange behaviors as representing behavioral "reminiscences" of unconscious memories—which Claparède found congenial to his way of thinking—was applied, as we have already noted, by Freud to his hysterical patients (Breuer & Freud, 1895/1955). In the modern experimental literature, such body memories or dramatizations of unconscious memories have come to be designated "implicit," or "procedural memories" (Cohen & Squire, 1980; Tulving, 1985; 1989; Schacter & Graf, 1986; Squire, 1987).

It is both sad and ironic that the person who perhaps contributed more than anyone to the science of memory in the 20th century was a profoundly amnesic patient known as H. M. (after his death in 2008, his actual name, Henry Molaison, was made public). In his early 20s H. M. suffered from intractable epileptic seizures and the experiment was undertaken by the neurosurgeon William Scoville (see, Dittrich, 2016; Scoville & Milner, 1957) to excise the epicenter of the attacks, in this case, the hippocampus and surrounding temporal-lobe tissues. The results were mixed. The epileptic seizures were diminished but a tragic side effect was that H. M. suffered for the rest of his life from profound anterograde amnesia. Even after years of interactions with his doctors and nurses in the hospital he was unable to recognize any of them. His preoperative memories were well preserved (he continued to do cross-word puzzles) but he could not remember where he was and who the people were who took care of him.

A striking additional fact was soon appreciated, one which led to the reformulation of the concept of "memory." H. M. could not remember his whereabouts or his caretakers, even after decades of interactions, but it became obvious that he was able to remember some things, for example, how to get to the bathroom or to the cafeteria. Psychologists and neuroscientists felt compelled to abandon a unitary conception of "memory" and proposed the existence of different kinds of memories. One of these, variously designated, "declarative," "episodic," or "explicit" memory, involves memory of life episodes that can be explicitly, or consciously remembered; another kind of memory, suggested by H. M.'s residual memory, was "implicit memory" (unconscious memory), a subset of which was "procedural memory," that is, memory for procedures, for example, how to get to the cafeteria (Cohen & Squire, 1980; 1987; Schacter & Graf, 1986). Later experimental research on H. M.

(Gabrieli, Corkin, Mickel, & Growdon (1993) showed that H. M. could learn and remember sensory-motor tasks, such as mirror drawing (drawing a star from its mirror image). The more practice sessions with the task, the better he got at it. Yet, H. M. could not remember ever practicing such a task. His performance improvement with practice was the proof that he could learn and remember the procedure of mirror drawing, even if he could not consciously remember learning and practicing the procedure. Another anterograde amnesic patient was given protracted chess lessons which resulted in clear improvement at the game, yet the patient could not consciously remember having been given any lessons. Asked to account for his ability to play chess, the patient suggested it was beginner's luck.

An important elaboration of this class of findings was the demonstration that the different memory systems could be selectively accessed by different testing methods. For example, Graf, Squire, and Mandler (1980) showed that amnesic patients who were given the first few letters of target words as memory cues were not able to benefit from the prefix cues in trying to remember the full target words. And yet, if the prefix cues were given to amnesic patients with no reference to memory but only the simple request that they make up a word that completed the prefix letters, the subjects managed to produce most of the words that they were not explicitly able to remember. It is as if free-associations worked where formal recollection failed.

Similarly, Zizak and Reber (2004) presented college students with a very difficult linguistic task in which they had to extract the "artificial grammar" of letter strings on the basis of a long series of grammatical exemplars (e.g., TXS, TSXS, TSSXXVV, TSXXTVPS, PVV, PTTVPS, PTVPXVPS, PTVPXVPS, PTVPXVPS, ...). The students, of course, thought this was an outrageous task and could not explicitly articulate the grammar that generated the exemplars. And yet, when the students were asked to discriminate between a set of grammatical exemplars (e.g., TSSX, PTV, SPSTVP, ...) from nongrammatical exemplars (e.g., SXS, SXTV, PVXXTVP, ...), they significantly exceeded chance-level performance (50%), achieving 60%–80% correct discriminations. Similarly, if the students were merely asked to say which test items they "liked" most, they significantly preferred the grammatical items. Thus, while the students appeared to have no conscious/explicit grasp of the artificial grammar, they could nevertheless discriminate grammatical strings from non-grammatical stings and showed an affective preference for the grammatical items.

We can now connect these dissociation effects (presence of implicit/procedural memory in the absence of explicit memory) to two aspects of dreaming. First, dreams, as has been emphasized, involve concretistic representations—imagery, dramatization—and it is likely that procedural/implicit aspects of memory are implemented in dreams, even if some of the episodic aspects are inaccessible to consciousness. The implicit/procedural representations may, moreover, yield reasonable interpretations of the inaccessible episodic contents, e.g., in the case of Claparède's subject, that she must have experienced a nasty event in shaking hands with him or, in the case of H. M., that he had been practicing mirror drawing. Also, the ability of Zizak and Reber's subjects to discriminate between grammatical and non-grammatical strings of letters in the absence of conscious insight into the underlying grammar, intersects with Deirdre Barrett's claim (see Chapter 3, pp. 86–88) that puzzles of various sorts (brain teasers, musical compositions, chemical structures) that are refractory to awake consciousness may be solved during sleep.

The Klüver–Bucy Syndrome

Classic Findings. The Klüver–Bucy Syndrome, named after the psychologist Heinrich Klüver and the neurologist Paul Bucy, was a discovery presented in a series of reports in the beginning of 1937 of research which originally sought to determine the regions of the brain which mediated drug-induced visual hallucinations (a subject close to dream phenomenology). The research, based on the ablation of the temporal lobes of monkeys—the more precise locus of the effective ablations has been shown by Pribram (1971) to be the amygdala (which is contained within the temporal lobe), yields a complexity of symptoms involving sexuality, orality, aggression, and fear. Informed by Freudian psychology and the work of James Papez (1937), the Klüver-Bucy syndrome was foundational in the development of the modern conception of the "limbic system" (LeDoux, 1996, p. 92).

Klüver and Bucy illustrated the clinical syndrome by reference to one of their monkey subjects:

> The animal does not exhibit the reactions generally associated with anger and fear. It approaches humans and animals, animate as well as inanimate objects without hesitation and although there are no motor [or visual acuity] defects tends to examine them by mouth rather than by the use of hands ... the monkey seems unable to recognize objects by the sense of sight. The hungry animal ... will ... indiscriminately pick up a comb, a bakelite knob, a sunflower seed, a screw, a stick, a piece of apple, a live snake, a piece of banana, and a live rat. Each object is transferred to the mouth and then discarded if not edible.
>
> *(Klüver & Bucy [1937], in Le Doux, 1996, p. 91)*

In addition to *loss of fear and aggression* and the striking *hyperorality*, animals with excised amygdalas also show marked and aberrant *hypersexuality*, attempting copulation with other monkeys, including monkeys of the same sex (which they had not done previous to their operation), or attempting copulation with members of other species. In sum, animals suffering from Klüver–Bucy syndrome exhibit: *loss of fear*, *loss of aggression*, *increased orality*, and *increased sexuality*.

Long-term research on the Klüver–Bucy syndrome has shown some surprising variability of effects which render any simple summary statement suspect. For decades, for example, the loss of aggression resulting from the ablation of the amygdala was observed often, but not invariably. Thus, the received view that the amygdala incited aggression (since its excision typically reduced aggression) was never free of doubt—or puzzlement. We are here, after all, dealing with a hard science, neurology, and it should be possible to state confidently that the ablation of the amygdala results in diminished aggression. Usually this was the case, but not invariably.

Interaction of Amygdalectomy Effects with Dominance Status (Karl Pribram). Karl Pribram and his colleagues (Rosvold, Mirsky, & Pribram, 1954) proposed a solution that entailed a deeper insight about ablation effects: The consequence of amygdalectomy may interact with the social and personal context of the experimental animal. Pribram and his colleagues noted that, for convenience's sake, animals in the past were mostly studied in isolation. Yet, monkeys are highly social creatures for whom dominance hierarchies play a crucial everyday role. Pribram and his colleagues suggested—and then provided supportive experimental evidence for the notion—that the dominance status of the monkey above and below the experimental monkey's played a role in the effect of an amygdalectomy.

Rosvold, Mirsky, and Pribram (1954) systematically studied a colony of 8 male rhesus monkeys, the three most dominant of which, starting with the most dominant, were subjected to successive amygdalectomies. First, the amygdala of the most dominant monkey, Dave, was excised. The animal was then given a sufficient postoperative recuperation period and then returned to the colony. If the amygdala supports aggression, which presumably is an important component of dominance, then the loss of the amygdala should result in the collapse of the experimental animal's dominance status. This is what happened to Dave; from top-monkey, he now became the lowest-status member of the colony. Zeke, who had been # 2 in dominance status, now ascended to the top of the hierarchy. Once his dominance was clearly established, Zeke, in turn, was subjected to an amygdalectomy and, as had Dave, suffered a collapse of his dominance status. Riva, now the top monkey, was amygdalectomized but, unlike Dave and Zeke, did not lose his dominant status but stayed at the top of the dominance hierarchy, becoming, surprisingly, a particularly aggressive and harsh # 1 monkey. How could this be? By dint of losing his amygdala, Riva should also have become less aggressive and, therefore, less dominant. Pribram and his colleagues thought that the key fact was the character of Herbie, the monkey immediately below Riva in dominance status. Herbie was less aggressive and seemed not that embroiled in the dominance struggles that animated the previous monkeys, Dave, Zeke, and Riva. In a whimsical cartoon sketch of the members of the colony (Pribram, 1991, pp. 203–204; Rosvold, Mirsky, & Pribram, 1954), Herbie was rendered as something of a flower-child artist-monkey who (we might conclude) had better things to do than constantly harass Riva for dominance, allowing the unchallenged Riva to stay on top of the dominance hierarchy. Thus, as in dreams, the context may be crucial. The critical point for us, however, is that a simple brain-mind isomorphism," so favored by Hobson (Hobson, 2002, p. 3), would not work, as the dominance status of the other monkeys in the colony would not show up in any gross imaging of Riva's brain.

Interactions Involving the Hypothalamus: Dominance, Sex, and Friendship (José Delgado, Bullfighter and Neuroscientist). Pribram and his colleagues' results with their monkey colony was not fool-proof. Maybe Riva stayed on top of the dominance hierarchy for other reasons than Herbie's personality. One methodological issue was the possibility that excisions in different animals did not remove exactly the same brain tissue (though Pribram [e.g., 1991] claimed that experimental data showed that slight variations in the locus of excisions was not critical). The decisive experiment, a beautiful methodological breakthrough, was achieved by José Delgado at Yale, and later at the University of Madrid. It had been previously determined that the amygdala produced its aggression-enhancing effects by stimulating the aggression center in the ventromedial nucleus (VMN) of the hypothalamus. Delgado decided to bypass the middleman amygdala and implant electrodes directly into the VMN and determine how stimulation of the VMN might be moderated by social and personal context.

Delgado, in general, was interested in remote-controlled electric brain-stimulation through electrodes permanently implanted in the animal's brain. His basic research goal was the medical use of such remote stimulation to control malfunctioning brain areas. He did garner much popular attention (and a 1965 spread in the *New York Times*) for his application of implant technology to a passion of his, bull-fighting, showing that he could dispense with the bullfighter's sword and cape to tame a ferocious charging bull by remote stimulation of an implant in the bull's brain. In the less flamboyant context of the Klüver–Bucy syndrome, involving the direct stimulation of the aggression center in the hypothalamus (the ventromedial nucleus, or VMN), Delgado showed that stimulation of the VMN *reliably* produced aggression—but only against monkeys lower in dominance status. When in the presence of more dominant monkeys, the same stimulation *reliably* produced not aggression but fear and an effort to back away from a confrontation. Although the effects of VMN stimulation were reliable, they were also nuanced, showing interactions with the social and personal environment: The subject monkey would not attack a less dominant monkey who happened to be his "friend," nor did he attack female rhesus monkeys who, in rhesus monkey society, are lower than males in dominance. Thus, there is no simple mind-brain isomorphism. The social and personal context of the subject monkey critically moderates behavior resulting from stimulation in the same brain location.

The Neural Default Network: Mind-Wandering, Fantasy, Daydreams, Dreams (Marcus Raichle, Randy Buckner, Jessica Andrews-Hanna, Dan Schacter, Bill Domhoff, et al.)

> [O]ne of the most intriguing neuroscience findings of the past decade has been the observation that certain regions of the brain become increasingly recruited with decreasing external task demands. This group of brain regions has collectively been termed the "default network" ... and includes, most prominently the medial prefrontal cortex [MPFC], posterior cingulate cortex [PCC]/precuneus region, and the temporoparietal junction.
>
> *(Christoff, Gordon, Smallwood, Smith, & Schooler, 2009)*

The recent discovery of the neural default network was quite accidental and arose from the mundane methodological need to have a base-rate level of brain activity against which to compare experimental activations of interest. It soon became evident, however, that the "resting brain" (like the sleeping brain) is actually a very busy brain, on par with the lively brain activity associated with the experimental task for which it was meant to serve as a control. Ironically, given the broad-brush description of the REM state as involving "hypofrontality" (pp. 105, 107) (true for *some* prefrontal regions, especially the DLPFC), the brain work now associated with the default network, which has been linked to dreaming, has been characterized by *hyper*fronality—a hyperfrontal pattern of high neural activity—which applies to other prefrontal regions, such as the MPFC (the medial prefrontal cortex) (Ingvar, 1979). Thus, in line with the paradoxical nature of dreaming, the REM state involves both hypofrontality *and* hyperfrontality.

The neural default network is broadly associated with the phenomenon of "mind-wandering," subsuming a range of internally directed spontaneous cognition such as fantasy, imagery, daydreaming, and according to some recent proposals, dreaming itself (Domhoff, 2011, 2018a; Domhoff & Fox, 2015; Fox, Nijeboer, Solomonova, Domhoff, & Christoff, 2013; Wamsley & Stickgold, 2010). Table 4.1 provides a compendium of default network characteristics culled from some of the more influential works in the literature.

One of the noteworthy features of the default network—though it has not been noted in the literature—is its overlap with many of the psychological, behavioral, and stimulus characteristics of psychoanalysis—both as theory and therapy. In many respects, the default network could be meaningfully described as the "Freud Network." A quantitative content-analysis (the technique is discussed in our next chapter) would no doubt reveal Freud's work, compared to the works of other major figures in psychology—from Fechner to James to Pavlov to Watson to Skinner to Piaget to Neisser to Bruner to Tulving to Tversky and Kahneman—to feature, to an unparalleled extent, the key phenomena of the default network. The quantified content differences would likely be so large as to require no fancy statistics—simple sign tests would likely do the trick ($p < 0.00$ ...).

Even without formal quantitative analysis, the content overlaps between the features of the default network and those of psychoanalysis are striking. Table 4.1 makes this plain. The "reclining position in a moderately lighted room" (Domhoff, 2015, p. 4) is, of course, a standard feature of psychoanalytic psychotherapy (Freud's psychoanalytic couch), as is the psychoanalytic "basic rule" of free-association which finds, as can be readily garnered from Table 4.1, ubiquitous counterparts in the default network, for example, "decline in vigilance" (Domhoff, 2015, p. 15), "unconstrained, spontaneous cognition" (Reichle & Snyder, 2007), "reduction of conscious suppression," "mind-wandering," and "abundance of 'SIT' (stimulus independent thinking)" (Reichle & Snyder, 2007, pp. 393–395); "freethinking," "not focus[ing] on the external environment," "internally directed cognition," "drifting waking thoughts," "fantasy" (Buckner, Andrews-Hanna, & Schater (2008, pp. 1, 1, 2, 5, 15); "self-reflection," "facilitation of insight," "internally focused thought,"

TABLE 4.1 Characteristics of the Default Network

Raichle, MacLeod, Snyder, Powers, Grusnard, and Shulman (2001); Raichle and Snyder (2007); Raichle (2015)

- ⋆ "a baseline or default state" active "in the absence of specific goal-directed activity" (2001, p. 680)
- ⋆ "intrinsic brain activity" vs. "evoked activity" (2007, p. 1087)
- ⋆ "unconstrained, spontaneous cognition" (2007, p. 1087)
- ⋆ "daydreams" (2007, p. 1087)
- ⋆ "stimulus independent thoughts" (2007, p. 1087)
- ⋆ "maintenance of information for interpreting, responding to and even *predicting* environmental demands" (2007, p. 1087)
- ⋆ "the brain's dark energy" (2015, p. 8)

Mason, Norton, and Wegner (2007)

- ⋆ reduction of "conscious suppression" (pp. 393-395)
- ⋆ "mind-wandering" (p. 393)
- ⋆ abundance of "SIT" (stimulus independent thinking) (p. 393)

Buckner, Andrews-Hanna, & Schacter (2008)

- ⋆ "freethinking" (p. 1)
- ⋆ "remembering the past and envisioning future events" (p. 1)
- ⋆ "considering thoughts and perspectives of other people" (p.1)
- ⋆ "not focused on the external environment" (p. 1)
- ⋆ "unconstrained states" (p. 2)
- ⋆ participants "subjectively describe their mental experiences" (p. 3)
- ⋆ internally directed cognition" (p. 2)
- ⋆ "free-wheeling" state (p. 4)
- ⋆ "spontaneous cognition" (pp. 14, 15)
- ⋆ "fantasy" (p. 15)
- ⋆ "imagination" (p. 15)
- ⋆ "daydreams" (p. 15)
- ⋆ "stimulus independent thoughts" ("SITs") (p. 15)
- ⋆ "mentalizing" (from the theory of mind: thinking about the beliefs and intentions of other people" (p. 20)

Andrews-Hanna (2012)

- ⋆ *"introspective state" (p. 251)*
- ⋆ "manipulation of mental images" (p. 258)
- ⋆ "reminiscing of past experiences" (p. 258)
- ⋆ "making plans," "mentally" planning "alternate scenarios" (p. 260)
- ⋆ "introspection about affective, personally significant information" (p. 261)
- ⋆ "retrieve contextual associations" . . . "simulate future outcomes" (p. 262)
- ⋆ "reflect on personal preferences, beliefs, values, feelings" (p. 263)

Christoff, Gordon, Smallwood, Smith, and Schooler (2009)

- ⋆ "internally focused thought" (p. 8719)
- ⋆ "mind-wandering" (p. 8719)
- ⋆ "absence of meta-awareness" (i.e., absence of awareness that mind wandering is taking place) (p. 8722)
- ⋆ "insight," "facilitation of insight" (pp. 8723-8724)
- ⋆ "self-reflection" (p. 8723)

(continued)

TABLE 4.1 Cont.

Domhoff, 2018; Domhoff & Fox (2015)
⋆ *"mental imagery" (2018,* p. 171)
⋆ *mentalizing" (2018,* p. 184)
⋆ *reclining position in a moderately lighted room (*2015, p. 4)
⋆ *spontaneous thoughts vs. task oriented thoughts" (p. 5)*
⋆ *"drifting waking thought"* (p. 5)
⋆ *"waking mind-wandering/daydreaming"* (p. 7)
⋆ *"internal cognitive processes about significant past and future events"* (p. 9)
⋆ *"decline in vigilance"* (p. 9)
⋆ *"loss of volitional control"* (p. 9)
⋆ *"prominence of alpha waves"* (brain correlates of trancy states, deep relaxation) (p. 9)
⋆ "waking dreams" (p. 8)

"mind-wandering" (Christoff, Gordon, Smallwood, Smith, & Schooler, 2009, pp. 8719, 8723–8724); "manipulation of mental images," "reminiscing of past experiences," planning "alternate scenarios," introspecting "about affective, personally significant information" (Andrews-Hanna, 2012, pp. 258, 260, 261).

In sum, the suppression of executive (ego) control of cognition leads not to a null state but to the "release" of less-constrained, less rational, more concretistic substrata of the overall psychological system—and, consequently, as may be argued, to greater creativity, greater artistic expression, and more out-of-the-box solutions to problems.

Release Phenomena: Meaning and Implications

The idea of"release" is of classic vintage, going back to Freud's favorite 19th century neuroscientist, Hughlings Jackson, who proposed that damage to higher order brain structures results in a "retrogression" to evolutionarily more primitive subsystems and, therefore, to the release of more primitive functions. The idea is used in modern neurology (Hobson, 2002, p. 145) and captures the Freudian notion (see Erdelyi, 1985; Fisher, 1960) that the relaxation of ego control (in dreams, daydreams, psychoanalytic therapy) releases inhibited substrata of the mind, revealing deeper truths about our thoughts and emotions than are accessible to everyday, focused executive functioning.

"Release" is an apt descriptive term, used by both Freudian and non-Freudian researchers (Fisher, 1960; Hobson, 2002; Solms & Turnbull, 2002), but it is also a unifying theoretical rubric that integrates a sweep of superficially disparate phenomena, among them, dreams, daydreams, free-associative fantasy, subliminal perception, paranoid delusions, art, paraphasias, jokes. Dreams are release phenomena by dint of the substantial relaxation of ego control that shifts the psychological mix from *secondary-process functioning* (linear, temporally constrained, logical, realistic, and abstract cognition) to *primary-process functioning* (primitive, irrational, nonlinear, temporally disordered, unrealistic, and concretistic cognition) (Freud, 1900/1953, pp. 597–609; 1901a/1953, pp. 676–677; 1915/1957, pp. 186–187; 1917/1963, pp. 34, 62–63). Similarly, but to a lesser extent, daydreams and free-associative fantasy yield cognitive regression to more primary-process modes of functioning, as do poetry, subliminal perception, and aphasia.

Thus, Freud's dream theory constitutes a subset of a wider all-encompassing theory of release phenomena. Neurotic symptoms, paranoid delusions, *parapraxes* (Freudian slips), jokes, are all cognate dialects arising from the same underlying reality and are understood and interpreted in the same manner (see Breuer & Freud, 1895/1955; Freud, 1900/1953; 1901b/1960; 1909b/1955; 1911/1958; 1917/1963; Erdelyi, 1985). Freud takes a hodge-podge of one-pointed phenomena and parlays them into a vast pointillist canvas. This is not widely appreciated.

In closing, we might note that release is actually an old story. In Chinese mysticism, it is doing-by-not-doing (*wei-wu-wei*); in martial arts (e.g., Tai-Qi-Quan), prevailing by yielding; in Freudian insight therapy, free-associating instead of concentrating; in neuroscience, stimulating by not inhibiting. In the end, "Dreaming is intrinsically the not-doing of sleep" (Castañeda, 1981, p. 28).

5

QUANTITATIVE CONTENT-ANALYSIS

Quantitative vs. Qualitative Analysis

Content-analysis refers to a wide range of possible techniques for extracting meaning from psychological materials such as dreams, fantasy, aphasic responses, jokes, and art. Content-analysis can be very simple, entailing subjective judgments or plain counts of elements, or involve complex clinical evaluations or technical mathematical treatments of data. When content-analysis involves quantification, it is designated *quantitative content-analysis*; when no quantification is involved—when it is based on subjective or clinical judgment—it may be referred to as *qualitative analysis* (e.g., Hall & Van De Castle, 1966, pp. ix–x; Domhoff, 1996, p. 7). "Interpretation," as used by classic theorists such as Freud, constitutes qualitative content-analysis employed for extracting meanings from complex materials (often from clinical cases). Thus, the interpretation of Freud's Irma dream (pp. 63–67) uncovers Freud's anxiety about Irma's treatment and, also, his anger at his skeptical colleagues. In the same vein, Jouvet's interpretation of the 18,000-year-old cave painting (see pp. 6–8) yields the information that the reclining man is dreaming and, further, that the dreamer is wishfully conjuring up a successful hunt.

The distinction between qualitative and quantitative analysis need not be ironclad. A qualitative analysis can shade into quantitative analysis through adjectival elaboration (e.g., "rare," "slight," "substantial") or through the use of temporal adverbs (e.g., "now," "recently," "later"), which can be turned into numbers. In the case of Fisher's study of the recovery of the subliminal snake-swastika stimulus (pp. 38–40), we can discern that "snake" increasingly emerges in the subject's successive fantasy productions and we could, although Fisher did not, assign progressively higher numerical scores for "snakiness" to each successive drawing (with the last drawing, which features an explicit snake, garnering a perfect score). This tack, of assigning numerical scores to the subject's productions, is precisely the

DOI: 10.4324/9781003300441-6

one taken by Haber and Erdelyi (1967), as will be elaborated below in the section, "Recovery of Subliminal Stimuli in Dreams, Daydreams, and Fantasy."

Before we proceed, we might note a strange disjunction that has persisted in the content-analytic literature. The classic clinicians, especially the Freudians and Jungians, invariably focused on deep semantic contents (latent contents) whereas modern quantitative analysts, almost as invariably, have focused on surface contents (manifest contents). The impression might be drawn that quantitative content-analysis must necessarily be consigned to surface meanings, but there is no reason why interpreted latent contents cannot be quantified. Quantification in content-analysis is, actually, orthogonal to psychological depth. Further, as will be seen, quantification of interpreted latent contents yields *reliable* measures. Psychologists are often surprised at this claim but, fortunately, the typical high levels of reliability (easily, $r = .85$) are readily replicable, and so we can conclude that quantification can work for both manifest as well as for latent contents.

Recovery of Subliminal Stimuli in Dreams, Daydreams, and Fantasy (Pötzl, Fisher, Haber and Erdelyi, Hilgard, Giddan, Shevrin and Luborsky, Leuschner et al., Schredl et al.)

In 1917, Otto Pötzl, a professor of psychiatry and neurology at the University of Vienna and, also, for many years, a member of the Vienna Psychoanalytic Association, published a research paper on the question whether some of the strange phenomena he was encountering in his brain trauma patients could be duplicated experimentally in neurologically intact dreaming subjects. Some of the brain-trauma patients evidenced paradoxical visual effects—too little and too much vision. For example, a patient who was virtually blind for central visual stimuli might also suffer from maladaptive excesses of perception such as double vision ("physiological diplopia") and, sometimes, awareness of the blind spot. Also, the presumably blind patient might eventually recover into consciousness stimulus materials that he had claimed not to have seen, a phenomenon Pötzl referred to as "delayed piecemeal delivery into consciousness." Such recoveries were invariably distorted versions of the stimulus which, "just like dream images, undergo all sorts of condensations (Pötzl, 1917/1960, p. 44).

In Pötzl's 1917 laboratory study, a dozen neurologically intact psychiatric patients (tested individually), were flashed a complex picture for 10 ms. The subjects were then required to produce an exhaustive drawing of whatever they had managed to see (usually very little beyond some shadows and vague shapes). They were then instructed to have a dream that night and to return to the laboratory next day to report (and draw) their dream. The basic finding was that the subjects' dreams tended to recover materials from the subliminal stimulus although, invariably, in distorted form.

Freud was quite taken with Pötzl's study, which Pötzl presented to the Vienna Psychoanalytic Society, and added a long footnote about it in his 1919 revision of *The interpretation of dreams* (pp. 181–182). Pötzl's results had at least two important theoretical implications: First, that unconscious materials may indeed be recovered in dreams and, second, that such recoveries are subject to a variety of distortions of the sort Freud had identified in his treatment of the dream-work. As will be seen, such distortions are universal features of impoverished cognition.

Notwithstanding Freud's favorable footnote and a number of experimental follow-ups by others (Allers & Teler, 1924; Malamud & Linder, 1931), Pötzl's work drifted into obscurity until it was revived by Charles Fisher in the 1950s, at the height of the "New Look" movement in psychology (arguably, a precursor to the now-mainstream "cognitive revolution" (Erdelyi, 1974, 1985)). Fisher translated Pötzl's study into English and carried out a number of experimental probes of his own (Fisher, 1954, 1956, 1960a, 1960b, 1988; Paul & Fisher, 1959). Fisher was able to replicate and extend Pötzl's findings by showing that subliminal contents could be recovered in dreams as well as in awake fantasy. He produced, as we have seen, some striking instances of such recoveries and, also, introduced some preliminary attempts to control for the possibility that the obtained "recoveries" were chance effects. Fisher tested a handful of control subjects (six in all) who were flashed a *blank* stimulus and then required to produce free-associative images, just as the experimental subjects had done. None of the control subjects generated any bird-like drawings, as had the experimental subjects (see pp. 36–40).

Although Fisher had produced some impressive instances of recoveries, which presumably were not chance artifacts, Fisher was not an experimental psychologist and never progressed to a formal, quantitative treatment of the effects. This effort was undertaken by subsequent experimenters (Erdelyi, 1970, 1972; Giddan, 1967; Haber & Erdelyi, 1967; Hilgard, 1962; Leuschner & Hau, 1992; Leuschner, Hau, Brech, & Volk, 1994; Schredl, Dombrowe, Bozzer, & Morlock, 1999; Shevrin & Luborsky, 1958). We shall focus here on the Haber and Erdelyi (1967) study, which developed into a programmatic project that eventually linked up with more general experimental traditions in memory psychology, especially *reminiscence* and *hypermnesia* (the opposite of *amnesia*) (Erdelyi, 1970, 1972, 1996, 2010). Some of this work will be examined in our next chapter, "Dreaming as Noisy Remembering."

Haber and Erdelyi's (1967) study sought to place Fisher's work on a firmer methodological footing. Two specific questions were pursued: (1) Could subliminal elements from a stimulus flash be recovered in fantasy? (No dreams were probed, on the common assumption that fantasy would yield similar findings as dreams—of this more later); and (2) If subliminal elements were recovered in fantasy, would fantasy be followed by enhanced post-fantasy recall?

The stimulus (depicting a cotton-gin complex that included a loading platform, bales of cotton, workers, carts, mules, hats, and trees in the background) was flashed for 100 ms. The subject was then asked to produce an exhaustive, labeled drawing of everything he had seen (the subjects were Yale undergraduates, who at this time were all males) and was prodded to include everything, even if uncertain about his percepts. This first report is designated, R_1. The subject's stimulus drawing, R_1, was then collected and never again shown to him. At this point, the subject was requested to produce fantasy (a mix of daydreams and free-associations) for some 40 minutes. After the fantasy session, a second recall drawing (R_2) of the original stimulus was elicited. The recorded fantasy productions were transcribed and numerically scored in a number of ways for fidelity to stimulus content. One of the scoring methods used with the free-associations (120 per subject) involved the assignment to each of the free-associations a numerical score from 0 to 1, in increments of .1 (thus, 0, .1, .2, ..., .9, 1), with 0 representing no semantic relation to the target item and 1 a perfect relation to the target item. For example, for the stimulus target, *mule*, the response "T.V," would get a score of 0; a free-association response, "mule" (or "mules"), a 1.0; a close response, for example, "horse," might be given a score of .8 or .9; and, some intermediate or vague response, such as "animal," a score of .2 or .3.

As for the pre- and post-fantasy drawings, R_1 and R_2, the scorers were trained on the scoring procedure by reviewing a short booklet that contained a range of examples of the kinds of drawings they might encounter and the scores that the experimenter would assign to them. (Once they were doing the actual scoring, the scorers were, of course, "blind" to the groups or conditions—R_1 or R_2, experimental or control—from which the drawings were selected for scoring.) It should be emphasized, given some of the more elaborate scoring schemes we shall encounter, especially for the quantitative content-analysis of dreams, that the whole training session required little over half-an-hour and yet produced high inter-judge reliabilities, in the order of $r = .85$. In related studies since then, the lowest inter-judge reliability ever obtained was .77, and the highest, .99. The .85 value is probably a conservative estimate of the reliabilities we might expect to obtain with such simple scoring procedures.

With the reliability of the scoring established, we may proceed to ask whether the free-association scores confirmed Fisher's findings of recovery of subliminal stimuli in fantasy. A control group is needed to ascertain that the positive recovery scores were not just chance correspondences. Fisher had sensed this methodological need, but his blank-flash control group is not really satisfactory. To the extent that the initial response (R_1) contained at least some of the stimulus items, it can be assumed that the ensuing free-associative fantasy would elaborate these initial percepts. Thus, perceiving a *mule* might yield related free-associations—cart, road, driver, hat, trees—which a blank stimulus would not as likely elicit. With this in mind, a *yoked-control* group was tested which was never exposed to the stimulus but, instead, copied, as faithfully a possible, the R_1 (post-flash) drawings of an experimental counterpart (each control subject was yoked to a different experimental counterpart). The basic finding was in agreement with Pötzl and Fisher: Subliminal (unreported) elements from a stimulus flash may be recovered, often in distorted form, in the content of fantasy ($p < .01$).

Furthermore, it was demonstrated that, unlike two control groups (one of which threw darts instead of producing fantasy for 40 minutes), the recall of the stimulus flash was invariably better *after* fantasy (i.e., in R_2) than *before* fantasy (i.e., in R_1, right after the stimulus flash). There were 20 fantasy subjects and since *all* of them improved their recall from before fantasy to after fantasy, no fancy statistics were required; a simple sign-test yields above-and-beyond statistical significance: $p = (1/2)^{20}$.

Signal Detection Theory (SDT) and Fantasy

The study generated some interest but, also, some questions. *Signal detection theory* (SDT), a highly quantitative contribution of psychophysics, with roots in applied engineering work on radar detection in WWII, had begun to penetrate mainstream psychology around this time and posed an alternative conceptualization of the types of findings reported by Pötzl, Fisher, Haber and Erdelyi, and others. (The Appendix at the end of our book, adapted from Erdelyi (1996, pp. 193–207), provides an accessible exposition of SDT and, also, an original methodological application of SDT to narrative recall, including dreams. It will come into play in our next chapter on dreams-as-memory.)

The SDT question for this family of research (see our Appendix for a more comprehensive treatment) is whether the reported stimulus "recoveries" in dreams, fantasy, and in post-fantasy recall entail true *recoveries* of subliminal materials or, merely, the *reporting* of previously unreported materials in free-wheeling dreams and fantasy. When we are asked to report what we have seen in a stimulus, we normally wish to give a reasonably accurate rendition of what has been seen and we tend to withhold uncertain possibilities and hunches. But, what is our criterion for what constitutes a "reasonable and accurate rendition," as opposed to uncertain hypotheses, hunches, or even outright guesses? If we were offered an incentive, say money, for each produced hit, would we not likely relax our standards, that is, our criterion for reporting, and produce more hits, even if, also, more false-alarms? Similarly, if we were penalized for false-alarms, would we not adopt stricter criteria for reporting and generate fewer false-alarms but, also, fewer hits. This, actually, is what research shows (Adams, 1957; Bricker & Chapanis, 1953; Green & Swets, 1966; Erdelyi, 1996; Macmillan & Creelman, 1991; Swets, 1964; Swets, Tanner, & Birdsall, 1961).

Thus, might it not be reasonable to suppose that in disinhibited cognition, like dreams and fantasy, the subject is less concerned than usual about false-alarms and therefore produces more hits, but also more false-alarms. If so, we might wish to distinguish between *recovery of unconscious percepts* and the *reporting of unreported percepts.*

ROC Curves, d′, and β

SDT, as our Appendix elaborates, offers a formal, quantitative approach to disentangling the two possibilities. Drastically, SDT makes away with the concept of "limen" (a threshold that supposedly divides conscious from unconscious) and, instead, extracts two parameters, (1) *sensitivity* (d') and (2) *response criterion* (β)—the subject's criterion for responding positively (saying "yes" or producing a recollection). Perceptual or memory responses are invariably imperfect, involving both *hits* (correct positive responses) and *false-alarms* (false positive responses), and so, simply counting hits *or* false-alarms does not measure sensitivity to the stimulus or memory trace. *Both* need to be considered, and in tandem. SDT provides a formal index of sensitivity in terms of the functional relation between hit-rates and false-alarm rates. The famous "ROC" (receiver operating characteristic) curve is the geometric representation of this function. The more bow-shaped it is (see Figure A.1 in our Appendix), the higher the sensitivity (*d'*) extracted. Moreover, and this is a major achievement of SDT, *motivation* (from monetary rewards, defensive needs, experimental pressure) does not affect sensitivity estimates (*d'*), as they do classic limen estimates, but only show up as criterion effects (β). As the subject adopts laxer and laxer response criteria, the ROC curve remains the same; what changes are the locations of the hit- and false-alarm points on the ("isosensitive") ROC curve, which are shifted rightward on the ROC function (again, see Figure A.1 in our Appendix).

SDT does not tilt against true recovery effects, which would entail increases in sensitivity, for sensitivity may, in fact, increase in fantasy, in dreams, or in post-fantasy reports. But increased sensitivity is not necessarily demonstrated by increased stimulus recoveries, since increases in the number of stimulus items in dreams, fantasy, and in post-fantasy recall could be due to (a) increased sensitivity to such items, (b) laxer response-criteria, or (c) both. This is an empirical question. The author undertook to untangle these possibilities experimentally in his PhD dissertation many years ago.

After three years and six formal experiments, all results converged on the dismal conclusion that, although the recovery effects were easy enough to replicate, they constituted mere response-criterion effects and not increases of sensitivity (Erdelyi, 1970). One could get as much recovery of unreported stimulus materials by forcing subjects to produce guesses as by inducing them to produce fantasy. (Actually, one study found that guessing was more effective than fantasy in producing recoveries (Erdelyi, 1972).)

It turned out later—we examine some of this work in our next chapter—that genuine recoveries (sensitivity increments, and not just criterion effects) are indeed possible, but not for subliminal *stimulus flashes*. What is not only possible but easy to demonstrate is the recovery of subliminal (inaccessible, unconscious) *memories*. Freud, actually, in his 1895 book with Joseph Breuer, had emphasized, on the basis of his empirical experiences with his patients, that unconscious memories can be recovered with protracted retrieval effort and, he added later, in the content of dreams (hence his conclusion, in *The interpretation of dreams*, that "dreams are hypermnesic" (Freud, 1900/1953, pp. 11–21, 589)). Some of these recovered memories turn out to be false-memories (false-alarms) but many, also, are true-memories (hits). Experimental work on memory, as we have already seen in Chapter 1 (pp. 22–26) and as will be seen further in our next chapter, shows that substantial memory improvement, beyond false-memories, are easy to obtain over time and that therefore memory can be *hypermnesic* and not just *amnesic* over time.

Quantitative Content-Analysis in Literary Criticism (Franco Moretti, Matthew Jockers, and the Stanford Literary Lab)

Quite independently of quantitative approaches to content in dream psychology or, for that matter, psychology in general, a surprising recent development in literary criticism has been the emergence of quantitative approaches to literary materials. This new movement, centered at the Stanford Literary Lab, founded in 2010 by Franco Moretti and Matthew Jockers, is known by various designations, including, "computational criticism" (Moretti, 2017, pp. 97, 203), "quantitative formalism" (Moretti, 2017, p. 33), "digital humanities" (Jockers, 2013, pp. 13–16; Moretti, 2017, p. 97), "macroanalysis" (Jockers, 2013, title, pp. 28–29); and "distant reading" (Jockers, 2013, pp. 17–18, 31–32; Moretti, 2013, pp. 47–49).

This new development in a field traditionally dedicated to the qualitative analysis of literary texts is both relevant and of interest to the quantitative content-analysis of dreams. It is relevant because, habits of thought aside, there really is no substantive difference between dream narratives and art narratives such as segments of novels or fairy tales; it is of interest because we have here the sudden emergence of a new and independent strand of quantitative analysis of texts, and it may be instructive to learn to what extent the quantitative analysis of literature and of dreams parallel each other and whether productive synergies might arise from their intersection.

Some of the quantitative approaches to literature entail little more than laborious counting (although computers now usually do this work) and, then, the graphing of the data (also, typically, by computer). In this respect, as we shall see, there is much overlap with quantitative approaches to dream content.

One of many examples, a preliminary step in the exploration of "style at the scale of the paragraph" (Algee-Hewitt, Heuser, Moretti, 2017, p. 69), is the determination of the frequency distribution of paragraph length (Figure 5.1). Regardless of whether the generated function is fruitful theoretically or not, at the minimum we can see a remarkable orderliness in the data. Psychology too has functions of this

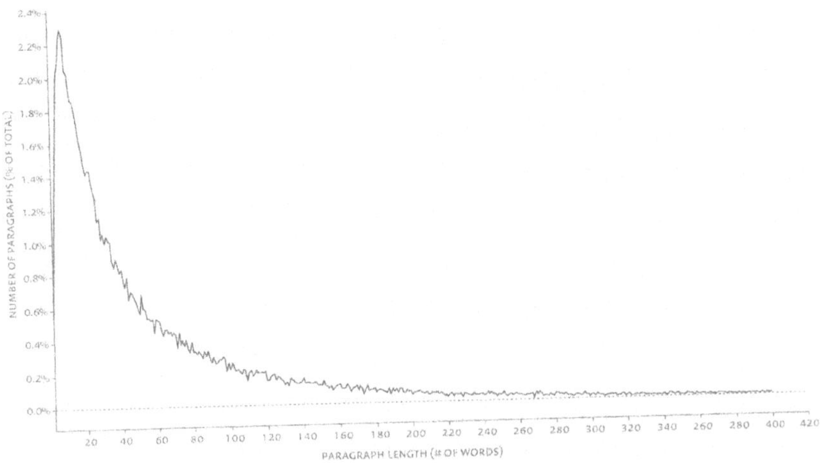

FIGURE 5.1 Paragraph length: Frequency of the number of words in a paragraph (Algee-Hewitt, Heuser, Moretti, 2017, Figure 3.4, p. 72) [Reproduced with the permission of Franco Moretti.]

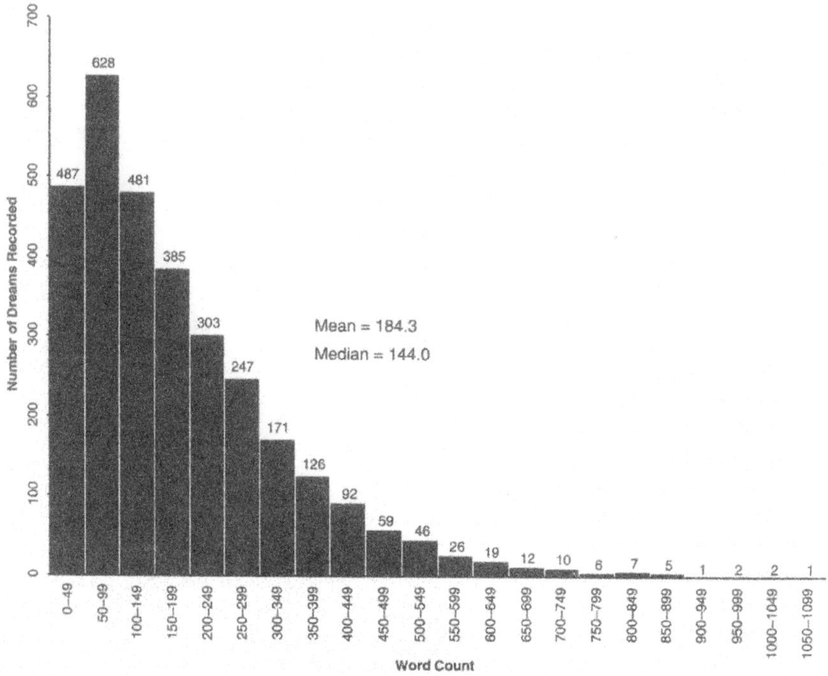

FIGURE 5.2 Dream lengths: Frequency distribution of number of words in Barb Sanders' dreams. (Domhoff, 2003, Figure 56.2, p. 1143) [Reproduced with the permission of Bill Domhoff.]

kind. For example, Figure 5.2 shows the frequency distribution of dream length for a long-term subject, Barb Sanders, extensively studied by Bill Domhoff, one of the foremost quantitative content-analysts of dreams. Clearly, the same type of function describes frequency distribution of text length across different venues. This itself may constitute a discovery of a (perhaps obvious) psychological law.

A different flavor of quantitative analysis of literary materials is the mapping of data (Moretti's 2005 book is titled, *Graphs, maps, trees*). An example (see Figure 5.3) is a quantification of "the emotions of London," a question that brings to mind the quantification of emotions in dreams (are they preponderantly happy? sad? fearful?). The literary mapping deals with "fictional London," the London of, for example, Sherlock Holmes, and not the real London, which actually yields different results (see Heuser, Moretti, & Steiner, 2017, pp. 227–250). We might note that, unlike dreams, which are preponderantly negative or fearful (see our next section), fictional London shows more happiness than fear (Heuser, Moretti, & Steiner, 2017, p. 237).

In a chapter on "Bankspeak" that was recently featured in *The New York Times* (J. Schnessler, October 30, 2017), Moretti and Pestre (2017, pp. 195–250) subject the Annual Reports of the World Bank, from 1946 to 2012, to a variety of quantitative

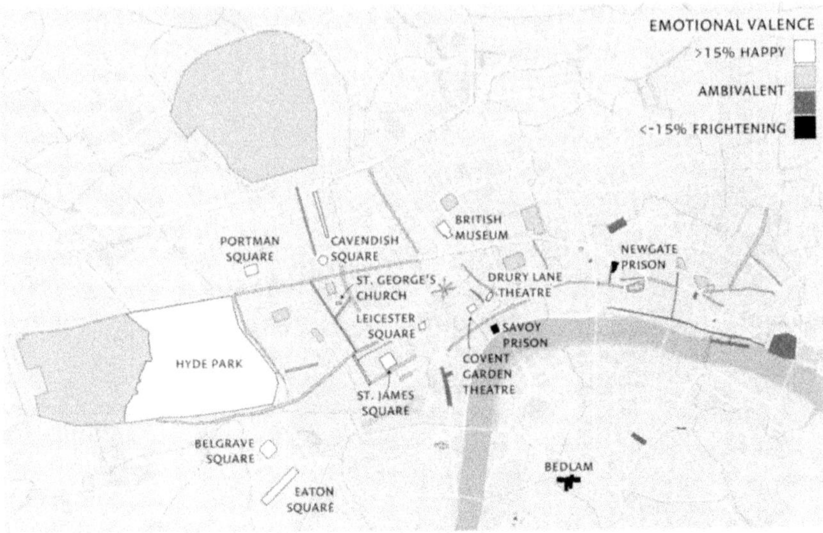

FIGURE 5.3 "The emotions of London" (Heuser, Moretti, & Steiner (2017, p. 237). In F. Moretti (Ed.), *Canon/Archive: Studies in quantitative formalism from the Stanford Literary Lab* (pp. 223–250). n+1 Books [Reproduced with the permission of Franco Moretti.]

analyses. It is clear that for the authors the Reports constitute a genre of ugly art, formulated in "almost another language, in both semantics and grammar" (p. 196). One striking finding is the sudden eruption in Bank texts of the word "governance," which is documented in Figure 5.4. An interesting yield of the analysis is its uncovery of a virtual universe of positive contents associated (by the Bank) with "governance." According to Moretti and Pestre:

> [In] its irresistible rise, "governance" has been invariably associated with words of a positive, even euphoric nature: *reforms, assistance, growth, efforts, capacity, transparency, education effective/ness, progress, stability, protection, health, access, implementation, human, new, sound, sustainable, strong, better, more,* and *most*. The same message is conveyed by verbs, which often appear in the progressive form, as if to identify the notion of governance with a tireless ongoing activity: *improve/ing/ed, strengthen/ing, support/ing, including, building, promoting, help/ing, restructuring.*
>
> *(p. 202)*

We have here the "Pavlovian subliminal message" (Erdelyi & Zizak, 2004, pp. 22–24) that governance is good and on the up and up morally. Logically, of course, "governance" (the method of governing) may be good, bad, or indifferent.

The quantitative analysis of World Bank texts also shows a propensity for self-congratulation. For example:

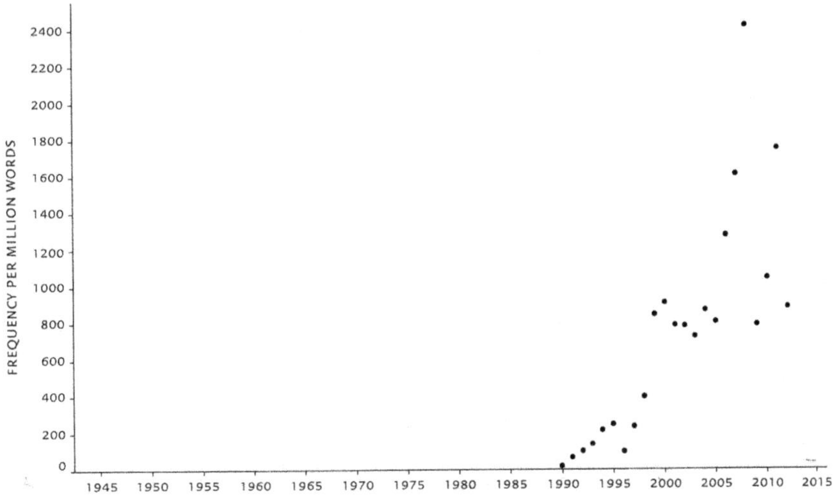

FIGURE 5.4 The sudden eruption of the word "governance" in World Bank reports (Moretti & Pestre, 2017, Figure 7.3, p. 202) [Reproduced with the permission of Franco Moretti.]

> In its ongoing dedication to overcoming poverty and creating opportunity for people in developing countries, the Bank is making progress both internally and in the field, and it continues to improve the way it serves its client countries.
>
> *(Opening of the 2012 Report, in Moretti & Pestre, 2017, p. 205)*

The point is cinched quantitatively in Figure 5.5, which shows that self-congratulation has been a growing trend for many decades.

In tandem with the increase of self-congratulation is a decline in coherence and temporal organization. As evidence, the authors cite the "grammatico-political monstrosity" (Moretti & Pestre, 2017, p. 214) from the 1999 Report, in which the conjunction "and" is sprinkled promiscuously throughout the text to create an illusion of coherence among the enumerated string of items:

> Promote corporate governance *and* competition policies *and* reform *and* privatize state-owned enterprises *and* labor market/social protection reform.
>
> *(Passage from the 1999 Report, quoted in Moretti & Pestre, 2017, p. 214)*

This is not just a one-time event but a relentless trend in World Bank Reports over the past many decades, as Figure 5.6 demonstrates. Not only does logical coherence break down but so does linear time, as suggested by Figure 5.7. It is as if Bankspeak is inexorably devolving into primary-process functioning, with the loss of logic and of linear time.

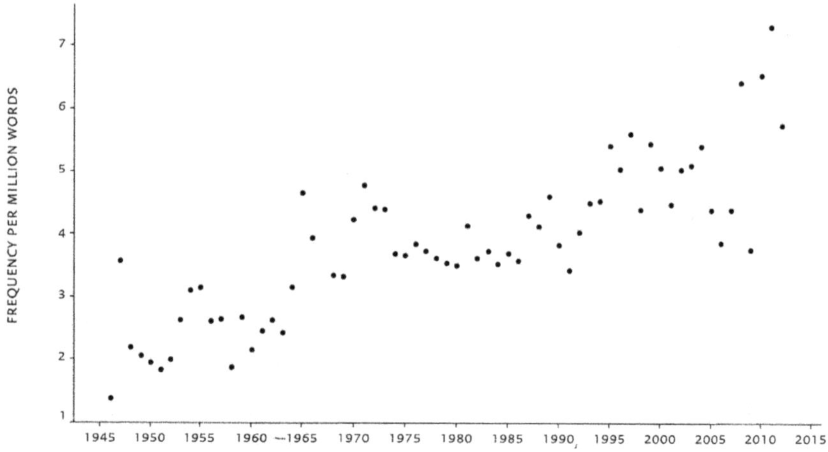

FIGURE 5.5 The increased frequency of self-congratulatory words that include *outstanding, key, stronger, better, more, significant,* and *critical* (Moretti & Pestre, 2017, Figure 7.7, p. 205) [Reproduced with the permission of Franco Moretti.]

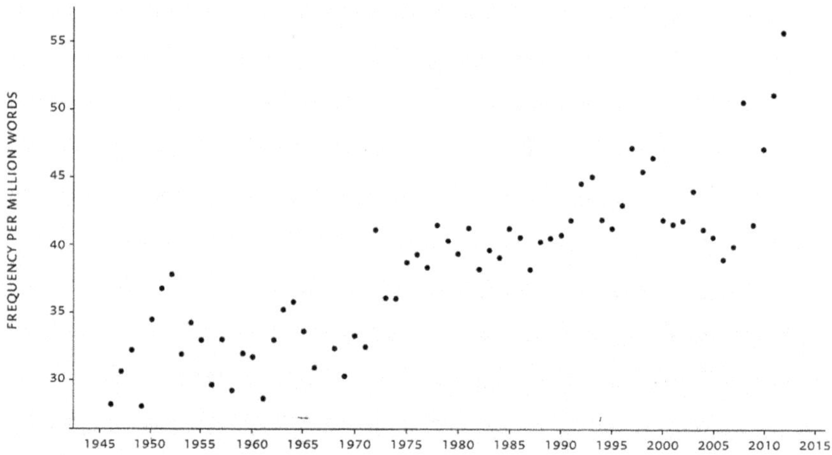

FIGURE 5.6 The relentless march of "and" in Bankspeak over decades. (Moretti & Pestre, 2017, Figure 7.10, p. 215) [Reproduced with the permission of Franco Moretti.]

These types of analyses might well be applied to the content of dreams over lengthy time periods to assess changes that may follow (or precede) landmark events in the dreamer's awake-life. What happens to logical coherence, temporal order, self-congratulation, joy and fear, following (and, perhaps, preceding) a marriage, a death, a rape, a professional breakthrough?

A noteworthy convergence between quantitative literary analysis and psychological approaches to meaning is the appreciation that elements of a text are not

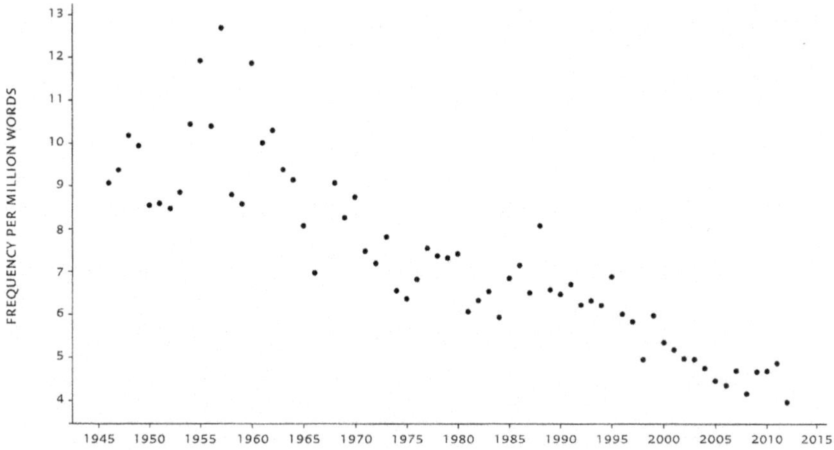

FIGURE 5.7 The breakdown of linear time in Bankspeak over six decades (1946–2008), as indexed by the decrease of temporal adverbs such as "now," "recently," and "later" (Moretti & Pestre, 2017, Figure 7.13, p. 219) [Reproduced with the permission of Franco Moretti.]

isolated units but constituents of broader networks of relations. We encountered an early version of this idea in Freud's (1891/1953) treatment of errors in aphasia (paraphasias), which Freud carried over from neurology into psychology in his treatment of errors in dreams, symptoms, jokes, and so on. As we have already noted (in our Chapter 2, pp. 34–40), aphasic errors are not random but semantically related. Freud made this clear in his treatment of paraphasias, which he defined as distortions "in which the appropriate word is replaced by a less appropriate one, which however, still retains a certain relationship to the correct word" (Freud, 1891/1953, p. 22). Thus, in Freud's example, the aphasic patient might respond with "**pen**" when the correct response would be "**pencil**" or say "**Potsdam**" instead of "**Berlin**" (p. 22).

More than half a century later, Heinz Werner (1956) independently expanded on the meaningful structure of aphasic errors, which he repeatedly showed to be semantically related to target materials and, therefore, to belong to a common "sphere of meaning" (see Chapter 2, pp. 34–40). We also saw (in Chapter 2, p. 37) that modern cognitive psychologists have (again, independently) elaborated the basic idea of the non-random "associative structure" of memory (Anderson, 1983; Anderson & Bower, 1983; Collins & Quillian, 1969; Collins & Loftus, 1975; Llewellyn, 2013; Rummerlhart, McClelland, & the PDP Research Group, 1986), which sometimes they have formalized mathematically (Andrews, Vigliocco, & Vinson, 2009; Landauer & Dumais, 1997), to the point of being able to extract "semantic representations" (meanings) from associative "neighborhood structures" (context, spheres). They have also been able to simulate behavioral phenomena such as *lexical substitution errors* in which, as in the case of paraphasias, "one word mistakenly replaces the intended word"—shades of Freud?—exhibiting "meaning resemblances to the intended word" (Andrews et al., 2009, p. 479).

Quantitative literary analysts have independently converged on many of these same ideas and may have even gone beyond the more established quantitative dream literature. Jockers (2013), for example, in a chapter on "Influence" (among large aggregates of literary works) emphasizes "macro patterns in style and theme" among different authors over substantial time-spans, seeking to demonstrate "subtle spheres of influence"—shades of Werner, this time?—that can be quantitatively demonstrated (Jockers, 2013, p. 155). Before we examine some of his studies of aggregates of works, we first turn to the corresponding "Network Theory" approach by Moretti (2013, pp. 211–240) to individual works, such as Hamlet.

A network deals with connections among a group of objects. The objects analyzed may involve virtually any complex system—bank reports, neurons, characters in a dream, the Danish Court in Hamlet. The elements of the network are called *nodes* or *vertices*; the connection among nodes, *edges*. Figure 5.8 depicts Moretti's rendition of the "Hamlet network." (In Moretti's treatment, an edge is defined as the occurrence of a verbal interaction between two characters.)

It is clear from just a cursory glance that a handful of individuals are the most central characters in the play plain dash in order, Hamlet, Claudius, Horatio, The

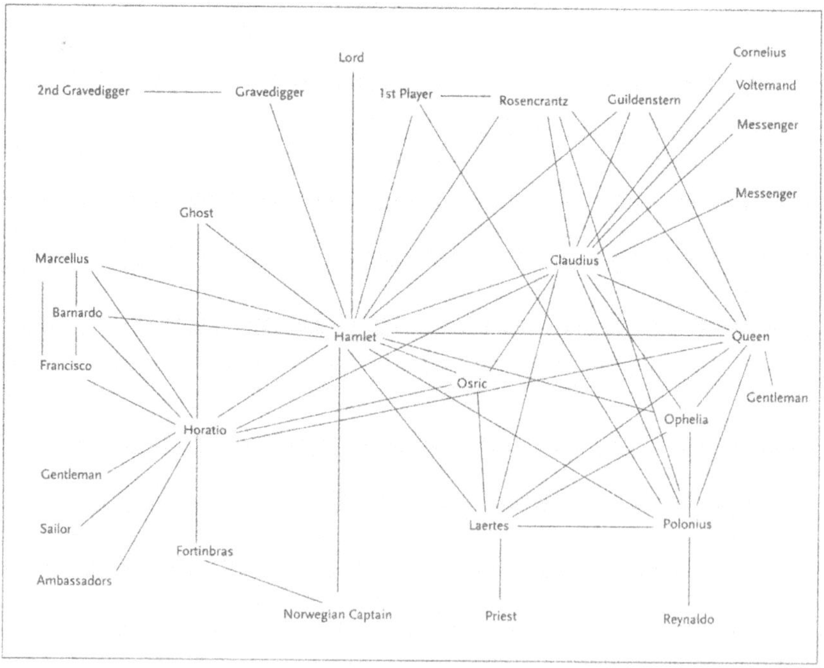

FIGURE 5.8 The Hamlet network (Moretti, 2013, Figure 1, p. 213) [Reproduced with the permission of Franco Moretti.]

Queen, Polonius, Laertes. Beyond some of the surface details, Moretti suggests (p. 218) that the network allows us to see—as in an "X-ray"—"underlying structures" ensconced in the network. (We might recall that Robert Van De Castle (p. 11) also used the X-ray metaphor to suggest the power of dreams to reveal unfolding biological events of which the dreamer might not yet be conscious.)

The quantitative treatment of literary texts allows "experiments" (p. 220) to be carried out on the data that may yield new insights—or corroboration of past insights. For example, what happens if Hamlet, the central character in the network, is removed from the play? The network virtually "splits in half" into a subnetwork of the Court, on the right, and the subnetwork bunched around Horatio, to the left (see Figure 5.9). This duality, according to Moretti, "emerges in all the great court scenes" (p. 223) and even features "different uses of language ... in different network regions" (p. 229).

This type of quantitative analysis might prove fruitful when applied to real-life individuals, both in their awake experiences and in their dreams. We might note that in psychology, "splitting" or "dissociation," is often observed in perturbed individuals or groups (see, Ellenberger, 1970; Erdelyi, 1985; Freud, 1940/1964b; Janet, 1889) and it might be revealing if quantitative approaches, such as Moretti's, could codify such splits in the clinical data. We could, moreover, quantitatively assess clinically relevant "experiments"—"experiments of nature," in this case—and determine what would happen to real-life networks if a member of a family, say the

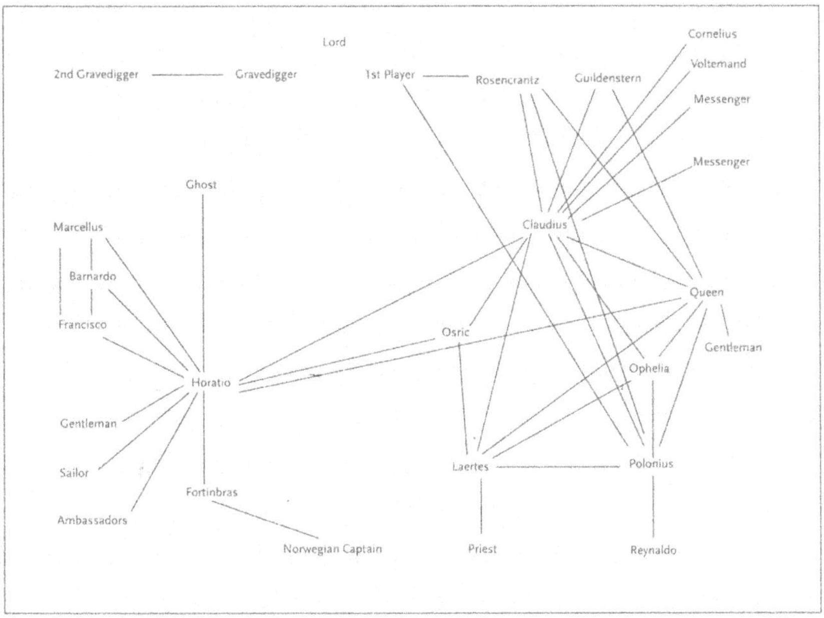

FIGURE 5.9 "Hamlet without Hamlet" (Moretti, 2013, Figure 7, p. 221) [Reproduced with the permission of Franco Moretti.]

father, is removed from the family network through death or divorce. Would the awake networks and the corresponding dream networks split into subnetworks (as a function, perhaps, of family pathology)? Importantly, could some of these quantitative approaches to networks reveal latent structures that remained hidden to the subject, the family, and, even, to the discerning clinician?

Matthew Jockers' (2013) book, *Macroanalysis*, deals not with the fine structure of individual works, such as Hamlet, but with the wider structure of aggregates of many works, distributed over decades. For this reason the approach is termed "macroanalyis," and involves not the "close reading" of a target text but "distant reading" (the title of Moretti's (2013) book) of patterns involving many texts.

This approach became possible only in recent years, with the increased availability of massive computational power and accompanying "massive digital-text collections" (Jockers, 2013, p. 7). The analyses are bound to be recondite to readers not conversant with a palette of statistical packages (e.g., "the R statistics package" (p. 160); "Google Exchange XML Format (GEXF)" (p. 163); "the Force Atlas 2 algorithm" (p. 164); "Gephi," (p. 163); "Gephi's PageRank Statistic (pp. 167–168), based on algorithms developed by Google founders, Sergey Brin and Lawrence Page, for gauging the relative importance of a book within a larger set of other books).

The basic idea in this statistical thicket is to determine (and visualize) "distances" among a set of objects (e.g., books) on some dimensions, in this case, literary *theme* and *style*. A small distance reflects close similarity between works (in theme, style) and a larger distance, greater dissimilarity. Thus, the "Eucledian distance" between Herman Melville's novel, *Moby-Dick or, the Whale* and his novel *Omoo: A Narrative of Adventures in the South Seas* is smaller than the distance between Melville's Moby-Dick and Edgar Allan Poe's, *The Narrative of Arthur Gordon Pym of Nantucket*, meaning that Melville is more like Melville than Poe, at least in this instance. (In some cases quantitative analysis demonstrates that an author's work is more similar to another author's work, e.g., Charles Dickens' *A Tale of two Cities* is closer to George Payne Rinsford James's *The False Heir* than to his own work, *Dombey and Son* (Jockers, 2013, p. 161).)

When the analysis is applied to a massive corpus (3,346 British novels in the 19th century), it is perhaps not surprising that visualization of the analysis yields a correspondingly massive looking network, as in Figure 5.10. The network is based on *thematic* and *stylistic* features—"books are being pulled together (and pushed apart) based on the similarity of their computed stylistic and thematic distances from each other" (p. 164). The computer program (Gephi) can, however, superimpose a temporal gradient on the network through "coloring or gray-scaling" (p. 164) in which the lighter-gray nodes and edges reflect earlier works from the century and darker gobs, later works. Figure 5.10 "reveals a clear time-signature to the stylistic-thematic data" (p. 164). Jockers reminds us that the novels are *not* being clustered in the network according to their publication dates but solely on their similarity in style and theme, which means that styles and themes in novels are "tethered in time" (p.165).

FIGURE 5.10 Nineteenth-century novel network (based on *style* and *theme*) with date shading ("beginning in the lighter, western, section of the graph ... and moving eastward through time" (Jockers, 2013, p. 164).) (Jockers, 2013, Fig. 5.3, p. 165). [From Macroanalysis: Digital Methods and Literary History. Copyright 2013 by the Board of Trustees of the University of Illinois. Used with permission of the University of Illinois Press.]

To shift to a different question, would we expect *gender* to be signaled by the style-theme network—that is, would we expect male and female novelists to write differently, and about different things? Is the answer obvious? Figure 5.11 gives the verdict of quantitative analysis:

> A clear boundary can be seen dividing the network into male [light gray] and female [black] regions. Works by female authors are more stylistically and thematically similar to each other, and they cluster together in the south and southeast portions of the main network. Males are drawn together in the north.
>
> *(Jockers, 2013, p. 165)*

The networks, though they look clearly bounded thanks to the large data set, are still statistical depictions. What look like mere wisps at the periphery (e.g., in the southeast outer border of Figure 5.11) may actually be informative, indicating meaningful "outlier communities." Also, anomalies masked by the sprawl of data, may be pointing to interesting facts. For example: "Maria Edgeworth's *Belinda* is mapped to a place in the network that puts her book twenty years ahead of its time" (p. 167); Harriet Beecher Stowe's books are "firmly rooted in the male sections of the network and many of James Payn's in the female half" (p. 167). Evidently, macroanalysis leads back to close reading. As Jockers makes clear, "macroanalysis ... is not offered as a challenge to, or replacement for, our traditional mode of inquiry. It is a complement" (Jockers, p. 171). This stance might also be urged for quantitative dream-analysis.

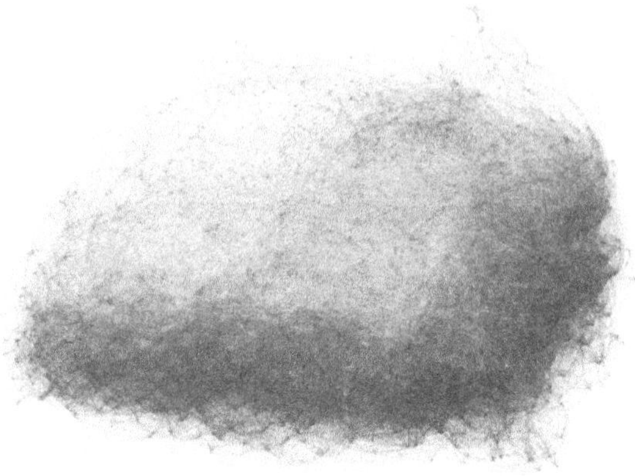

FIGURE 5.11 [Jockers, 2013, Fig. 9.5, p. 166.]. Nineteenth-century novel network (based on *style* and *theme*) with gender shading (Jockers, 2013, Figure 9.5, p. 166) [From Macroanalysis: Digital Methods and Literary History. Copyright 2013 by the Board of Trustees of the University of Illinois. Used with permission of the University of Illinois Press.]

There has been one research program thus far on the application of associative network analysis to dreams. This is the work of the memory researcher, Richard Schweickert, who produced the beautiful figures (Figures 5.12 and 5.13) (Schweickert (2007), pp. 272, 273) that depict the social associative networks of two dreamers, "Arlie" (a female subject) and "The Engine Man" (also called "The Natural Scientist"). Here the associations (the edges in the figures) represent the co-occurrences of characters in dreams; in Moretti's (2013) similar analysis of Hamlet, the edges represent verbal interactions among characters. The data points for the many dreams are more numerous than those for Shakespeare's single play, Hamlet, and yielded aesthetically striking representations. (Jockers' too, with his vast data set, produced impressive structures that look like streaking asteroids, neural networks, and whimsical clouds.) The associative networks, moreover, suggest psychological meanings. Moretti, as we have seen, subjected his data to quantitative "experiments," which produced information about the characters in Hamlet and how they related to one another—and to their likely fates (e.g., where they resided with respect to "killing zones"). Jockers' associative clouds, as he shows, are also seeded with meanings. Schweickert's two figures, for their part, suggest psychological differences between the dreamers. The Engine Man (Figure 5.13), whose constricted emotional life-style seems to place him somewhere in the autism-Asperger spectrum, yielded a constricted social network that is short of branchings and is substantially linear, while the associative network for the socially engaged Arlie (Figure 5.12) opens up, branches out, and appears to bloom into abstract flowers. Future research might explore further the potential psychological meanings that could be extracted from such associative networks.

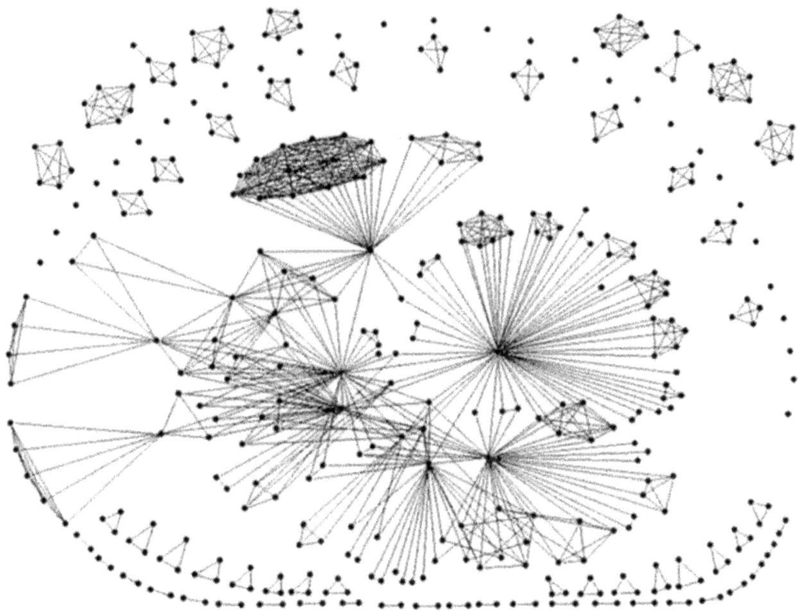

FIGURE 5.12 Social network for characters in Arlie's dreams. (Schweickert, 2007, p. 272) [Reprinted by permission of Psychonomic Bulletin & Review, Springer Nature. © 2007.]

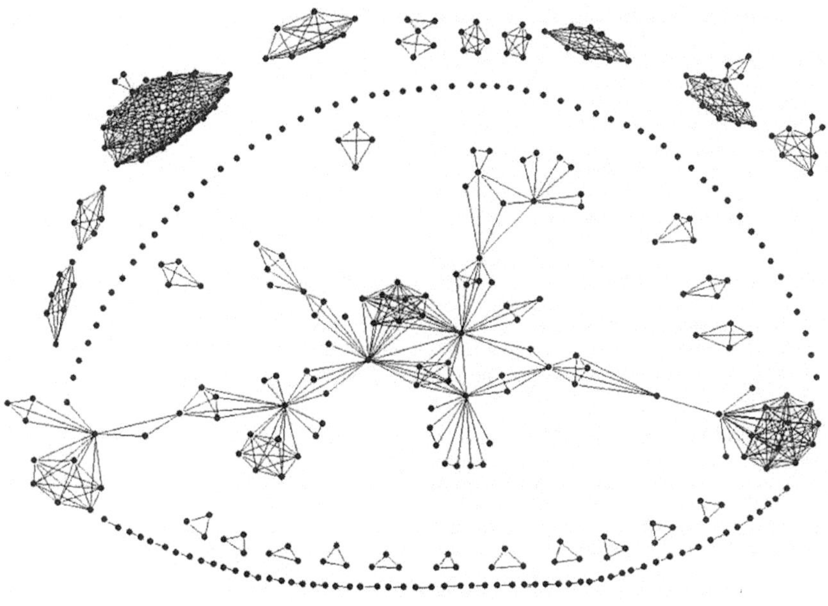

FIGURE 5.13 Social network for characters in the dreams of the "The Natural Scientist" (Schweickert, 2007, p. 273) [Reprinted by permission of Psychonomic Bulletin & Review, Springer Nature. ©2007.]

Quantitative Content-Analysis of Dreams (Hall, Van De Castle, Domhoff, Hartmann, Schredl, Bulkeley)

As suggested in the beginning of this chapter (p. 119), a basic disjunction has persisted for over a century in psychology's approach to meaning in dreams. Freud's *The interpretation of dreams* challenged lingering notions that dreams might be "mere froth" (Freud,1900/1953, p. 634)—an idea that briefly resurfaced and then quickly receded again in modern psychology—and insisted that dreams were not only meaningful at face value but also ensconced meanings at deeper levels that required interpretation. Freud's Irma Dream (pp. 63–67) illustrates this point. The dream report was a narrative that obviously carried meaning ("A large hall—numerous guests, whom we were receiving. Among them was Irma. . . .") and was clearly connected to events in Freud's personal and professional waking-life. Freud's project, as his title suggests, was to delve deeper and extract meanings (latent contents) that underpinned the surface (manifest) dream contents (e.g., what was the meaning of Dr. M.'s absurd declaration, "There is no doubt it's an infection, but no matter; dysentery will supervene and the toxin will be eliminated.") The title of Freud's book, placing interpretation at the center of his project, suggests his fundamental distinction, mostly absent in modern content-analytic approaches, between manifest and latent contents (see pp. 8–9, 41–42, 47–49, 57–58, 141–142).

What was abandoned by modern content-analytic approaches to the meaning of dreams was supplanted by the espousal of quantification of meanings, something entirely absent in Freud's own work. Modern content-analysts focus not on *interpreting* deep meanings but on *counting* meanings (characteristically, surface meanings). The most influential approach to quantitative content-analysis was developed by Calvin Hall and Robert Van De Castle (Hall, 1951, 1953; Hall & Van De Castle, 1966; Van De Castle, 1977) and extensively elaborated by Bill Domhoff (1996, 2003, 2018).

What does the quantitative Hall–Van De Castle system count? Table 5.1 lists the 10 meaning categories which, according to Domhoff (1996), "encompass virtually

TABLE 5.1 The 10 scoring categories of the Hall-Van De Castle Scoring System

- ⋆ CHARACTERS (subdivided into animals, humans, mythical figures)
- ⋆ SOCIAL INTERACTIONS (subdivided into friendly, aggressive, and sexual)
- ⋆ ACTIVITIES (physical, nonphysical)
- ⋆ STRIVING (success, failure)
- ⋆ MISFORTUNES and GOOD FORTUNES
- ⋆ EMOTIONS (anger, apprehension, confusion, happiness, and sadness)
- ⋆ PHYSICAL SURROUNDINGS (settings and objects)
- ⋆ DESCRIPTIVE ELEMENTS (modifiers, temporality, and negativity)
- ⋆ FOOD and EATING
- ⋆ ELEMENTS FROM THE PAST

Source: Domhoff, 2003, p. 67 [Adapted with the permission of Bill Domhoff].

all elements to be found in dreams" (p. 24). A little reflection suggests that the 10 meaning categories are rather broad, even if they are sometimes qualified, as in the subdivision of the SOCIAL INTERACTIONS category into *friendly, aggressive,* and *sexual* or the subdivision of EMOTIONS into *anger, apprehension, confusion, happiness,* and *sadness.* The Hall–Van De Castle system further refines meaning categories to allow for finer-grained analyses. Domhoff, for example, lists eight scorable varieties of *aggression* (itself a sub-class of SOCIAL INTERACTIONS), which include, in descending order of gravity: "An aggressive act resulting in the death of a character," "an aggressive act involving an attempt to harm a person physically" ... and, finally, "a covert feeling of hostility or anger without any overt expression of anger."

Table 5.2 provides empirically derived norms for some male–female differences, a major yield of the Hall–Van De Castle program. The first item under CHARACTERS is the "male/female" ratio which shows that about two-thirds (67%) of male dreams involve males but only about half (48%) of the dreams of females involve males. Why is this interesting? For one, it is a solid fact extracted from the subjective medium of dreams which, moreover, holds cross-culturally (with one possible problem with a Japanese study). Also, the results are counter-intuitive, with most students who are unfamiliar with the results incorrectly predicting that males dream more about women and women more about males. Calvin Hall devoted at least two articles to this obtained gender difference, which he designated the "ubiquitous sex difference in dreams" (Hall, 1963; 1984).

Note from Table 5.2 that the "ubiquitous sex difference" is highly significant statistically ($p < .0001$) but the magnitude of the effect, the *effect size* (Cohen's h), is .39, only a mid-range value. (Domhoff, 2003, p. 88, suggests that $h = .20$ is a small effect size, $h = .40$, a medium effect size, and $h = .80$ a large effect size.) A number of other significant, if not always large gender effects, are reported in Table 5.2. Females, compared to males, dream more about the *familiar*, about *friends*, and about *family* (all $p < .0001$) but the dreams of males, compared to those of females, include a larger percentage of *animals* (6% vs. 4%) and *physical aggression* (50% vs. 34%), and the *proportion of aggression to friendliness* (A/F%) is higher in the dreams of males that in those of females (59% vs. 51%). Males dream substantially more about *sex* than females (12% vs. 4%; $h = .31$. $p < .0001$) and more about *striving, success, and failure*.

The Hall–Van De Castle normative data could be used for clinical inferences through the comparison of a particular subject's percentages with the normative percentages. Barb Sanders (Domhoff, 2003, p. 116) significantly exceeds the female norms on aggression (aggression/character, $h = .21$, $p < 0001$; Aggressor Percent, $h = .36$, $p < 0001$) and yet she also exceeds the norms on Friendliness/Character and Sexuality/Character. She might, therefore, without any direct clinical contact, be described as aggressive, sexual, friendly—at least in her dreams. (Note, however, that, as discussed in the last section of this chapter, there exists a basic continuity between the contents of dream-life and of awake-life, and so what applies to dreams probably—although not certainly—also applies to awake-life.)

TABLE 5.2 A Comparison of the Male and Female Norms for the Hall–Van De Castle System (Domhoff, 2003, p. 73)

	Male norms (%)	*Female norms (%)*	*Effect size*	*p*
Characters				
Male/female percent	67	48	+.39	.000**
Familiarity percent	45	58	–.26	.000**
Friends percent	31	37	–.12	.004**
Family percent	12	19	–.21	.000**
Animal percent	6	4	+.08	.037*
Social interaction percents				
Aggression/friendliness percent	59	51	+.15	.014*
Befriender percent	50	47	+.06	.517
Aggressor percent	40	33	+.14	.129
Victimization percent	60	67	–.14	.129
Physical aggression percent	50	34	+.33	.000**
Social interaction ratios				
Aggression/character index	.34	.24	+.24	.000**
Friendliness/character index	.21	.22	–.01	.852
Sexuality/character index	.06	.01	+.11	.000**
Self-concept percents				
Self-negativity percent	65	66	–.02	.617
Bodily misfortunes percent	29	35	–.12	.217
Negative emotions percent	80	80	+.00	.995
Dreamer-involved success percent	51	42	+.18	.213
Torso/anatomy percent	31	20	+.26	.002**
Other indicators				
Physical activities percent	60	52	–.38	.000**
Indoor setting percent	48	61	–.26	.000**
Familiar setting percent	62	79	–.38	.000**
Percentage of dreams with at least one				
Aggression	47	44	+.05	.409
Friendliness	38	42	+.08	.197
Sexuality	12	4	+.31	.000**
Misfortune	36	33	+.06	.353
Good fortune	6	6	+.02	.787
Success	15	8	+.24	.000**
Failure	15	10	+.17	.007**
Striving	27	15	+.31	.000**

Note. The p values are based on the formula for the significance of differences between two proportions.

The effect size derives from Cohen's h. The h statistic is determined by the following formula

$$h = \cos^{-1}(1–2P_1)–\text{Cos}^{-1}(1–2P_2)$$

P_1 and P_2 are proportions between 0 and 1, and the $\cos^{-1}$ operation returns a value in radians.
* significant at the .05 level
** significant at the .01 level
[Reproduced with the permission of Bill Domhoff.]

TABLE 5.3 Barb Sanders' Social Interactions with Family and Friends Compared with a Baseline 250 Sample (Domhoff, 2003, p. 116) (Reproduced with the permission of Bill Domhoff)

	N	*A/C index*	*F/C index*	*A/F (%)*	*Aggressor (%)*	*Befriender (%)*
Baseline	884	.33	.32	49	50	53
Mother	239	.70	.27	72	46	48
Father	213	.36	.37	50	47	42
Oldest daughter	81	.51	.65	44	73	77
Middle daughter	165	.92	.52	64	79	70
Youngest daughter	83	.36	.81	31	63	61
Favorite brother	97	.23	.69	25	59	60
Friend Ginny	96	.26	.89	23	52	53
Friend Lucy	59	.39	.63	38	78	78

Other clinically relevant contrasts in Barb Sanders' dreams are the frequency differences involving her circle of friends and family. Barb Sanders admits to having fraught relations with her mother but to be on better terms with her father. As shown in Table 5.3, her dream content is consistent with her claim: 70% of her mentions of her mother in her dreams involve aggression (her Aggression to Character ratio, or "A/C Index," is .70). The corresponding A/C Index for her father is only 36%, about half the aggression rate for her mother. The Friendliness per Character ratio (the F/C Index) for her mother and father—.27 and .37, respectively—are also consistent with Barb Sanders' friendlier feelings toward her father in awake-life.

The dream content frequencies also mirror Sanders' different feelings toward her three daughters, revealing her negative emotions toward her (disturbed) middle daughter (A/C% = .92) and her more positive feelings toward her younger and older daughters (respectively, A/C% = .36 and .51). Her favorite brother garners the lowest A/C% (.23) of all the characters in her dreams. The dream data parallel the dreamer's awake emotional dispositions and so could be used as an indicator of awake emotional valences.

A serious interest in clinical aspects of dream contents would, however, require more than a demonstration of continuity between the content of dreams and the content of awake life, for if continuities were the only concern, we might dispense with dreams altogether and turn directly to reports from the subject's waking life. The crucial missing dimension is the X-ray aspect of dreams (pp. 11, 131), the possibility that dreams might be more revealing of certain covert events than awake-reports. As suggested in later pages of this chapter, the characteristic neglect of deep meanings and of unconscious contents in contemporary quantitative approaches to dreams likely accounts for this lacuna.

Personality in Dreams

Dreams have been probed for possible leads to the personality of the dreamer (Bell & Hall, 1971) but the early efforts had little success, and some major modern quantitative content-analysts appear to have given up on the venture (e.g., "Dreams do not tell us much if anything about personality" (Domhoff, 2017, p. 51)). As noted by the author in a recent article (Erdelyi, 2017, p. 340), scientific personality psychology was itself experiencing repeated failures around Bell and Hall's time in its efforts to predict behavior from personality traits. The problem was that personality-behavior correlations (except for cognitive dimensions and psychopathological traits) refused to exceed what Walter Mischel (1968, p. 78) disdainfully dubbed the "personality coefficient," the small to trifling correlation coefficient of $r \leq |.30|$ invariably found between traits and behaviors.

The story had a happy ending, however, with a surprisingly obvious solution that had largely evaded the field for several decades. The problem, according to the breakthrough insight, was that while personality tests contained a large number of questions (e.g., 566 in the MMPI [the Minnesota Multiphasic Personality Inventory], 57 in the Eysenck Personality Inventory, 94 in the Myers-Briggs Type Indicator), the behavior tests, which are expensive in terms of time and research funds, characteristically involved only one behavioral observation. An *n* of 1, it finally dawned on the field, was simply insufficient. When the behavior reports were increased by only a little, even to half a dozen, the straightjacketing personality coefficient gave way and the correlation coefficients triumphantly soared to $r > |0.80|$—and, with larger *n's*, to stratospheric correlations in the .90's that sometimes approached 1.00 (Epstein, 1977, 1979; Epstein & O'Brian, 1985; Fleeson, 2001, 2004; Moskowitz, 1982). The issue of inadequate sample sizes, as discussed at the end of this chapter, has independently become a concern in quantitative dream research.

For now, we might note that some work has been done showing a potentially high correlation between the personality trait dimension of *thin-thick boundaries* and the frequency of dream recall (Hartmann, 2011; Hartmann & Kunzendorf, 2006–07; Schredl, 1996; 1999; Schredl & Piel, 2003; Schredl, Kleinferchner, & Gell, 1996; Schredl, Schafer, Hoffman, & Jacobs, 1999). People who have thin boundaries have relatively loose mental borders, tending to mix emotions and thoughts, fantasy and reality, conscious and unconscious mentation. Such people spend a lot of time daydreaming, are very sensitive to other people's feelings, and when getting involved with another person tend to get too close. They are intuitive and dreamy. People with thick boundaries are the opposite, tending to be orderly and well organized, to separate their emotions from their reasoning, and to like relationships that have clearly spelled-out rules and well demarcated borders. Women tend to have thinner boundaries than men (by about half of a standard deviation, on the average). The dimension correlates highly ($r = .73$) with the well-known Big-5 personality dimension of "Openness" (Hartmann, 2011, p. 97).

The Hartmann and the Schredl research groups have expended some effort to establish a relation between thin boundaries and dream-recall frequency. Positive correlations were obtained but they were modest initially, in the order of the personality coefficient in most cases. Hartmann and his colleagues (Hartmann, 2003; Hartmann & Kunzendorf (2006–2007) sought to establish a more powerful prediction of dream recall frequency from boundary scores. They sensed that "noise" was undermining the predictive power of the thin-thick dimension and in the vein of the aggregation solution to the weak trait-behavior correlations, attempted to show stronger correlations with larger *n*'s, in this specific case by correlating not individual scores but the aggregated scores of well-defined groups that tended to differ on thinness. The results were striking: The thinner the (group's) boundaries, the greater the dream recall frequencies. The correlations, as in the case of the breakthrough personality research involving aggregation, yielded outstanding correlations, for example, $r = .92$. It appears that individuals with thin boundaries do not lose contact with their dream experiences on awakening as much as individuals with thicker boundaries. The high correlation coefficients obtained document the high predictive power of the thin-boundaries trait. Note, however, that a single individual's score would predict far less well. Only when error of measurement, or noise, is reduced by aggregation (since as *n* goes up, error variance goes down), does the relation approach a perfect value. Here, then, we have an extremely robust personality-dream connection.

Problems with Current Quantitative Content-Analytic Approaches to Dreams

Neglect of Deep Meanings and of Unconscious Contents

Modern quantitative content-analytic schemes, such as the Hall–Van De Castle system, count meanings but often fail to count the meanings that count. For example, the Hall–Van De Castle system would not "get" the meaning of any joke (e.g., pp. 52–58). It would be stumped by the dreams presented in Chapter 3, even the simpler ones such as, "The Picture Dream of Dolores P." or the "Elephant Dream" of John Nemiah's subject (pp. 67–70). It would miss the target meanings of paraphasias (see pp. 34–40) and thus miss the rich associative structures ("spheres of meaning") implied by such errors, as it would miss the meanings and associative structures of their psychological counterparts, the *parapraxes* (Freudian errors). It would fail to grasp the meaning of much poetry (e.g., "Freud Dreams Chinese Poetry" in Chapter 3). In every case, the problem is that such content-analysis counts surface contents but fails to count latent contents.

This neglect of latent contents is an unforced error. There is no reason why latent contents should not be quantified (as was done, for example, by Erdelyi and Stein (1981) and Bergstein and Erdelyi (2008) with jokes). When no latent contents are involved, as in the stimulus of Haber and Erdelyi (1967) (p. 120), then, of course, latent contents need not concern us. But complex, real-life stimuli are suffused with deep meanings and quantitative dream-analysis, as currently practiced, will tend to miss the action.

Unconscious contents pose a more refractory problem since even the most exacting content counts do not gauge unconscious contents. The long-term hypermnesic memory functions of Erdelyi and Kleinbard (1978) (see our pp. 22–26) show that a first recall test drastically undercounts (by more than 50%, on the average) the recall counts eventually obtained a week later after multiple testing. For the present, we must acknowledged that current quantitative content-analyses give us counts of only contents that are conscious at a given time. In our next chapter, "Dreaming as Noisy Remembering," we shall consider how we might mitigate the problem and access some of the unconscious content of dreams.

Although both Calvin Hall and Bill Domhoff emphasize the cognitive thrust of their approach to dreams (Hall, 1953; Domhoff, 2003, 2018a), it might be useful to note that the neglect of latent contents is a behaviorist throw-back. The fact of quantification does not alter this observation. B. F. Skinner, after all, introduced mechanical cumulative-response recorders that produced beautiful quantitative stimulus-response functions. Nor does the subject matter that is being quantified serve as a counterargument, for Skinner (e.g., 1957) also concerned himself with cognitive subject matters, e.g., language (which, however, he called "verbal behavior"). The behaviorist program precisely sought to shed the burden of interpretation for the doubting-Thomas certitude of palpable behavior. Don't ask if the man is "angry" (an interpretation), ask what is the man's blood pressure? Or, ask whether he is shouting (and how loudly and for how long), or whether he is breaking furniture. The Hall–Van De Castle system is not as extreme as Skinner would have it be, for it does involve some low-grade interpretation for its content categories—for example, "friendly," "aggressive," "anger," and "apprehension," but it stays too close to the surface to grapple with significant latent contents.

Where does this leave us? It would be a mistake to embrace an either-or answer, as different questions call for different answers. If we wish to "get" a joke—or a dream—we do not launch a quantitative Armada—a sprawling count of "characters," "misfortunes and good fortunes," "elements from the past," "successes and failures," and so on. It would not get us there. On the other hand, if our objective is to count the manifest contents of dreams in a subject population or in a series of dreams, an exhaustive approach, such as that of the Hall–Van De Castle system, is indicated. Such manifest-content counts might be supplemented by counts of latent contents to avoid merely superficial counts. Broad-swath content analytic approaches, such that of Hall–Van De Castle, would give us essential background information which would point to important facts about dream contents (e.g., male–females differences) and, also, forestall errors such as Freud's wish-fulfillment hypothesis, since dreams, as quantitative content-analysis shows, pitch negatively toward fearful and upsetting contents and not toward wishes.

Problems with Generic (One-Size-Fits-All) Content-Analytic Schemes

The Hall–Van De Castle system, the most widely used quantitative content-analytic scheme for dreams, has many strong features: It is highly reliable; it has produced a variety of noteworthy counts of manifest dream contents which, for the most part, seem to hold across cultures; it supports an impressive (and publicly accessible) website (DREAMBANK.NET) developed by Domhoff's associate, Adam Schneider, that contains a large number of dreams for analysis and various analytic tools for such analyses. Nevertheless, it is not the appropriate analytic approach in many cases. We often are concerned with some specific content category and need not launch a wide-net probe to capture all conceivable dream-content categories.

A good example of this point is the already discussed subliminal perception study of Haber and Erdelyi (pp. 120–122), which required quantitative content-analyses to assess the emergence in drawings and free-associative fantasy of *specific stimulus contents* (mules, carts, workers, platforms, buildings, bales of cotton, and so on). It would not have been sensible to deploy the Hall–Van De Castle system, for this broad-gauge scheme counts categories that belong, mostly, to a different universe of contents. The simple, targeted content-analytic approach of Haber and Erdelyi easily yielded reliable as well as significant effects. Similarly, in our next chapter on "Dreaming as Noisy Remembering," we discuss various approaches to quantifying repeated recalls of Bartlett's famous stimulus, the Native American folk tale, "The War of the Ghosts." These scoring methods are extremely simple, including straightforward counts of word-correspondences between the recalls and the 334 words in the story. The overall reliabilities were extremely high, in the mid .90's. Again, since the contents of "The War of the Ghosts" do not neatly fit the Hall–Van De Castle categories (although here Hall–Van De Castle scoring would pick up some of the narrative strands), the Hall–Van De Castle system would not have been the most efficient counting scheme. The key point is that we need to fit the counting scheme to the contents of interest.

Many of the questions addressed by wide-net probes of content, such as that of the Hall–Van De Castle system, could actually be answered with simpler and more narrowly focused assays. If, for example, we were interested in gender differences in dreams, we could study this single dimension effectively without committing ourselves to large samples and irrelevant content categories. The simpler targeted approaches would presumable replicate the "ubiquitous sex difference" found by Hall (1963, 1984) with the Hall–Van De Castle system, and, possibly, discover new wrinkles in the effect with latent contents taken into account. Or, a more targeted (and simpler) approach to counting sexual content in dreams should, again, yield the Hall–Van De Castle results—but also, with more probing for latent contents, produce a new estimate that would show—as the author predicts—a significant undercount (perhaps by 100%) of sexual content in dreams by the Hall–Van De Castle system.

A highly automated word-count approach to dreams—"digital dream analysis"—has been developed by Kelly Bulkeley (2014, 2018) which does not even require the reading by the human experimenter of the computer record of the subject's dream series. The computer analysis picks up 40 categories of word usage that are organized into 8 classes (perception, emotion, cognition, characters, social interactions, elements, movements, and culture) and delivers word-counts for each of the category classes. The obtained frequencies for the eight classes are then compared to baselines which allow clinical inferences to be made about the dreamer (which, typically, are confirmed by the dreamer (see Bulkeley, 2018, pp. 341–344)). As with Jockers' approach to distant reading (pp.

132–134), digital reading is complemented by the eventual close reading by the interpreter.

Mechanical Stances toward Statistical Power

As with content-counts, our statistical analyses should not be mechanical applications of familiar procedures but be tailor-made to suit our statistical needs. For example, Domhoff (2018a) often urges the use of a large sample of dreams ($n \geq 120$) to ensure statistical significance in dream-content research. This may well hold for his type of work (the counting of a wide range of meanings by the Hall–Van De Castle system)—just as it would be correct to insist on a very large sample size, for example, $n = 600$, in conducting polling during a presidential campaign, where small margins of error could be crucial. There is much noise (error variance) in such data, which, as we have noted, a large *n* reduces. However, when dealing with more targeted counts, we may need far smaller *n*'s.

If there were no cost to using large samples there would be no reason to resist using large samples. But there invariably is a cost, and the effort expended on large samples is the effort that might not be expended on focused interrogation of the data—for example, for latent contents or, even, for unconscious contents. This type of issue has been a classic concern in personality psychology, often under the heading of *idiogrphic* vs. *nomothetic* strategies of research. Idiographic refers to the in-depth study of one or a few subjects (as in in-depth clinical case-histories). Nomothetic refers to the simple evaluation of some personality characteristic, usually with a personality test, which takes little time and easily generates large-*n* data that can then be evaluated through standard statistical analyses. For some decades these poles were thought to be antagonistic but, more recently, both strategies have begun to be recognized as valid and complementary. There is no one correct approach. A single subject ($n = 1$) can have a seminal impact on an entire discipline—for example, Paul Broca's patient, Tan (see p. 32), led to the systematic study of aphasia and the amnesic H.M. (Henry Molaison, pp. 109–110), who, though he could not remember the people who took care of him for decades, transformed the field of memory in the 20th century (Scoville & Milner, 1957; Squire, 1987, 2009). In other cases it is necessary, as we saw with the aggregation tactic for resolving the personality-behavior connection, to shift to larger sample sizes, although even here only a few observations were necessary to break the back of the nefarious personality coefficient.

Ironically, the success of large-sample data in producing positive results that small-*n*'s could not achieve has a conceptual underside. By managing to achieve statistical significance through the brute-force use of larger *n*'s to reduce noise, we might neglect to reduce noise through the better understanding of the phenomenon we are studying. *Statistical power* (the probability that a test will detect an effect—when there is an effect to be detected) is boosted by *both* sample size and effect size (the magnitude of the effect) (Cohen, 1998; Cumming, 2012; Ellis, 2010). By achieving a greater understanding of our phenomenon, we can produce stronger effects and, therefore, greater statistical power, without resorting to an inflation of *n*.

Before concluding this section, we should consider briefly the subject of "statistical significance" and "effect size," which play important roles in quantitative content-analysis (note, Domhoff's Table 5.2 in p. 138 lists *both* significance levels *and* effect sizes). The significance-level, *p*, is well known to experimental psychologists. It refers to the probability, *p*, that an obtained effect—or larger—resulted merely by chance; thus a value of *less than p* (e.g., $p < .05$) is an effect that is conventionally accepted as too improbable to have resulted by chance; that is, it is concluded that the effect is *not* due to chance. We are in effect trying to reject the *null hypothesis*, which usually is defined as the hypothesis that our effect was a mere chance effect. Thus, the male-female difference in animal content in dreams (6% vs. 4% in Table 5.2, p. 138) is 2%, a small difference that might easily have been a chance result. The *p* value listed, $p = .037$, indicates, however, that the probability of getting this difference (or larger) by chance alone is .037, and thus, $p < .05$, which by convention is small enough to reject the null hypothesis that all we found was a chance effect. This roundabout way of supporting our effect by rejecting the null-hypothesis—which the author's graduate statistics professor, the late Robert Abelson, once referred to as "the ritualized exercise of devil's advocacy" (1995, p. 9)—enables us to make crisp yes or no decisions. In this case: No, the effect was not likely to have been a chance occurrence, so, yes, we are willing to conclude that the male-female difference is real.

The null-hypothesis testing approach yields significance values which, notwithstanding their ubiquitous use, have been widely criticized over the last several decades for giving very little of the information we really want. It is nice to know that our results were not likely due to chance, but "significance" is a misnomer since we don't known how large or how important ("significant" in the common sense of the word) the outcome might be. Modern statisticians (Cohen, 1998; Cummings, 2012; Ellis, 2010) have advocated the reporting of the actual size of the effect—the *effect size*—which, it should be noted, Domhoff frequently includes along with his *p* values. The reader will not be surprised to learn that the concept is not without nuances—Ellis (2010, p. 6), citing Kirk (2003), notes that "there are more than 70 varieties of effect size." The essential idea, however, is straightforward: Any data that reflect actual magnitude, such as the arithmetic mean ($\bar{X}$), a percentage (%), a frequency (*f*), a correlation coefficient (*r*), is an effect size; some effect sizes, however, for example, Cohen's *d* or Cohen's *h* (the percentage counterpart of Cohen's *d*) are standardized in some way (e.g., Cohen's *d* is rendered in standard scores, or *z*-scores) and are not always obvious to all readers and, for this reason, are often designated (to the consternation of some statisticians) as "small," "medium," or "large" by Cohen—and by Domhoff, following Cohen. Note that "statistically significant" effects (e.g., $p < .05$) can be associated with small effect sizes. For example, as we saw in Table 5.2, the 2% male–female difference in the frequency of animal dreams was statistically significant ($p = .037$), but the effect size was quite small ($h = .08$). This simply means that very small effects can be real.

The Continuity Hypothesis (Freud, Jung, Calkins, Hall, Domhoff, Schredl, Bulkeley, Erdelyi, Jenkins)

Ever since the 19th century, the theoretically important view has been crystallizing in dream psychology that, notwithstanding some differences in degree, dream-life is more or less continuous with awake-life. Freud, in the first dozen pages of *The interpretation of dreams*, summarizes various articulations of this view:

> "dreams carry on waking life."
>
> *Haffner, 1887; in Freud, p. 2*

> "the majority of dreams ... usually lead us back to ordinary life instead of freeing us from it."
>
> *Weygandt, 1893, p. 6; in Freud, pp. 7–8*

> "*Nous rêvons de ce que nous avons vu, dit, désiré ou fait*" [We dream of what we have seen, said, desired, or done"]
>
> *Maury, 1878, p. 51; in Freud, 1900, p. 8*

> "The content of a dream is invariably more or less determined by the individual personality of the dreamer, by his age, sex, class, standard of education and habitual ways of living, and by the events and experiences of his whole previous life."
>
> *Jessen, 1885, p. 330; in Freud, 1900, p. 8*

Contrary to some modern treatments of Freud's position, to which we shall presently turn, Freud matter of course embraced the basic continuity between dream-life and awake-life: "All of the material making up the content of a dream is in some way derived from experience, that is to say, has been reproduced or remembered in the dream. . . " (Freud, 1900/1953, p. 11).

Quantitative content-analysis has led to the same place. Mary Calkins, the first female president of the American Psychological Association, reported in her 1893 article, "Statistics of Dreams," that there is "an essential congruity and continuity of the dream life with the waking life" (p. 323). Hall and his early associates (Bell & Hall, 1971; Hall & Nordby, 1972) reached the same conclusion—"there is a continuity between dreams and waking life" (Bell & Hall, 1971, p. 117)—a position they labeled, "the continuity-hypothesis." Hall and Nordby (1972) fleshed out the hypothesis as follows:

> [D]reams are continuous with waking life; the world of dreaming and the world of waking are one. The dream world is neither discontinuous nor inverse in its relationship to the conscious world. We remain the same person, the same personality with the same characteristics, and the same basic beliefs and conventions whether awake or asleep. The wishes and fears that

> determine our actions and thoughts in everyday life also determine what we will dream about.
>
> *(p. 104)*

A puzzling error, however, which has no bearing on the fact of continuity itself, was piggy-backed onto the continuity hypothesis, namely, the claim, alluded to by Hall and Nordby's quote above, that Freud and Jung were opposed to such continuity and thus were "discontinuity theorists" (Domhoff, 2017; Hall & Lind, 1970). This claim involves a basic misunderstanding of Freud's position, as Freud's brief quote already suggests. For Freud, the importance of dreams lay precisely in their power to shed light on the awake behaviors and thoughts of his patients. (We shall briefly return to Jung's position after we deal with Freud's.)

The misunderstanding of Freud's view arose, apparently, form his emphasis of *censorship* as a major component of the dream-work (see Chapter 2, p. 42), which ostensibly disconnects the dream from awake-consciousness. Freud's position, however, is that

> [I]t would be a mistake to suppose that a connection of this kind between the content of a dream and reality is bound to come to light easily . . . . The connection requires ... to be looked for diligently, and in a whole quantity of cases may long remain hidden.
>
> *Freud, 1900, p. 11*

Thus, Freud is not arguing against the "connection" between dream content and awake "reality." He is merely saying that we have to look for it "diligently" and that it might take some time to find the connection. An important nuance here is that it is *not the manifest content* that poses a problem for continuity, as the congruence between the manifest dream and events in the dreamer's life is palpably clear to all concerned. It is the dream's *latent-content* that may not be fully continuous with awake consciousness, although even the latent-contents of dreams are not fully disconnected from awake experience but may merely need more effort to bring to light. In statistical terms, the correlation between the manifest-content of dreams and the manifest-content of awake experience is high; the counterpart correlation between the latent-content of dreams and the manifest-content of awake experience is lower thanks to censorship—although not absent.

Censorship, actually, cuts both ways, for awake-consciousness is also subject to censorship, although the usual term assigned to the process in awake-life is *repression* or *suppression* (see Erdelyi, 1985, 1990, 2006a). Consequently, the repression or suppression to which awake cognition is subject will also undermine to some extent the continuity of awake-life, which may be conceived of as a Swiss Cheese continuity, a kind of continuity with holes. Indeed, as emphasized by the author (Erdelyi, 1985, 1990, 2014) and also by some others, for example, the neuropsychoanalysist, Mark Solms (Solms & Turnbull, 2002, pp. 214–215), the censorship of dreams is actually *less* than the censorship (repression, suppression) of awake consciousness, hence the enhanced sensitivity of dreams to normally inaccessible thoughts and emotions.

Returning briefly to Jung, we again encounter a major misunderstanding, although a different one than the misunderstanding that applied to Freud. Jung (e.g., 1968; 1974) often claimed that dreams were *compensatory* in function and brought out aspects of personality that waking-consciousness had neglected. Apart from the truth value of this position, which the author does not champion, the compensation position is, nevertheless, not contrary to continuity. What is involved here is a *negative correlation* rather than a *positive correlation*, which, as in a mirror image of ourselves, is continuous but inverse to the manifest reality. Thus, an "inverse ... relation" (see Hall & Nordby's quote above) does not spell discontinuity; what would be required to show discontinuity is not a negative correlation but a correlation of zero.

One final controversy about the continuity hypothesis, which may have been finally settled in the very recent literature, concerns a version of the continuity hypothesis forcefully promoted by Bill Domhoff (see the 2017–2018 discussions in the journal, *Dreaming*, of Bulkeley, 2018; Domhoff, 1917, 1918; Erdelyi, 2017; Jenkins, 2018; and Schredl, 2017). A decade after Bell and Hall's (1971) promulgation of their continuity hypothesis, other colleagues, notably Bill Domhoff, urged a more constricting formulation of the hypothesis:

> The continuity hypothesis states that dreaming is continuous with waking life. That is, people will manifest in their dreams the *concerns and preoccupations of their waking life.*
>
> *(Hall, Domhoff, Blick, & Weesner, 1982, p. 193)*

The first part of this updated definition is, of course, a restatement of the original Bell and Hall proposal (see above, pp. 146–147). The qualifying second part, however, is the emphasis that Domhoff has sought to impose on the simple continuity hypothesis. The problem with the add-on is not that it is wrong—it certainly captures an important subset of the broader principle—but that Domhoff has sought to exclude, as if by ownership of the term, other types of continuities between dream-content and awake life-content as valid versions of the continuity hypothesis (see, Erdelyi, 2017; Jenkins, 2018; Schredl, 2017). For Domhoff, *cognitive* continuities ("conceptions," "preoccupations," "interests") extending over temporal windows of "months, years, decades" (Domhoff, 2017, p. 27) are the continuities that define "the continuity hypothesis." To other continuity theorists, who might focus on short-term correspondences or emotional congruencies, Domhoff urged a change in nomenclature. Not surprisingly, this suggestion provoked some blow-back.

The good news is that this tempest in a tea-cup is yielding a resolution, with Domhoff accepting the usage of "the continuity hypothesis" by proponents of other types of continuity. Further, in line with the author's voiced concern (Erdelyi, 2017,

p. 342) that a "hypothesis" in science has a limited shelf-life, requiring timely confirmation or disconfirmation, Domhoff has now moved on to declare the continuity hypothesis to be "an established generalization and no longer a hypothesis" (p. 358).

Still, even if continuity has moved past the stage of "hypothesis," more work is called for on the continuity between dream-life and awake-life (see Erdelyi, 2017). Although continuity undoubtedly exists, it is not a perfect continuity. We may think of it as involving a substantial, but not perfect overlap between dream-life and awake-life. For example, dreams are more primary-process in character (they are more visual, less logical, less realistic, and less time-structured) (see our Chapter 2, p. 41). Also, certain aspects of awake-experiences are not likely to be represented in dreams. For example, dreams tend not to feature "close-knit, over-learned" awake activities such as "the three R's" ("reading," "riting," and "rithmetic") (Hartmann (2011, p. 45)) or common waking-life contents from politics, sports, entertainment, international affairs, religion (Bulkeley, 2018, p. 338; Domhoff, 2018a, p. 4).

Thus, continuity between dream-consciousness and awake-consciousness is a fact, but so is discontinuity. The reality is a mixed picture; the correlation is positive but not perfect. From a statistical standpoint, we are bound to obtain continuity with large enough samples, since instances of continuity combined with instances of discontinuity will average out as continuity. With further work we may ascertain, more comprehensively than now, when we may expect continuity and when discontinuity.

Application of Signal Detection Theory to Dream Recall (Erdelyi et al.)

A substantive area of psychophysics, SDT, has been assimilated by mainstream scientific psychology for many decades now but has not yet been touched by dream science. Yet the subject is obviously relevant for dream interpretation—and content-analysis in general—since what is involved in both cases is the detection of information embedded in noise. We have already briefly considered the subject-matter in our discussion of the Haber and Erdelyi (1967) study of the recovery of subliminal stimuli in fantasy (pp. 120–122). In a dedicated Appendix at the end of our book a more detailed exposition of the subject-matter is presented, along with an original technique for controlling response criteria in narrative free-recall, including dreams.

6

DREAMING AS NOISY REMEMBERING

We begin our chapter on a perverse note by considering, as some dream scientists have (Hartmann, 2011), why dreaming is *not* a form of remembering but is, instead, a creative activity which frequently deals not with past events, as memory does, but with made-up scenarios, sometimes about the future. According to Hartmann (2011, p. 23), "[a] dream is a creation, not a replay ... it is somewhat like a work of art."

We can happily agree with Hartmann and others that much dream content is not strictly veridical but involves constructive, creative products. What we can confidently add, however, is that modern memory psychology has abandoned its video-recorder notion of memory and now conceives of memory not as a faithful, if fading trace of past events but as a constructive elaboration of events retained from the past (Bartlett, 1932; Bransford & Franks, 1977; Erdelyi, 1996; Loftus & Palmer, 1974; Neisser, 1967; Roediger & McDermott, 1995). We shall encounter below many concrete examples of this type of memory artistry, notably in the dream-incorporation of drastic body-events (e.g., an amputation) and in the long-distance recalls of "The War of the Ghosts" by two little girls, Karina and Maya, at the end of this chapter (pp. 164–179). It will be seen that we do not have an either-or situation. True, memory is riddled with distortions of omission and commission but it is also true that our memories—as well as our dreams—are positively, even if not perfectly correlated with our experiences from the past. Thus, it would be quite accurate to conceive of dreaming, as we do in this chapter, as a form of "noisy remembering." This is not a new precept. Freud, actually, over a century ago, had already suggested that "dreaming is another kind of remembering (Freud, 1918/1955, p. 51).

DOI: 10.4324/9781003300441-7

Incorporation of Awake Experiences in Dreams over Time (Freud, Jouvet, Nielsen, Blagrove, Brugger)

If dreaming is a form of remembering, we might ask the classic memory question, first posed by Ebbinghaus (1885/1984), the father of the experimental study of memory: What is the course of dream-memory for events from the awake-past? Ebbinghaus asked the same question of awake-memories and, on the basis of his experimental work (on himself as the sole subject), produced the negatively accelerated amnesic function depicted in Figure 1.5. This graph is probably the best known figure in experimental psychology, even though Ebbinghaus never actually published the figure but, instead, provided the mathematical function fitting his data points (namely, $M = (100k)/[\log t^c + k]$), where M = % Retained, t = time, and k and c, constants of proportionality).

Short Term Intervals (0—Around 1 Month)

Figure 6.1 reproduces a memory function published by Jouvet (1999), also based on research done on himself, depicting incorporation in dreams of awake experiences as a function of the time elapsed between the dream and the awake experiences. For the moment, let us consider only the left half of the graph (incorporation "latencies" of 0 through 6 days). Visual inspection suggests an Ebbinghaus-like decay function, with day-event incorporation progressively decreasing over time from

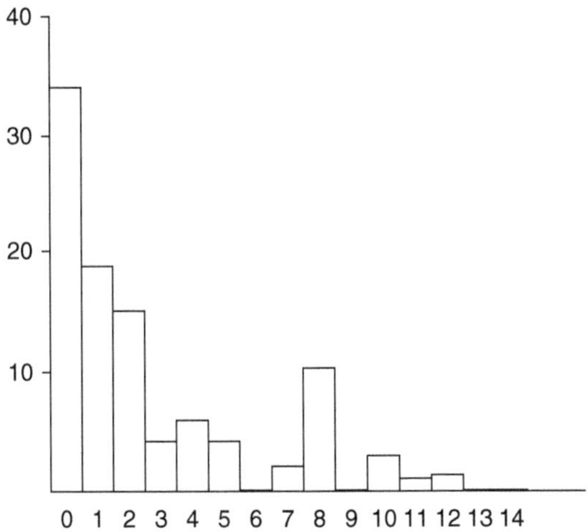

FIGURE 6.1 Dream incorporation of awake experiences as a function of elapsed time (Jouvet, 1999, Figure 12, p. 68).

an initial 34% incorporation rate to zero by week's end. The first day (Latency 0) produces, roughly, Freud's *day-residue effect* (the maximum incorporation rate that ostensibly occurs for events of the day preceding the night dream), which we shall presently consider in more detail.

But first, let us note the surprising uptick of dream incorporation for awake experiences at a latency of 8 days (Day 9 by modern convention; Jouvet treats the day before the dream as Latency 0, and so, to bring Jouvet's "latencies" into alignment with modern practice, we simply add 1 to Jouvet's latencies to get the number of days before the dream—thus, Latency 0 becomes Day 1; Latency 1, Day 2; Latency 2, Day 3; and so on.) We might be tempted to ascribe the upward jump to mere error-of-measurement but, it turns out, other investigators have obtained up-trends in dream-memory at around 7 ± 2 days after the awake-events, which has come to be known as the *dream-lag effect* (after Nielsen and his colleagues (Nielsen & Powell, 1988, 1989, 1992; Nielsen, Kuiken, Alain, Senstrom, & Powell, 2004)). If both the day-residue and the dream-lag effects are real, we have something of a *U-shaped temporal relation* between real-life events and their incorporation into dreams.

The Day-Residue Effect. In *The interpretation of dreams*, Freud proposed, based on his observations of the dreams of his patients and also on some of the extant literature, that "Dreams show a clear preference for the impressions of the immediately preceding day" (p. 163). The observation—often referred to as the "day-residue" effect (after Freud, e.g., 1900/1953, p. 555)—turns out to be roughly correct, as the highest percentage of dream incorporations of awake-events do come from the previous day, but calls for some qualification since often none of the events from the preceding day make an appearance in our dreams of the same night. Freud acknowledged this fact some 20 years later and seems to revise his stance: "[It] would be something if it could be asserted of all dreams without exception ... [that they] are recollections of daily life ... but that is out of the question; this characteristic ... belongs only to a minority of dreams. In most dreams we find no connection with the day before ..." (Freud, 1917/1963, p. 87).

The recency of dream memories turns out not to be an easy question, as the modern literature yields highly variable estimates. Nielsen and Powell (1992) provide a review in which incorporation rates from the preceding day (Day 1) range from 94% (Hartmann, 1968) to 52% (Epstein, 1985) to 34% (Jouvet, 1999) to 22% (Verdone, 1965). Averaging these values, the probability of some event from the day before the dream being incorporated is around 50.5%. There is an Ebbinghausian lilt to the data, as dream incorporations do seem to decline over time.

The Dream-Lag Effect. What can be said about the uptick in day-event incorporations at Day 9 (Jouvet's 8-day latency)? Freud did consider the question "whether the point of contact with the dream is invariably the events of the *immediately* preceding day, or whether it may go back to impressions derived from a rather more extensive period of the most recent past" (p. 166). He was inclined, in *The interpretation of dreams*, to favor the immediately preceding day, although the modern research literature tends to point (inconsistently) to a curvilinear relation (Nielsen, & Powell, 1989; Eichenlaub et al., 2019).

If the U-shaped component of the incorporation function is real, it would suggest the important theoretical conclusion (first advanced by Jouvet (1999)) that the activities of two different memory systems are being indexed, one associated with the day-residue effect and the other with the dream-lag effect. Some dream scientists (Nielsen & Stenstrom, 2005; Stickgold, 2005; Walker 2005) have suggested that the dream-lag effect might be indicating the consolidation of memories from awake-experiences and that, within the first week, memories are undergoing major relocations from the hippocampus to the neocortex (Nielsen & Stenstrom, 2005).

The consolidation hypothesis is provocative but also calls for caution, given the variability of the research data, especially for the dream-lag component of the posited U-shaped function. Eichenlaub, van Rijn, et al. (2019, pp. 6–7) discuss several studies that failed to replicate the dream-lag effect, with possible reasons for these failures. Even the more solid day-residue effect is not always found. Jouvet (1999), whose Figure 6.1 results were used to introduce the dream-residue effect, also reported data he collected on trips away from home in which he repeatedly found no day-residue effects but, instead, delayed incorporations of vacation events starting at around 7–8 days and continuing for about 2–3 weeks. One theoretical explanation provided by Jouvet (1999) is that the temporal course of incorporation interacts with the awake stimuli being recovered (as is the case with regular memory interacting with the stimulus being recalled—see our Chapter 1, pp. 22–26 and, for more comprehensive overviews, Erdelyi (1996, 2010)). Jouvet connected his findings to anecdotes about prisoners' memories: "At the beginning of their detention, prisoners' dreams take place in locations associated with their previous life of freedom, whereas after leaving prison their dreams continue to take place in their cell" (Jouvet, 1999, p. 70). We shall see below (pp. 154–155) that drastic body events, such as an amputation, often are *never* incorporated into dream consciousness.

Ebbinghaus Meets Freud. A profusion of interactions seems to moderate the course of dream-incorporation of awake-experiences over time. The often qualified nature of the results points to the need for more research or for theoretical reorientation (or perhaps both). Since dreams are repeatedly shown to incorporate events from the awake-past, they are forms of remembering. However, it is possible that the Ebbinghaus model of memory smoothly decaying over time is not the best model for dream-memory—or indeed, as soon as we venture past nonsense syllables—for awake memory.

A pertinent point, brought to the foreground by Freud's distinction between *primary-* and *secondary-process* functioning (see p. 41), is that the more primitive primary-process, which characterizes dream cognition more than regular awake-cognition, fails to abide by linear time. If linear time is unreliable in cognitive venues such as dreams, it makes sense that the relation between dream incorporation and time should not be altogether reliable either. The primary- vs. secondary-process distinction, however, involves not a dichotomy but a continuum (Erdelyi, 1985; Fisher, 1956, 1960, 1988; Freud, 1917/1963; Hartmann, 2003, 2011). An examination of the dream samples in Chapter 3 shows that dreams are not as primary-process in nature as often supposed, and are, in fact, substantially secondary-process except for some startling outcroppings (e.g., the sudden appearance of the dead Mozart in Hobson's dream (p. 71)). Thus, we might expect some noise in our dream functions involving time, but not an outright disappearance of temporal regularities.

Further, the associative structure of memory, implied early on by the phenomena of aphasic errors (paraphasias) (pp. 32–40; 181–184) and since then amply corroborated by laboratory work on memory (see pp. 181–184), suggests that we *should* have problems with a simplistic notion of temporal intervals. We encounter many relevant examples in our examinations of dreams. Zelda, a few pages below (pp. 156–158), dreams of her deceased friend, Jean, from *15 years* before but, after some psychological work, discovers the relation between Jean and a Jean-look-alike, with whom her last interaction occurred only *2 weeks* before. She then further remembers that five colleagues, who included Zelda and the Jean-look-alike, had gone out to a Sicilian restaurant *5 years* before her dream where they all ordered an eggplant stew for dinner. Zelda, Jean, and the Jean-look-alike had apparently become parts of a semantic configuration ("semantic network," "neighborhood structure"). If we wished to pin-down the temporal lag between the awake-stimulus "Jean" and the appearance of "Jean" in Zelda's dream, we would be stuck with three possible temporal lags—15 years, 5 years, and 2 weeks. Nonsense syllables, by design, largely eliminate associative structure and avoid such complications, yielding simple amnesic functions. Unfortunately, the simple findings are about nonsense.

Very Long-Term Intervals

No systematic research has been reported on the incorporation of awake experiences in dreams over *very long-term intervals*, although it is obvious from individual dream reports (such as the dreams of Zelda or of Nemiah's patient, Alice V., in Chapter 3, and also the various dreams reported further below) that life-events from the distant past do often emerge in current dream contents. Systematic assays of dream incorporation of different type of awake experiences over very long-term time intervals is indicated.

Incorporation of Drastic Body-Events in Dreams

A small research literature has accumulated on the incorporation of drastic body-events, such as a limb amputation, into dreams. Here too the data are variable.

Mulder, Hochstenbach, Dijkstra and Gareetzen (2008) reported that a large percentage (31%) of long-term amputees fail to adapt their body-image in their dreams to their current awake-reality, even though, on the average, they had been amputees for over 10 years. Alessandria, Vetrugno, Costelli, and Montagnam (2011) actually found *no* dream-incorporation of amputation among their six amputee subjects. It was suggested that the altered body-schema in awake-life was being "suppressed during sleep" (Alessandria et al., 2011, p. 1831)—something we might not have expected from the disinhibited medium of dreams. Even more striking is the finding that congenital paraplegics fail to reflect their paraplegias in their dreams: "Subjects who had never walked or stopped walking 4-64 years prior to this study still experience walking in their dreams . . . . Paraplegics walk, run, dance, swim, drive a car and ride a bike in their dreams" (Saurat, Agbkou, Itagui, Golmard, & Arnulf, 2011, p. 1425). Surat et al. suggest (as did Moulder et al., 2008) the possible existence of a "genetic cerebral walking program" (p. 1425) that controls dream representations of some motor behaviors or, alternately, the possibility that the subjects are reflecting learned schemas arising from the activation of mirror neurons from the observed behaviors of intact others. Obviously, this family of findings pose problems for both the day-residue and the dream-lag effects, constituting one more case where interactions between the stimulus and dream incorporation seem to subvert straightforward main effects.

In a brief but important commentary, Brugger (2008) shows that the broader literature on the incorporation of drastic body-events is quite mixed. For nine studies surveyed, 50% of the amputees showed intact bodies in their dreams, 24% showed mostly amputated bodies, and 14% produced a mixed picture. (The percentages do not add up to 100% because some of the required information was not reported in some of the studies.) These simple counts, however, underestimate subtle incorporations. For example, in a case drawn from Frank and Lorenzoni (1992, p. 77), a 24-year-old man who had lost a leg in an accident at the age of 14, had recurrent dreams around the time he was taking driving lessons. In his dreams, he invariably experienced himself as having both his legs but, also invariably, he would lose control over the car because his foot would mismanage the breaks. So, at one level there was no incorporation of the amputation of his leg but, at another level, there apparently was some incorporation of the amputation. Similarly, Setter (1950), himself a leg amputee, found that a patient's phantom foot pain was "symbolically represented as induced by a rat, which was gnawing at the foot while he was swimming" (in Brugger, p. 5). Also, two women with spinal cord injury studied by Alkadhi et al. (2005) showed anosognosia (denial) of their incapacitation in their dreams while producing signs of "implicit knowledge" (p. 9) of their condition: Both women noted the regular presence of their wheelchair in their dreams but almost always pushed their empty wheelchairs rather than sitting in them.

As to the temporal course of incorporations, Mulder et al. (2008) found that the incorporation of an amputation in the dreams of amputees had a variable course: About one-third of the subjects started to dream of themselves as amputees "more or less immediately," another third took longer times (e.g., 6–12 months or more than a year), and the remaining third (31%) maintained their previous, intact body in their dreams till the end of the study. Obviously, there are significant individual differences. Also, there are age effects, with older amputees being less likely to adjust their dream representations to fit their current anatomical reality. Delayed incorporations are not restricted to grim events like amputations. Brugger (p. 6) cites MacDonald's (1984) finding that it took some 18 months for a newly grown beard to be represented in his dreams.

Hypermnesic Dreams

"No one who occupies himself with dreams can, I believe, fail to discover that it is a very common event for a dream to give evidence of knowledge and memories which the waking subject is unaware of possessing." (Freud, 1900/1953, p. 14)

As noted earlier, Freud (1900/1953, pp. 11–21, 589) specifically suggested that "dreams are hypermnesic," meaning that dreams can reflect enhanced memory for past events that are inaccessible to consciousness. Zelda (see below 156–159), who is a prodigious dreamer, reported that she frequently experienced hypermnesic dreams. Three brief examples from her dream life are presented below (rendered the way she had typed out her experiences).

Zelda's Hypermnesic Dreams (As Reported by Zelda)

The Watch Lost at the Beach and Found in a Dream

This event happened many years ago, when I was a teenager. I had lost my watch somewhere and was repeatedly searching for it throughout the house. It was a simple Timex, but I really liked it a lot and missed having it. After approximately a week or two of not finding it, I had a dream: I dreamt that the watch was sitting at the bottom of a beach bag. When I awoke, I went straight to the beach bag that I had brought home, but not emptied, from my last trip to the beach—and there it was, right under all of my other things at the bottom of the bag. (Zelda, 2016, personal communication)

Cutty Sark

Many years ago, I had the experience of waking one morning with the words "Cutty Sark" on my lips. I had absolutely no idea what those words meant. They haunted me for many weeks. I tried to guess if they were foreign words, or perhaps distortions of other words, but try as I might, I could not figure out their meaning. (This was before the days of the internet, so I did not have the simple recourse of just Googling them.) Then, one day, as I was riding the subway to school, I noticed from the corner of my eye one of the many billboards that lined the elevated train line. Sure enough, there it was: "CUTTY SARK—an ad for a whiskey! Evidently I had been exposed to this billboard as it flitted by my line of vision during one of my previous commutes, but neither the meaning nor the source of these odd words registered in my waking consciousness." (Zelda, 2016, personal communication)

The Ratatouille Dream

This dream occurred approximately 3 years ago (sometime in 2013). I was sitting somewhere (a kitchen?) and talking with my friend, Jean. It was a very casual and nonchalant scene, which is very odd, because Jean has been dead for some 15 years. I was enthusiastically telling her about this fantastic dish I had just had at a restaurant, and I wanted very much for her to try it. I remember being almost able to taste it in my dream. I described it as an eggplant and pasta dish, and I was sure Jeannie would love it! (She was Greek, and she and her mother made many eggplant dishes when I knew her.)

I believe it was at this point that she started telling me in the dream that what I was describing was "ratatouille"—which sounded exotic (French? Greek?), but I did not know the term. I told her I did not know what that was, but that in any event, I wanted her to go to the restaurant with me and try this eggplant dish.

I woke up with the word "ratatouille" on my lips. I still did not know what it was, but I had a general idea that it was some sort of French dish. I looked it up in a cookbook, and discovered that it was, in fact, an eggplant stew. I found it amusing that my dream had "taught me" the name of the dish, but I was perplexed as to why I would be dreaming of Jean at this point in time, and, even more bizarre, that I would be casually discussing food with her. Then, I started to make the following associative connections:

> Approximately 2 weeks prior to this dream, I was attending a professional conference during which I ran into an old colleague. She greeted me warmly and we chatted briefly. I was quite embarrassed because I could not remember her name & I was afraid she would realize that during the encounter. I tried to remember her name but all I could do was make a mental note that she looked quite a bit like my old friend Jean back when I knew her some 15 years ago.

It bothered me that I could not recall this person's name. We had not been that close, but we had crossed paths professionally on many occasions. We had almost never socialized outside of work, but we had been in the same training program years earlier. Since then, we worked in different schools and had no further contact. Then, I recalled the last time I saw her: A group of us from that program decided it would be nice for all of us to get together, so about 5 of us made plans to meet. (This get-together occurred some 5 years before my dream and my meeting of the Jean-look-alike.)

We chose a Sicilian restaurant in the area, and we met there for dinner one evening. None of us really knew each other that well; we had only worked together on occasion, meeting when our paths crossed at professional workshops. What I remember about that evening is that when the waiter took our orders for dinner, it turned out that all five of us had selected the exact same dish: a pasta dish with sautéed eggplant—Sicilian style. The waiter was very amused and tried to encourage us to choose different dishes so that we could share and taste each other's selections. He found it funny that we all wanted the same thing and kept trying to suggest other dishes we should try. But no, we were all very adamant about wanting that particular dish! We all joked about how resolved we were in our dinner selection. Everyone laughed about it and it was a bit of a running joke with the waiter.

Of note is that I did not make these connections to the dream immediately after waking. I thought that it was a bit bizarre that I should be dreaming of my old friend Jean. I could not figure out why she should be on my mind; it was not her birthday or the anniversary of her death. The dream did not have a morbid or sad tone to it. It all seemed so "random." I was pondering the dream for a couple of days before it all came together in my mind, and then, only after retelling the dream out loud. Then I found the whole dream event quite funny. (Zelda, 2016, personal communication)

Commentary on Zelda's Hypermnesic Dreams

The hypermnesic dream about the lost watch is straightforward. We might worry, however, about two methodological issues. The finding of the watch occurred in a dream, but was the dream necessary? Might the memory recovery have taken place anyhow in awake consciousness a week or two later because of protracted retrieval effort? Long-term repeated recall effort over periods of days or weeks does produce memory recoveries (Erdelyi, 1996, 2010; our book, pp. 22–26 and pp. 164–179). We shall return to the subject of long-term awake hypermnesia in the next section of our chapter. The other methodological question, which applies also to the Pötzl Phenomenon reviewed in Chapter 2, is the extent to which chance might account for the outcomes; Zelda might have gotten lucky in finding her watch in her beach bag.

The "CUTTY SARK" dream, for its part, seems to be a real-life instantiation of the Pötzl Phenomenon. It shows that subliminal stimuli can turn up in the content of dreams.

The "ratatouille" dream is more complex than the first two examples but it nicely instantiates the modern distinction in cognitive psychology between *accessible* and *available memories*, which roughly corresponds to the classic *conscious–unconscious* distinction ("accessible" corresponding to conscious, and "available-but-inaccessible" to unconscious). Zelda does not recognize the term "ratatouille" and has to look it up in her cook book upon awakening. Yet, although the information was not accessible, it was obviously available to Zelda since the dead Jean in Zelda's dream produces the term. Also, the colleague whose name Zelda could not remember but who looked like her deceased friend, Jean, apparently primed a dream about Jean which also connected the unanimous menu choice of an eggplant dish to the inaccessible term, "ratatouille."

Hypermnesic Dreams Reported by Freud

Laboratory work on very old memories going back, for example, 15 years, is obviously not practicable. It is therefore useful to note that the phenomenon has been reported by other dreamers than Zelda. We consider here two examples reported by Freud (1900/1953)).

Delboeuf's Fern: Applenium Ruta Muraria

The first case, which has surprising overlaps with Zelda's "Ratatouille Dream," involved the hypermnesic dream of J. Delboeuf (1855, pp. 107 ff). In his dream, Delboeuf saw the courtyard of his house, covered in snow. He found there two buried, half-frozen lizards, which Delboeuf proceeded to rescue by placing them in a warm place and providing them with a few leaves of fern that he knew the lizards liked to eat. A key detail is that in his dream Delboeuf knew the name of the plant—*Applenium Ruta Muralis*—which, however, was quite foreign to his awake-consciousness. Delboeuf did some research and was surprised to be able to confirm the name of the fern, *applenium ruta muraria* (note the slight distortion in the dream's rendering of the plant's name).

Additional relevant materials emerged a long time later. Sixteen years after the dream, Delboeuf visited one of his old-time friends and found an album of pressed flowers with the Latin name of each plant, including *applenium ruta muraria*, written under each plant—in Delboeuf's own handwriting! Although Delboeuf had no conscious recollection of the name of the plant that had returned to him in his dream, there could be no question, thanks to his handwriting, that he had known the name of the fern many years earlier. Freud remarks that "the fact that dreams have at their command memories which are inaccessible to waking life ... is remarkable" (p. 12).

The Recovery of "Kontuszówka" by Freud's Patient

Another hypermnesic dream reported by Freud calls to mind the Pötzl Effect and Zelda's real-life instantiation of it in the puzzling emergence of CUTTY SARK in her consciousness on awakening. Freud's case involved a patient who in a dream found himself ordering a *"Kontuszówka"* in a café. In his recounting of the dream to Freud the patient expressed surprise at the dream because he did not know what a *Kontuszówka* might be, just as Zelda did not know what CUTTY SARK might be. Freud was able to inform his patient that *Kontuszówka* was a Polish liqueur. Some days later, "after making his dream come true" in a café, he noticed the name on a [billboard] at a street corner which he must have gone past at least twice a day for several months" (p.14).

Leading, Lagging, and Concurrent Indicators

The notion of indicators, typically encountered in economics but also in other domains such as subliminal perception research (Goldiamond, 1958), comes into play when some target event of interest is in some sense invisible—because, for example, it is unconscious, because it has happened sometime in the past, or because it has not yet come to pass. Indicators, simply, are measures that correlate with some class of events of interest. Indicators have the terminological advantage of not committing us to a particular temporal orientation (as does "memory" or "remembering," which orient us toward the past). The correlates of indicators can be events from the past but they can also involve events from the present or the future.

We might ask here whether the notion of indicating events from the future constitutes a violation of standard canons of science. If we asked a scientifically rigorous dream researcher whether dreams can foretell the future, we might well get a dismissive rejection of the idea because we could be perceived as veering into the realm of parapsychology (in this case, *precognition*), which remains taboo in mainstream psychological science. There actually exist some sober efforts to evaluate positive evidence for parapsychological effects (e.g., Cardeña, 2018; Child, 1985; Krippner, 2019; Ullman & Krippner, with Vaughan, 2002; Storm, Sherwood, Roe, et al., 2017). Just as modern physics has embraced what Einstein once termed "spooky effects," psychological science may yet change its stance toward some "paranormal" phenomena (in which case, these phenomena will be recast as "normal"), but without taking such a leap at this juncture, we might simply underscore the fact that *there is nothing remotely unscientific about predicting the future*; indeed, prediction is a bedrock feature of the scientific enterprise.

In the social sciences prediction tends to be statistical (not perfect, but probabilistic). Three kinds of indicators are usually considered: (1) *Lagging indicators*, which are statistical assays of the past. Thus, in economics, the current employment rate tends to reflect the level of economic activity that was occurring in the past; (2) *Concurrent indicators*, which reflect economic activity taking place at the present (e.g., personal income); Of special interest to us are (3) *leading indicators*, which predict activity likely to take place in the future. The stock-market, for example, is a leading indicator of future economic activity.

Indicators, which are standard tools in economics, show clearly that there is nothing unscientific about seeking to predict the future in complex systems. Perhaps one of the most important questions for dreams is whether dreams can predict future events of potential significance to the dreamer. Such predictive dreams are sometimes designated *prodromal dreams* (Van De Castle, 1974) or, more dramatically, *prophetic dreams* (Bulkeley, 2018), and have been proposed by classic thinkers—such as Aristotle, Hippocrates, Galen—to foretell future illness (Van De Castle, 1974, p. 364). It helps clarify the subject if we distinguished between events that the subject might successfully predict from conscious knowledge (death and taxes, for instance) or psychological contents that might currently be unconscious (e.g., some aspects of one's feelings for another person or, perhaps, psychological derivatives of some somatic changes) as against fore-knowledge of random future events (e.g., tomorrow's winning lottery number). One type of prediction is obvious, the other, dubious.

Some leading memory and clinical scientists have in recent years begun to emphasize the "prospective" thrust of memory (Seligman, Railton, Baumeister, & Strirade, 2013; Schachter & Addis, 2007). Thus, memory is not only about the past but also about the future, as the past tends to predict the future as well as to guide it. A similar future-orientation is developing in dream science, with notions such as *predictive processing* and the view that the brain is a *Bayesian* or *inference machine* (Friston, 2018; Hobson, Hong, & Friston, 2014; Tuominen, Stenberg, Revonsuo, & Valli (2019).

Lexical Leakage and Its Prediction of Biopsy Outcomes (Donald Spence)

In striking research findings, Donald Spence and his associates (Spence, 1980; Spence, Scarborough, & Ginsberg, 1978) reported that "lexical choice" in women awaiting biopsy results for possible cervical cancer tended to predict later biopsy findings of malignancy *before* either the patient or the physician knew the outcome. The patient's mood (e.g., pessimism-optimism) or conscious appraisal of her situation did not predict the biopsy results. What did (statistically) predict the biopsy outcome were certain words the patient tended to use. The most predictive word, *death*, was usually produced in metaphorical language (e.g., "I was scared to death," "I love them to death," "I almost froze to death" (Spence, 1980, p. 122)).

Gayle Delaney (1990), independently from Spence's research, has suggested that metaphorical language might be an especially effective conduit to mental contents of personal significance. Delaney's work, which is much influenced by Jung's approach to dreams, assumes that we often miss out on important dream information for lack of systematic effort (e.g., *amplification*).

Spence, who came from a psychoanalytic background, proposed a defense hypothesis: "Metaphor provides a particularly useful hiding place for the taboo information" (p. 122) because the explicit meaning of the embedded word is not fully processed consciously. In either case, metaphor is seen as carrying covert meanings that are not immediately accessible to consciousness.

It would be highly desirable to replicate the Spence et al. (1978) findings and to extend the results to dreams. If this line of work pans out and generalizes to dreams, the implications would be basic, both theoretically and practically. It would suggest that we might, more than we suppose, have unconscious information about our developing somatic illnesses and, moreover, that this unconscious information can leak out into consciousness, much as in the Pötzl Effect subliminal stimuli leak out into consciousness in fantasy and dreams (see our Chapter 2). If such leakage into consciousness of illness-related information can be reliably detected (as has the emergence of subliminal stimuli in fantasy and dreams), such leakages would allow potentially life-saving predictions about some future illness, with obvious implications for medical practice.

Dream Correlates of the Ovulation Cycle (Robert Van De Castle)

In a promising but underdeveloped research program, Van De Castle (1971) reported systematic dream content changes in women (50 first-year nursing students) across their menstrual cycle. Menstrual dreams were found to contain more anatomical and room references as well as more babies, children, and mothers. Feelings were also found to vary over the cycle: "During menstruation the dreamer extends more friendliness toward other female characters, although ... males are less friendly with her at this time" (p. 40). During the pre-ovulative phase, however, males are "extremely friendly to the dreamer" (p. 40) while the dreamer is less friendly with other females. Also, the dreamer exhibits "heightened narcissism" during the post-ovulation phase. Thus, systematic somatic changes over time seem to be indicated by systematic changes in dream-content over time. Note that in this case, which involves repeating cycles of changes, any indicator can simultaneously serve as a concurrent, leading, or lagging indicator.

Van De Castle's research calls for replication and extension. It would be useful, for example, to get systematic content measures for each day of the roughly one-month cycle. Further, and this goes for other dream-research programs (see Erdelyi, 2017), it would be essential to collect parallel data on awake mental contents across the ovulation cycle to ascertain whether dreams yield more (or less—or different) information than awake mental samples.

Dreams as Predictors of Psychological Breakdowns

Although, to the author's knowledge, no systematic research has been published on the subject, there is anecdotal evidence that dream content can presage a psychological breakdown. We have already encountered the example of Nemiah's patient, Alice V. (see pp. 69–72), who developed unbearable obsessive thoughts involving her father which she could not suppress, resulting in her eventual hospitalization. The outbreak of the obsessions were presaged by a nightmare from the night before about "animals mating" and a struggling elephant.

Another example of dreams predicting psychological breakdowns is encountered in Freud's (1911) case history, "The Psychotic Dr. Schreber". Dr. Schreber (*juris doctor*) was a brilliant jurist who eventually succumbed to paranoid schizophrenia, which required his hospitalization. It was in the mental hospital that Dr. Schreber wrote his remarkable autobiographical memoir of his mental illness, on which Freud's case-history is based. (Freud never met Dr. Schreber.) After Schreber's prospective appointment as *Senatpräsident* of Dresden, which, he complained burdened him with overwork and stress, he experienced some dreams to which at first he assigned little significance, but which turned out to be premonitory. "He dreamed two or three times that his old nervous disorder had come back (Freud, 1911, p. 108), which it did, and with a vengeance, requiring his hospitalization.

Dreams as Predictors of the Course of an Illness

There is some, although only spare research on the question. For example, dreams collected from hospital patients months before their discharge predicted later deterioration (Smith, 1984, 1986; Van De Castle, 1994, p. 170). Interestingly, the dream themes that were the best predictors were different for males and females. *Death-related* dreams (e.g., graveyards, funerals, wills), predicted health deterioration in males, but *separation dreams* (e.g., disruption of relationships, displacement from one's home) predicted deterioration in females.

Parasomnias as Concurrent Indicators of Dreaming (Arnulf)

One imponderable in dream science is that, typically, we have no real-time access to the dreams of a sleeping subject and so usually can only infer a dream from the awake dreamer's subsequent recollection of the dream (Erdelyi, 2014). Thus, the title of Freud's classic work, *The interpretation of dreams*, should be, strictly speaking, *The interpretation of remembered dreams*. This qualification applies to all other major works on dreams—for example, Domhoff's (2003), *The scientific study of dreams*; Hall and Van De Castle's (1966), *The content analysis of dreams*; Hobson's (1978), *The dreaming brain;* Foulkes's (1978), *A grammar of dreams*.

For Freud, this issue would not have been of much import since he always assumed that dreams, both during and after they occurred, are subject to extensive distortions, and his theory bakes in these distortions. Freud's crucial findings, which focus on latent contents, would hold even if they were based only on the memory of the original event, whatever that event might have been.

Quantitative content-analysts, who try to establish correct counts of dream contents, do worry about the problem, since memory introduces not only forgetting but also a variety of distortions which would affect accurate counts of dream contents. It is sometimes suggested that laboratory dreams should be elicited as soon as possible after awaking from REM sleep to minimize the depredations of memory. Memory, however, is not always methodologically obliging, for, as we have seen, memory is not only amnesic but also hypermenesic over time. (One gifted dreamer, DMZ, has claimed to the author that if she keeps still on awakening and briefly reviews her dream, she is likely to remember significantly more dream material as she further ponders the dream in the course of the day. She has also found that important dream contents often return when she narrates her dream aloud.)

The quantum theorist, Fred Alan Wolf (1995), has a quite different take on the problem, challenging the very notion that dreams actually exists. Just as certain sub-atomic outcomes in quantum physics cannot be known before the "collapse of the wave function" that occurs with observation, the dream is only realized on awakening and not during sleep. According to Wolf: "All I have to verify my report is my memory of the dream . . . . Perhaps my report was made up at the instant I awoke, and in that state of awareness, I made up the whole thing" (p. 300). Thus, "there is no such thing as a dream!" (p. 298). Similar doubts have been voiced by prominent philosophers such as Jean Paul Sartre, Daniel C. Dennett, Norman Malcom, and Ludwig Wittgenstein.

Modern research, however, is beginning to refute such doubts about the substantive reality of dreams. The relevant data are being supplied by dream *parasominas,* which are "sleep disorders that involve abnormal movements, behaviors, emotions,

[and] perceptions" (Arnulf, 2019, pp. 238–249). We cannot elicit narrative reports of ongoing dreams but parasomnias can give us substantial clues. According to Arnulf:

> NREM and REM parasomnias constitute exceptional, direct window into the dreaming process. Because there is often an isomorphism between the observed behaviors and the dream content reported upon awakening, many parasomniac behaviors can be considered materialized indications of what is going on in the dream.
>
> *(Arnulf, 2019, p. 238)*

Sleep-talking is an interesting case in point, since in some sense it does provide a verbal record of the ongoing dream (see also, Domhoff, 2018, p. 8). Although about half of sleep-talking is unintelligible, the other half is understandable and even correct grammatically (Arnulf, 2019, p. 244). Some dream-talkers "exhibit turn taking, as if having a conversation" (Arnulf, 2019, p. 244). As with dream reports, in which a preponderance of the content is negative, the content of sleep talking is likewise negative and conflictual, involving a "high frequency of negations, exclamations, questions, and profanities" (p. 244), with swearing predominating during NREM sleep and insults and condemnations in REM sleep. "The observed vocalizations or behaviors during RBD often correlate with simultaneously occurring dream mentation, leading the patients to report that 'they are acting out their dreams'" (Arnulf, 2019, p. 246).

Not only are RBD (REM Behavior Disorder) parasomnias concurrent indicators of dream mentation but they are also leading indicators of brain pathology since some 92% of patients suffering from RBD develop Parkinson's Disease or Lewy Body Dementia in 10 years (on the average) after the initial RBD diagnosis (Arnulf, 2019, p. 246). Thus, while dream content is usually "off-line," both NREM and REM parasomnias suggest that mentation—dreaming—is occurring in real-time and is not an instant creation of awakened-consciousness.

Amnesia and Hypermnesia for "The War of the Ghosts" over Intervals of Weeks and Months: Quantitative and Qualitative Analyses (Matthew Erdelyi, Michael Halberstam, Merryl Feigen-Pfau, Joyce Finks)

In this section, we examine long-distance memory (spanning weeks and months) for a dream-like story, "The War of the Ghosts" (WOG), introduced into laboratory psychology by Sir Frederick Bartlett (1932). The 334 word-long American-Indian story (see Box 6.1) is very strange, even dream-like (it may actually have been a cautionary tale about telling one's dreams to others) and was originally used with Cambridge University students whose mental *schemas* (habits of thought, expectations, world view) were not likely to mesh with the alien story. This mismatch was an intentional feature, for Bartlett wished to demonstrate that memory is not a passive receptacle of past events but, instead, an active, creative construction shaped by our schemas.

BOX 6.1 "THE WAR OF THE GHOSTS" (WOG)

One night two young men from Egulac went down to the river to hunt seals, and while they were there it became foggy and calm. Then they heard war-cries, and they thought: "Maybe this a war-party." They escaped to the shore, and hid behind a log. Now canoes came up, and they heard the noise of paddles, and saw one canoe coming up to them. There were five men in the canoe, and they said: "What do you think? We wish to take you along. We are going up the river to make war on the people." One of the young men said: "I have no arrows" Arrows are in the canoe," they said. "I will not go along. I might be killed. My relatives do not know where I have gone. But you," he said turning to the other, "may go with them." So one of the young men went, but the other returned home. And the warriors went on up the river to a town on the other side of Kalama. The people came down to the water, and they began to fight, and many were killed. But presently the young man heard one of the warriors say: "Quick, let us go home: that Indian has been hit." Now he thought "Oh, they are ghosts." He did not feel sick, but they said he had been hit. So the canoes went back to Egulac and the young man went ashore to his house, and made a fire. And he told everybody and said: "Behold I accompanied the ghosts, and we went to fight. Many of our fellows were killed, and many of those who attacked us were killed. They said I was hit, and I did not feel sick." He told it all, and then he became quiet. When the sun rose he fell down. Something black came out of his mouth. His face became contorted. The people jumped up and cried. He was dead.

(Bartlett, 1932, p. 65)

Nine subjects, mostly college students but also a college professor and a nine-and-a-half-year-old girl, were tested individually over a period of some 3 months. After reading the story two times, a final written recall, designated R_1, was elicited, after which the subjects were dismissed. Without forewarning, the subjects were invited back to the laboratory about 10–12 weeks later. On their return to the lab, each (individually tested) subject was asked to produce three consecutive recall efforts, R_2, R_3, and R_4, and was then sent home for about a week of self-testing on the story, several times a day. (Note, the subjects never saw the story after the original two readings and did not review any of their recall productions, each of which, on completion, was placed in a coded envelope and sealed; for details, see Erdelyi, 1996, Chapter 6.) The subjects returned to the lab with their packet of sealed envelopes containing their at-home recalls and were then administered three final recall tests. Since the subjects did not produce the same number of recalls over the week of self-testing, the last three recall tests are designated generically as, R_{n-2}, R_{n-1}, R_n.

Each narrative recall was scored *subjectively* for fidelity to the story as well as *objectively* by word-counts of correspondences between recall texts and the story. To our surprise, since we worried that mere word-counts would miss the narrative thread of the story, the subjective scores and the objective word-counts turned out to be highly correlated ($r > 0.90$) and so the objective word-counts were used as indices of story recall. Figure 6.2 shows the number of story words recalled in each recall trial. It is readily seen that recall substantially declined from an initial 209.25 words recalled to only 87.08 words after an interval of around 10–12 weeks. Of interest, however, is the memory increase over the next week of repeated recall effort, from 87.08 to 113.74 words. This increase (of around 31%) was statistically significant (of the 9 subjects tested, 8 of the 9 produced increase in memory after repeated testing following the 10–12 weeks' fallow interval, which by a simple sign-test yields $p = 0.02$).

The study proves that even after substantial amnesia for the story, much story information remains in memory, some of which can be accessed with repeated recall over time. The data do not impose a limit on how much additional unconscious memory can be recovered, as still further testing might well yield additional hypermnesia.

As noted, one of the subjects was a nine-and-a-half-year-old girl (named Karina). She was used as a subject because of her high verbal competence, good memory, and her interest in the study. Her initial recall, R_1, was, impressive—actually, better than the average adult subject's—but twelve weeks later her memory of the story had collapsed and could be seen at a glance to be worse than that of any of the adult subjects. Karina's recall had deteriorated so much after twelve weeks that the surprised members of our laboratory wondered whether, with the passage of a little more time, Karina's recall might actually deteriorate to chance-levels. Michael Halberstam and the author decided to address the question by testing Karina 6 months after her last recall trial. Additionally, since we were doing more testing, Merryl Feigin-Pfau undertook the parallel multiple-recall testing of a new subject, Maya, Karina's younger sister, who was at the time six-and-a-half years old.

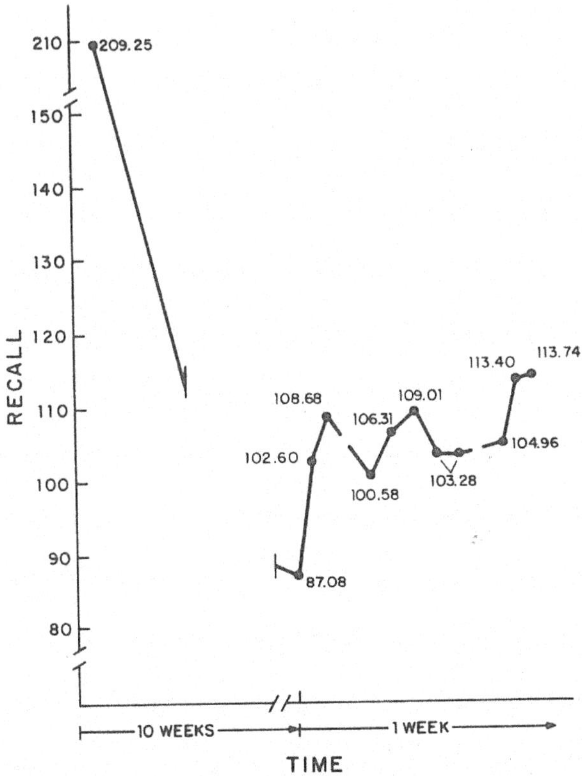

FIGURE 6.2 Average number of words recalled from "The War of the Ghosts" by the nine subjects over some dozen weeks, with repeated recall effort in the last week. (Erdelyi, 1996, p. 158) [© 1996 by the University of Chicago. Reprinted with permission from the University of Chicago Press.]

Quantitative and Qualitative Analysis of Karina's and Maya's Repeated Recalls

Even though it does not directly deal with dream memory, this work on the long-distance repeated recall efforts of the two little girls is relevant to us for several reasons. First, we shall see how *both qualitative and quantitative analysis* can provide unique but complementary information in the extraction of meanings from complex texts. The quantitative analysis demonstrates clearly—and objectively—that memory increases (hypermnesia) can occur over very long-term time intervals and after previous recall efforts seem to have exhausted accessible memory. There is more memory there than we might suppose, a fact that provides a memory foundation for reports of very long-term dream hypermnesias (see pp. 156–159).

The qualitative analysis, for its part, demonstrates that standard—perhaps universal—distortions invariably overtake even focused recall efforts, let alone dreams. These approximately dozen-and-a-half types of distortions—e.g., *omissions, elaborations, rationalizations, displacements, condensations, symbolizations* (discussed in more detail in our next section)—reveal how both Bartlett's and Freud's distortions are the same but for motive, potentially yielding a grand unification of two dissociated psychological traditions. These standard distortions also point to a necessary qualification of Freud's "dream-work" notion (see pp. 41–47; 179–181), which involves not so much "work" as relative *absence of work*.

Finally, the long-distance multiple recalls of Karina and Maya illustrate the need to consider not just *recalls* (hits) but also *false-recalls* (false-alarms, or false memories), which invariably accompany true recalls in memory and perception. This *unavoidable* comingling of "hits" and "false-alarms" in perception and memory reports has been treated in psychophysics for more than half a century under the aegis of "Signal Detection Theory" (SDT) (see, Green & Swets, 1966; Macmillan & Creelman, 1991; McNicol, 1972; Swets, 1964; Swets, Tanner, & Birdsall, 1961) but has not yet informed dream research. A new SDT-inspired technique ("Criterion-Controlled Free Recall," or CCFR) for dealing with *narrative recall*—SDT thus far has been almost completely restricted to *recognition memory*—was introduced by the author and his colleagues some years ago (Erdelyi, 1996) and is detailed in our APPENDIX. A special feature of the CCFR is that it can be applied retroactively to narrative materials that have already been collected (or published).

Quantitative Analysis. Before we focus on some of the qualitative aspects of the recalls, let us first consider the yield of the quantitative analyses of the little girls' productions. Karina's very long-term recall efforts are depicted in Figure 6.3. The leftmost section shows her performance after a first and second reading of the story.

The 82 | 47 designates 82 hits with 47 false-alarms and, likewise, 123 | 73 designates 123 hits with 73 false-alarms. The story was never shown again to Karina after the second reading and her recall after this second reading (123 | 73) is treated as R_1.

Karina appears to have remembered the story better after two passes (her hits increased from 82 to 123), although we might wonder whether we can consider recall improved if false-recalls also increased (from 47 to 73). This precisely is the problem which the CCFR technique was designed to resolve.

Before we apply the CCFR, let us first focus just on the hits obtained in each recall trial. After the passage of three months, Karina's hits precipitously dropped—from 123 to 39—and, unlike eight similarly tested adult subjects, failed to produce hypermnesia in the ensuing one week of repeated testing ($R_2 = 39$, $R_3 = 33$, $R_4 = 25$ ... $R_{n\text{-}2} = 25$, $R_{n-1} = 24$, $R_n = 23$). Since hypermnesia for effective stimuli is almost always obtained with multiple recall testing—all the eight similarly treated adult subjects produced it—Karina's failure to generate hypermnesia was a surprise.

Another surprise was the collapse of Karina's memory after the passage of 3 months. Although the adults' recalls also declined significantly after this interval, Karina's loss of memory was far more pronounced, which prompted the author and

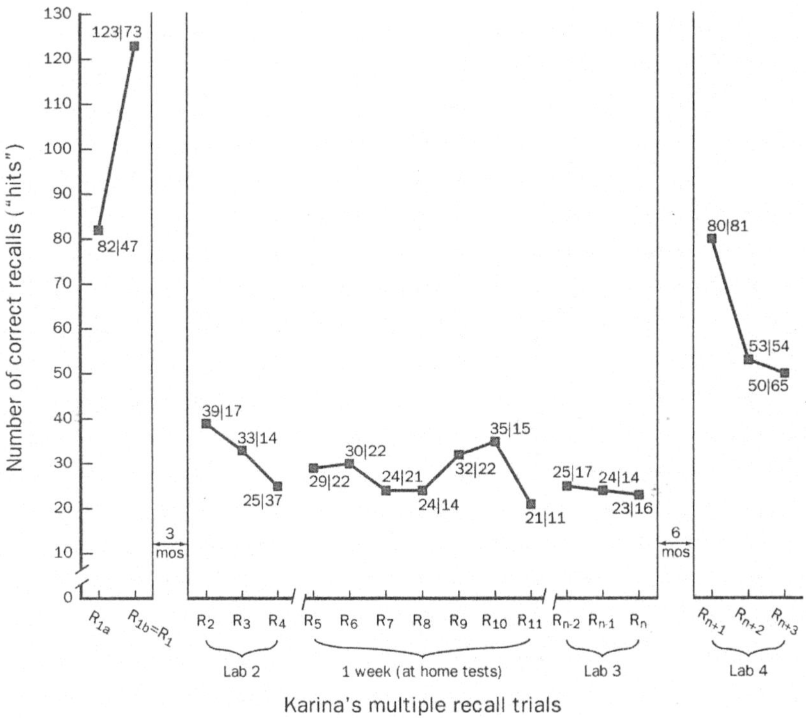

FIGURE 6.3 Karina's successive recalls, with the last three, R_{n+1}, R_{n+2}, and R_{n+3}, occurring some 9 months after last exposure to the story, "The War of the Ghosts." (Erdelyi, 1996, p. 170) [© 1996 by the University of Chicago. Reprinted with permission from the University of Chicago Press.]

his honor student, Michael Halberstam, to retest Karina six months after her last recall trial, R_n, to determine if her recall might deteriorate to chance levels (complete amnesia).

An exciting aspect of doing experimental work is that the experimenter can, on occasion, obtain quite unexpected outcomes. In this case, instead of getting further forgetting, let alone complete amnesia after the additional 6 months' interval, we were astonished to find that Karina's recall had jumped up dramatically, from 23 hits (R_n = 23 | 16) to 80 hits (R_{n+1} = 80 | 81). The reader might now appreciate the methodological need for dealing with false alarms, for it might be fairly wondered whether 80 hits with 81 false alarms is really superior to 23 hits with 16 false alarms.

If we could somehow equalize false-alarm levels for each trial then hit levels would unambiguously index relative memory level for each trial. This precisely is what CCFR technique accomplishes. Our APPENDIX spells out the rationale and details of the simple procedure. In the present study, each trial's recall score was adjusted to a preset false-alarm level of 10 (F = 10).

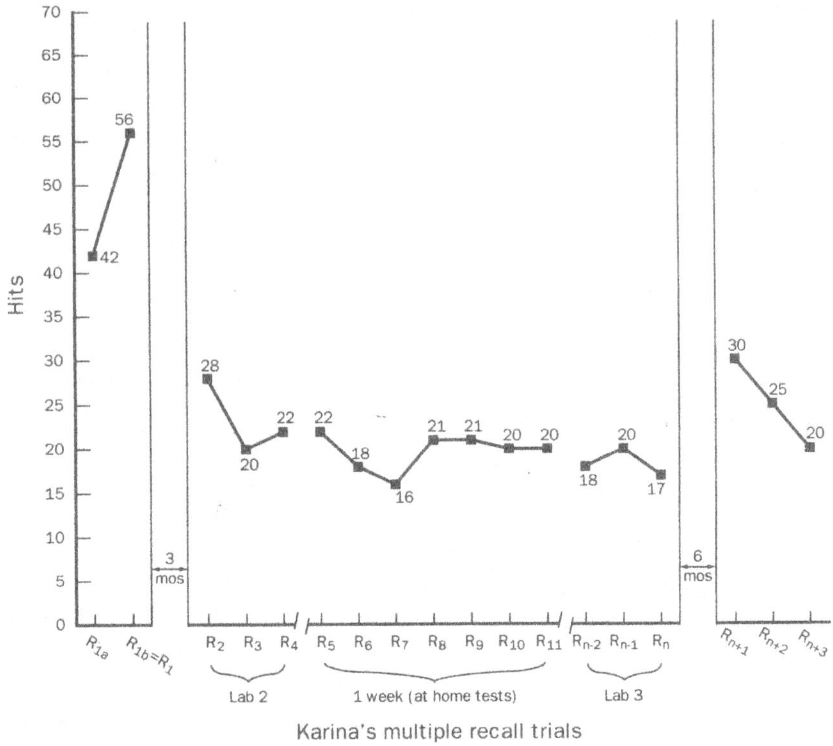

FIGURE 6.4 Karina's repeated recalls corresponding to Figure 6.3, with criterion control such that all hits are conditionalized on a fixed false-alarm level of 10 ($H|(F = 10)$. Erdelyi (1996, p. 175). [© 1996 by the University of Chicago. Reprinted with permission from the University of Chicago Press.]

Karina's criterion-controlled free recalls across all trials are shown in Figure 6.4. Since, all the recall trials were conditionalization on a false-recall level of 10, the false-recall level need not be repeated from trial to trial, as each trial is now associated with the same preset false-recall level ($F = 10$). Thus, the jump from $R_n = 17$ to $R_{n+1} = 30$, reflects a dramatic increase in recall over 6 months, as both of these hit levels are now associated with the same false-alarm level. In Karina's case, the criterion-controlled free recall seems to have produced essentially the same pattern across the 9 months of testing as the raw, uncontrolled recalls: There is learning during the learning trials ($R_{1a} = 42$, $R_{1b} = 56$), an amnesic decline with repeated testing for a week after the 3-month hiatus, from R_2 (=28) to R_n (=17), and then, an upward jump in recall 6 months later ($R_n = 17$ to $R_{n+1} = 30$).

Figure 6.5 summarizes Maya's repeated recall performance. She was treated essentially the same as her sister, Karina, but instead of reading the story, had it read to her and, instead of writing out her recalls, recited them into a tape-recorder. Also, the time intervals were shorter than Karina's (6 weeks instead of 3 months for the first hiatus, 3 days instead of a week for laboratory testing, and 3 months

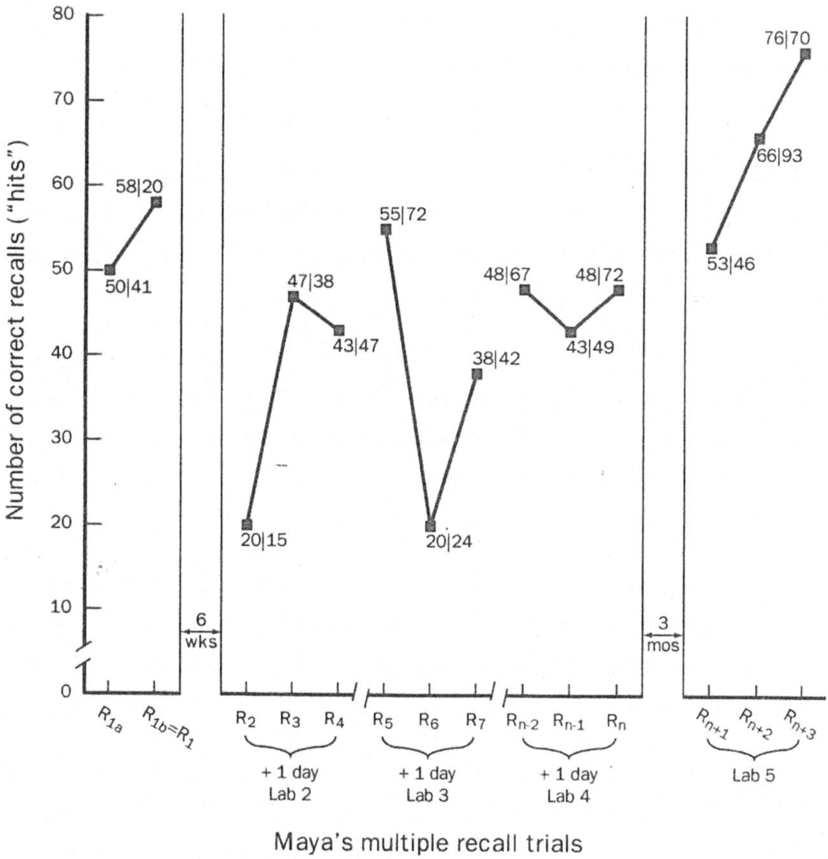

FIGURE 6.5 Maya's repeated recalls, with the last three, R_{n+1}, R_{n+2}, and R_{n+3}, occurring three months after the lab trials and four-and-a-half months after the last exposure to the story. (Erdelyi, 1996, p. 171). [©1996 by the University of Chicago. Reprinted with permission from the University of Chicago Press.]

instead of 6 months for the second hiatus). Her recall scores were quite variable but, unlike Karina, Maya did produce a hypermnesic recall pattern, improving from $R_2 = 20 \mid 15$ to $R_n = 48 \mid 72$. After a 3-month quiet interval, Maya's last three trials also show an upward swing: from $R_n = 48 \mid 72$ to, 3 months later, $R_{n+1} = 53 \mid 46$ to $R_{n+2} = 66 \mid 93$ to $R_{n+3} = 76 \mid 70$.

Maya's recalls were corrected for criterion effects with the CCFR and were also conditionalized on a false-recall level of 10 ($F = 10$). These criterion-controlled recalls produced a smoother pattern—see Figure 6.6—which nevertheless preserved the hypermnesic trend over the three laboratory days—from $R_2 = 15$ to $R_n = 21$. Moreover, there was also a marked upward jump after the quiet interval of 3 months (from $R_n = 21$ to $R_{n+1} = 29$). In this case, unlike in Karina's, the CCFR does change part of the repeated-recall pattern, eliminating the upward surge in Maya's last lab session (for the criterion controlled recalls, $R_{n+1} = 29$, $R_{n+2} = 28$, $R_{n+3} = 29$). Over

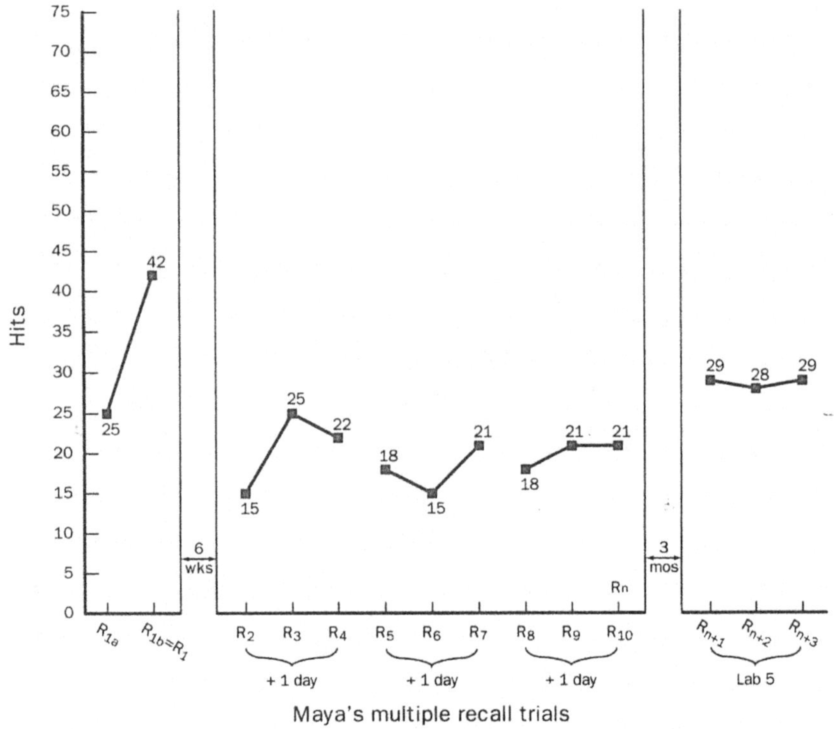

FIGURE 6.6 Maya's criterion-controlled free recalls, with the last three, R_{n+1}, R_{n+2}, and R_{n+3}, occurring three months after the lab trials and four-and-a-half months after the last exposure to the story. Erdelyi (1996, p. 176). [© 1996 by the University of Chicago. Reprinted with permission from the University of Chicago Press.]

all the delayed recall trials (from R_2 to R_n to R_{n+3}) Maya did produce a marked hypermnesic pattern ($R_2 = 15$, $R_n = 21$, $R_{n+3} = 29$).

In future research, it may well be asked whether, and to what extent, further recall efforts over additional time intervals might yield more recoveries of inaccessible memories. What is clearly established by now is that more information is available to the subject than is accessible to consciousness even after periods of weeks and months. It may be surmised that these long-term available-but-inaccessible memories—that is, unconscious memories—are drawn upon in dreams.

Qualitative Analysis. Let us now turn to some of the qualitative aspects of the data. Karina's first recall, R_1, is reproduced in Box 6.2 (without any corrections of grammar, spelling, or punctuation). It appears to be an impressively faithful rendition of the story, with the first few lines sometimes described by students as "photographic memory." However, even the first line of Karina's recall features standard distortions such as found by Bartlett in his Cambridge students' recalls.

BOX 6.2 KARINA'S FIRST RECALL (R_1) OF THE "WAR OF THE GHOSTS" (AS WRITTEN BY KARINA, INCLUDING ERRORS)

Karina's R_1

One day two young men went down to the river to hunt for seals. Suddenly they heard war cries. They heard the sound of paddles splashing in the water. The young men thought this was a war party and hid themselves behind a log. Soon they saw a canoe coming towards them. There was five Indians in the canoe, One of them asked the young men "What do you think?" Will you join us? We are going to war on the people. One of the young men said "I have no arrows"! The Indian replied "we have arrows in the canoe". Then one of the young men said, "I cannot go for my family does not know where I am; but you can go". Soon they departed one to war and one to his family. The soon arrived at a village further south than Kalama. The villager soon came to the waterfront and started a battle. Many people from both sides died. Soon the young man heard an Indian warrior say, "We better leave that man got hit", So they left for Egulac. The young man then went home and lit a fire and told his story when he was done he sat there to sunrise and then fell down. Something black came out of his mouth. His face was twisted. He was dead (Erdelyi 1990, 23)

(from Erdelyi, 1996, p.160) [© 1996 by the University of Chicago. Reprinted with permission from the University of Chicago Press.]

Karina's first recall starts (see Line 1), "*One day*," when the actual story begins, One night. Karina is a city girl, knows nothing about hunting seals, and apparently assumes that a day's work is sensibly done during the day. She continues, "*two young men went down*," omitting from Egulac. She imposes her speech habits by writing, "*to hunt for seals*," when the story does not include "for." As noted earlier, Karina's subsequent recalls were produced three months after R_1 (see Figure 6.3) and 13 successive recalls were elicited over a period of a week.

Box 6.3 reproduces Karina's R_2 and R_4 (produced 12 weeks after R_1) and R_n, produced at the end of the one-week period, that is, 13 weeks after R_1. Some obvious distortions may be noted: The two young men went "fishing," an activity with which she is more familiar than hunting seals. The warriors are described as "Soiix Indians," when no specific Indian group is designated in the story.

BOX 6.3 SOME OF KARINA'S RECALLS OF "THE WAR OF THE GHOSTS" AFTER A 12-WEEK INTERVAL

Karina's R_2 (some 12 weeks after R_1)

Two men went fishing. They saw some Soiixx Indians. The were not on the warpath. There were canoes full of Indians. One of the canoes came near the log where they were hiding. It was a very mossy log. The canoe that went by them didn't see them. This all happened out in the woods. The two men were fishing in a lake.

Karina's R_4

One day two men went fishing. They went to a lake in the forest. When they were in the middle of fishing some Souixx Indians on the warpath came along. The two men hid from the Indians behind an old mossy log. There were canoes full of Indians. One of these canoes went by the old, mossy log were the two men were hiding. But the Indians did not see the two men.

Karina's R_n

One day two men went fishing. While in the middle of fishing some Souixx Indians on the warpath came along. The two frightened men hid behind an old mossy log. One of the canoes went past the log but the Indians didn't see the two men.

(Erdelyi, 1996, p. 161) [© 1996 by the University of Chicago. Reprinted with permission from the University of Chicago Press.]

Some of the distortions in Karina's recalls appear to be defensive. She never mentions the title of the story, which contains "war." In R_1, the warriors in the canoe *didn't* see the two young men (*negation*). Also, the warriors in the canoe are described as "not on the warpath (negation, again). The two young Indians are "fishing," a less violent concept than "hunting" (*mitigation*).

There is some affective modulation across the recall trials. In R_2 the warriors are *not* on the warpath but by R_4 the Indians *are* on the warpath (Line 2). The rest of the recall trial, however, turns up nothing new. A week later, in her last recall of the series (R_n), Karina notes that the two young men were "frightened" (Line 2) but adds nothing to the narrative. In general, a cursory glance at the recall series, from R_1 to R_n, shows what the objective quantitative analysis showed: There was a drastic memory decline over 3 months (from R_1 to R_2) and, uncharacteristically, no hypermnesia (actually, amnesia) from R_2 to R_n.

After the passage of a very long time interval, 6 months, Karina was tested for a last three times for recall of the story (R_{n+1}, R_{n+2}, and R_{n+3}). Her last three recalls are reproduced in Box 6.4. Cursory inspection shows, as did the objective quantitative analysis, a dramatic jump in memory from R_n to R_{n+1}, 6 months later. This is not an Ebbinghausian result. Not only is Karina's recall hypermnesic after 6 months but it also shows that many of the memory recoveries are distorted versions of the story. In the original story, the warriors not only see the two frightened young men but challenge them with an invitation: "What do you think? We wish to take you along. We are going up the river to make war on the people" (Lines 6–8). In Karina's R_{n+1} rendition, "*the indian chief said, do any of you want to join the trib[e]*" (Lines 3–4), apparently a scary notion to Karina. In Karina's recall, the prudent young man, who refused to go along, sets out, in a successful version of the Orpheus legend, to rescue his lost friend and return him to his family.

BOX 6.4 KARINA'S LAST THREE REPEATED RECALLS AFTER THE PASSAGE OF 6 MONTHS

Karina's R_{n+1} (some 9 months after R_1)

There were two men and they went fishing one day. They went to a pond. They caught some fish, then an indian war canoe came and both men hid behind an old rotting moldy log. The indian chief said, "do any of you want to join the trib." Then one man got up and said yes it was, it was his friend. But the other man knew that he had children and a wife and they would be heartbroken if he left them. The other man seemed out of his mind his friend thought. Then he went to his friends home and told them what happened. The wife and the children were very heartbroken. Then his friend said, "I'll go join the indian chief and try to get your husband back the friend", said. So the friend went back to the pond where he had been fishing recently and found the indian chief still there and joined the tribe. He found his friend and told him and then he decided he would miss his wife so he went with his friend and lived quite happily ever on and erased this from memory.

Karina's R_{n+2}

There were two men who went fishing one day at the swamp. Then suddenly and Indian war canoe came down the stream of the swamp. The two men hid behind an old rotting log for they were scared. The chief asked if anyone wanted to join his tribe knowing people were there because they were always there. One of the two men said yes. But the other man persued him out of it saying that he would break his wifes and childrens hearts so the man didn't go. His friend the husbands story and told them never to mention it (the story) to him. So they his family did theat, and the family lived happily ever after and never mentioned it again. The End.

Karina's R_{n+3}

One day two peasant farmers went fishing in a swamp. They had caught a couple of fish. Then suddenly an indian war canoe came. The two men hid behind an old rotting moldy log. The chief knowing people were there asked if anyone wanted to join his tribe. One of the men was about to say yes but his friend peursued him not too by telling him how heartbroken his wife and children would be if he joined the tribe. The friend told the family and told them not to mention the incident again to him, so they never did and they lived happily ever after and never mentioned the incident again to him scared he might actually leave them and they would all be heartbroken. They all live *happily* ever after.

The End.

(Erdelyi, 1996, pp. 162–163.) [© 1996 by the University of Chicago. Reprinted with permission from the University of Chicago Press.]

Contrary to the original "War of the Ghosts story," Karina's rendition has a happy ending, with a hint of repression: "... and [they] lived quite happily ever on and erased this from memory" (R_{n+1}, Lines 13–14). Karina's last two recalls of the story (R_{n+2} and R_{n+3}) are similar, also ending on a positive, avoidant note: "and the family lived happily ever after and never mentioned it again. The End." (R_{n+2}, Lines 8–9).

The *undoing* of the dreaded outcome is reminiscent of the reconstructive revisions in the classic *Little Red Riding Hood* story over centuries—from the savage oral tradition, for example, "The Grandmother Tale," to Charles Perrault's [1697] more civilized though still fatal "Little Red Riding Hood," to the Brothers Grimm version [1812], in which the devoured grandmother and *Little Red Cap* are rescued by the hunter from the stomach of the "wicked" wolf.

The repeated recalls of Karina's younger sister, Maya, also illustrate the characteristic distortions uncovered by Bartlett—and by Freud, some decades earlier. Maya's R_2—see Box 6.5—produced 6 weeks after her R_1, suggests virtually no remaining recall of the story. Perhaps the one hint of recall is: "*they heard a crowd scream*" (Maya R_2, Line 1), presumably a distorted rendition of the story's, "Then they heard war-cries."

BOX 6.5 SOME OF MAYA'S RECALLS OF "THE WAR OF THE GHOSTS" (AS VERBALLY REPORTED BY MAYA, INCLUDING ERRORS)

Maya's R_1 (after two presentations of the story)

The War of the Ghosts

One night some men going hunting to hunt seals. While they were hunting they heard someone screaming for help. It was the Indians fighting with the young men. One of the Indians was shot. He did not know that he got shot. He told everything to the men. He said the people thought I got shot. Then the man was quiet. He went outside. He tripped over a rock. Something black from his mouth came out. He died. Everybody jumped up and cried.

Maya's R_2 (six weeks after R_1)

One night some men were walking. They heard a crowd scream. The men heard them screaming. They rushed and tried to find where the people were screaming. At last, they found them. They were on top of the highest hill.

Maya's R_{n+2}, 3 months after R_n and 4 ½ months after R_1)

One night three men wanted to go on a boat. So they did and they went through the woods to a short cut on the lake. Then they heard something. They tried to see what it was. They looked around. Then two of the men saw Indians coming with lots of feathers and very red skin. And they had very long, black, black hair. They had instruments in their hands and they made lots of noise in the forest. The three men did not like the noise and neither did the animals. The Indians were having a great big celebration party because it was the chief's birthday. They stayed all night until three o'clock in the morning. So the men slept far away from the Indians because they were making so much noise that they could hear them in the house. And so they walked a long way. They almost were in the country of New Jersey. They knew there was a big lake in the country so they went to the lake because they knew they could not hear the Indians and they were very happy.

Maya's R_{n+3}

One night three men were walking and they decided to go to the woods. They heard Indians coming and they ducked down because they were shooting things and they did not want to get hurt. So when they ducked down the Indians were not shooting. They were really having a big celebration. But they did not like the white people because their skin was a different color than theirs. Then they went back home to get something to eat. They went back outside to the woods and set down on a bench to eat. One of the Indians shot an arrow and the arrow got on one of the man's hats but did not get on his head. So the man took the hat off and took out the arrow and put the arrow on a tree. So the man walked back to the bench to finish eating and soon they went back home to throw the napkins away. But the Indians started to make lots of noise and so the three men went someplace quiet.

(Erdelyi, 1996, pp. 165–168) [© 1996 by the University of Chicago. Reprinted with permission from the University of Chicago Press.]

Maya's recalls are often dream-like. After her deeply amnesic performance on R_2, she produces, three months after R_{n+1}, R_{n+2}, R_{n+3}, substantial recoveries of the story, even though her recalls are often wildly confabulatory (see Box 6.5). Some of the story recoveries are straightforward and accurate, for example, "*noise*" (R_{n+2}, Line 6), "*went back*" (R_{n+3}, Line 6), "*quiet*" (R_{n+3}, Line 14). Other responses are distorted renditions of story elements. Thus, the story's "Maybe this is a war party" (Line 3) is construed by Maya in R_{n+2} as, "*The Indians were having a great big celebration party because it was the chief's birthday*" (Lines 7–8). In a *rationalization* (Bartlett, Freud) as ingenious as any of the Cambridge students', Maya both recovers and resolves the story's paradoxical, "He did not feel sick, but they said he had been shot" (WOG, Lines 15–16) ... "They said I was hit, and I didn't feel sick" (WOG, Line 20). Maya's solution: "*One of the Indians shot an arrow and the arrow got on one of the man's hats but did not get on his head.*" She adds the *displacement*, "*So the man took the hat off and took out the arrow and put the arrow on a tree*" (R_{n+3}, Lines 8–10).

Karina and Maya produced all the distortions of Bartlett's Cambridge students, and with a vengeance; in their childish way, their distortions were more flagrant, whimsical, and dream-like. Although Karina and Maya constitute only two subjects, there can be little doubt that the basic long-term hypermnesic outcomes are reliable. As noted before, Karina was only one subject among eight adults to be multiply tested for a week after a hiatus of 3 months, and all eight adult subjects produced hypermnesia after the fallow 3 months' interval. Although, surprisingly, Karina did not produce hypermnesia in the one week of testing after the 3-month hiatus, she did achieve a dramatic improvement in recall after the additional 6 months' interval, jumping from $R_n = 23$ to $R_{n+1} = 80$ correct recalls, for an improvement of 350%. (The criterion-controlled recalls produced a smaller but still hefty jump, from 17 hits to 30 hits.) At a later date, Joyce Finks, from our laboratory, was able to obtain similar hypemnesic outcomes with two children although a third child failed to produce long-term hypermnesia.

Merryl Feigin-Pfau, who had done the testing of Maya, also explored the question, which may be a key issue for dream memory, whether the emotionality of the stimulus might be crucial for hypermnesia. We prepared an alternate version of the "The War of the Ghosts" story, "The Sport of the Ghosts," which transposed the original into a sporting event. This alternate story, which retained a lot of the action but shed the scary elements of the original, also produced hypermnesia with multiple testing in a single laboratory session. Thus, story emotionality does not seem to be crucial for hypermnesia. Another story, however, "The Stone on the Road," which we found very boring, produced no hypermnesia. Apparently, nonsense syllables or boring narratives tend not to yield hypermnesia.

The author (Erdelyi, 1996) delved into the question, not so easy to answer simply, what is the effective stimulus for hypermnesia? Certainly, pictures almost invariably yield hypermnesia but, then, so do words that have been mentally transformed into images. Also, poetry and (interesting) stories reliably produce hypermnesia. To make things more complicated, Ballard (1913), in his classic experimental program, found that the meaning of Latin nouns (which had been learned in school in the past) produced more hypermnesia than any of his other effective stimuli. The author and his doctoral student Jackie Bergstein (Bergstein & Erdelyi, 2008; Erdelyi, 1996, pp. 115–119; 126–127) ventured to answer this simple but difficult question operationally, with a two-stage model of hypermnesia: Any stimulus that is both (1) *retrievable* (prone to being recovered in the course of multiple recall efforts—indexed objectively by cumulative recall performance over trials) and also (2) *recognizable* (recognized, once retrieved, as being a stimulus item), will yield hypermnesia.

Freudian Distortions are the Same as Bartlettian Distortions but for Motive: Implications for Freud's Dream-Work Notion

The multiple recalls of Karina and Maya treated in the preceding section showed a plethora of distortions of the story they were repeatedly attempting to recall. This too was the landmark finding of Bartlett with his adult Cambridge students. Distortions, as we have seen in Chapter 2, were also a major focus of Freud in his treatment of psychological products like dreams, aphasic errors, parapraxes, jokes. We have already reviewed his dream-work distortions (censorship/omission, condensation, displacement, plastic representation, symbolization, elaboration—see pp. 41–46), which, presumably, translate—or mistranslate—latent contents into manifest contents. If we included some of the other types of distortions Freud extensively examined (e.g., in Breuer & Freud, 1895/1955; Freud, 1891/1953; 1901b/1960; 1905/1958; 1909b1955/; 1911/1958; 1917/1963) it is clear that substantial overlaps exist between Bartlettian and Freudian distortions. The author and

TABLE 6.1 Overlaps between Freudian and Bartlettian Distortions

Freud (Various: e.g., 1900; 1901b; 1905; 1909b; 1911; 1917)	*Bartlett (1932)*
Omission, censorship, ellipsis	**Omission**
Rationalization	**Rationalization**
Secondary elaboration	**Elaboration**
Displacement of accent	**Change in emphasis**
Condensation, displacement, smuggled-in items	**Condensation, importations, transference**
Symbolization	Items are **symbolized**
Constructions	**Constructions**
Interpretation	**Interpretation**
Tendentious recall	**Bias in recall**
False connections, compulsion to associate	**Imposed links of connection,** striving after **associative links**
Distortion, falsification	**Distortion**
Transformations	**Transformations**
Reversal, reaction-formation	**Reversals** ("opinions and conclusions are reversed," p. 128)
Imaging, plastic representation	**Imaging**
Representation by triviality	**Curious preservation of the trivial** (p.184)

Note. Actual terms are bolded. Adapted from Erdelyi, M.H.(2006). "The Unifies Theory of Repression," *Behavioral and Brain Sciences,* 29, Table 1, p. 509. Adapted with permission, Cambridge University Press.

his student, Michel Halberstam, sought to determine the extent of this overlap. To our surprise, our systematic examination showed that *Freudian and Bartlettian distortions are not just similar but identical.*

Table 6.1 (adapted from Erdelyi, 2006, p. 509) lists the distortions ("constructions," "reconstructions") uncovered by Bartlett (1932) and the corresponding distortions elaborated by Freud decades earlier (Freud 1900–1920). Bartlett, who seems not to have known about Freud's work, discovered essentially the same distortions in his laboratory program. The actual terms used by Freud and Bartlett are bolded and reveal the remarkable overlaps in both terminology and concept. The only difference between Freudian and Bartlettian distortions is the *motive* for the distortions. For Bartlett, the distortions are cognitively motivated, arising from efforts to fit fragments of memories and percepts into the subject's mental schemas. For Freud, the distortions are emotionally motivated, arising from efforts to render the memories and percepts tolerable (defense). Thus, for Bartlett, omissions occur because there is no ready schema into which to fit the percept or memory; for Freud, omissions occur because of defensive efforts to expunge unpalatable materials.

We do not need to choose between one and the other since both types of motives—the need for emotional tolerability *and* the need for cognitive sense—could be at play in any given situation (although we might note that emotional tolerability is more of an issue in the clinic than in the academic laboratory). Freud, the clinician, almost surely overemphasizes emotion-motivated distortions but Bartlett, the laboratory researcher—along with most modern cognitive psychologists—almost surely overemphasize "cognitive" causes of distortion and neglect defensive distortions.

The operation of defensive distortion, which is difficult to prove in a brief text fragment—for example, Karina's "*they were not on the warpath*" (R_2, Lines 1–2)—is cinched easily in jokes (see our Chapter 2, pp. 53–59; Erdelyi, 1985), where it is obvious that some of the fancy footwork involving omissions and commissions manages the emotional force of the taboo contents. The evolution of fairy tales (over centuries), such as the story of "Little Red Riding Hood," also shows the defensive management of successive versions of the story, from the primitive and brutal oral-tradition version ("The Grandmother's Tale") to the more civilized Perrault version ("Little Red Riding Hood"), to the still further massaged Brothers Grimm iteration ("Little Red Cap").

The theoretical implication of the demonstrated overlaps between Bartlettian and Freudian distortions is that the "dream-work" notion is unnecessary for explaining distortions in dreams. It is sufficient to stipulate (the fact) that memory invariably entails errors of omission and commission, which are *more abundant in cases of impoverished cognition* (because of, e.g., fatigue, sleep, brain damage, or the immaturity of the subject) or because of impoverished stimulation (as in subliminal stimuli). The "dream-work" terminology leads to easy misunderstanding because, actually, *less work* is involved on account of the debilitated cognitive state of the dreamer (see Erdelyi, 1985, 2014; Solms & Turnbull 2002).

When the distortions are deployed for defense, the "dream-work" still constitutes "sub-work" (Erdelyi, 2014) because it involves less high-level cognitive work than is standard in awake cognition. Because the central executive system--the ego, the DLPFC--is in a weakened state during sleep (Freud, 1900/1953, 1917/1963; Hobson, & McCarley, 1977; Solms & Turnbull 2002) censorship is correspondingly weaker (but cruder, and therefore more obvious) and so more is revealed in dreams than in normal awake cognition. This is why "dream are the royal road to the knowledge of the unconscious" (Freud, 1900/1953, p. 608; see Chapter 2, pp. 40–41).

Ironically, the "dream-work" terminology fares better outside the venue of dreams, as in art, jokes, poetry, or fairy tales, where distortions are not the result of resource-poverty but are *intentionally* deployed for psychological effect. For convenience, we may continue to use "dream-work" to refer to the specific distortions enumerated by Freud for dreams (omissions/censorship, condensation, displacement, plastic representation/symbolism, and elaboration), regardless of whether less work or more work is involved.

The Associative Structure of Memory and Resulting "Spheres of Meaning"

A basic, increasingly appreciated fact about memory is that it does not comprise a random collection of elements but is, rather, a highly structured network of associations of elements (Anderson, 1983; Anderson & Bower, 1973; Andrews, Vigliocco, & Vinson, 2009; Collins & Quillian, 1969; Collins & Loftus, 1975; Landauer & Dumais, 1997; Llewellyn, 2013, 2020; Rummelhart, McClelland, & the PDP Research Group, 1986). The associative structure of memory has fundamental implications for dreams and, indeed, for cognition in general. We have already begun to consider this idea with aphasic errors (paraphasias), which are excellent analogs of dreams.

Freud, in his 1891 neuroscience monograph, *On aphasia*, articulates the notion that memory elements that are associatively close can easily be confused with one another or, even, merged with one another. Thus, when a patient is shown a *pencil*, and incorrectly responds with *pen* (Freud, 1891/1953, p. 22), the patient is implicitly reflecting an understanding that pencils and pens are close associatively, constituting implements for writing. Similarly, confusing *Berlin* with *Potsdam* (p. 22) reflects underlying knowledge that these items are cities in Europe. Further, a verbal "malformation" (p. 22) such as *Vutter* is a "fusing" (p. 22) of two allied concepts, *Vater* (father) and *Mutter* (mother). As already noted (Chapter 2, pp. 31-40), these aphasic errors turn up a few years later in psychoanalysis in the guise of the dream-work and other psychological distortions (e.g., "fusing" becomes "condensation"). Also, it is easy to conceptualize hypermnesia, whether in dreams or awake cognition, as arising from the eventual location of a memory item in a sprawling and (largely) unconscious associative network.

Werner (1956), in his classic paper, "Microgenesis and Aphasia," saw clearly the semantic implication of what he termed *spheres of meaning*, which some more modern scholars have called *neighborhood structures* (Andrews, Vigliocco, & Vinson, 2009). Items occupying the same sphere of meaning, or sharing neighborhood structures, are in some sense similar in meaning. Thus, when an aphasic patient responds to the stimulus word, "Zunge" (tongue, in German), with, "Something on the body, where and what I do not know" (Conrad, 1948, cited in Werner, 1956, p. 351), the patient shows his knowledge that the fugitive item, Zunge, is subordinately related to the broader concept of a body part. Similarly, when the same patient, trying to read "Eine flinke Katze kriegt die Mäuse" (a quick cat gets the mice), responds, "Fox and rabbit, or something; something to do with hunting," he clearly reflects knowledge of the basic concept but, because of his diminished mental resources, fails, toward the end-point of processing, to untangle the target item from other neighboring items—just as our mailman sometime mistakenly delivers mail from our neighbor.

Like paraphasias, dreams also reflect spheres of meaning. In Nemiah's case-history of Alice V. (pp. 69–70), the patient dreams, the night before her nervous breakdown, of an elephant who is struggling to get up. By itself, this isolated element is baffling and carries no interesting meaning. In the same dream, however, the scene is associated with sex, as the zoo keeper explains in the dream that the animals are "mating." A further associative link connects the elephant to Alice's traumatic experience, at the age of four, of witnessing her parents' lovemaking and her father's awkward attempts to get up and cover his nudity. There is more that could be added, but even this circumscribed sphere of meaning is enough to yield a straightforward interpretation of the meaning of the elephant (Who is he? What was he doing before? What is he trying to do now?)

Similarly, in Freud's Irma Dream (pp. 63–67), Dr. M., the senior figure in Freud's medical circle, to whom Freud turned for advice in difficult cases, made the ridiculous observation, "it's an infection, but no matter; dysentery will supervene and the toxin will be eliminated" (p. 66). The infection, moreover, is linked to Freud's younger medical colleague and friend, Otto, who had (in Freud's dream) thoughtlessly injected Irma with a preparation of trimethylamine—and to boot, with a syringe that had not been cleaned. Freud's group of medical friends do not fare well in his dream. Dr. M. is even burdened with health problems—"he was very pale and walked with a limp" (see p. 66) and is shorn of his manly beard. There are other failures—in others—that are touched on in the dream, leading to the overall interpretation (by Freud himself) that this was a dream of self-exculpation and of revenge against his friends (for their criticism of his treatment of Irma). There may be deeper meanings still, which Freud does not touch on (e.g., Freud's possible jealous feelings toward Otto with respect to the young widow, Irma, at whose home Otto stayed for several days—see the full discussion in pp. 64–67).

It is easy to show, as has been done above and in more detail in Chapter 3, that elements in a dream are associatively connected to each other and belong to a sphere of meaning. We should underscore, however, that spheres of meaning are not clearly demarcated and may not lend themselves to a brief exposition. The subject himself cannot access the full scope of his associative network and only with extensive effort (as in dynamic insight therapies, including, of course, psychoanalysis), can, over significant time intervals, uncover more comprehensive spheres of meanings. Additionally, in the process of extending the search through associative networks over time, elements may be discovered which have hitherto not been accessed and thus yield recoveries of memories, along with broader and deeper meanings. The task of exploring the subject's associative structure is made more laborious by the subject's emotional resistances (Breuer & Freud, 1895/1955; Freud, 1900/1953, 1917/1963), which delay and often derail the exploration of regions of associative structure. In our sample dream-analyses in Chapter 3, both Freud and Zelda explicitly admit to having withheld some of their associations.

Finally, it might be noted that the associative structure of memory, which we may assume is shared by both awake and sleep consciousness (Erdelyi, 2014, 2017; Han, 2014 [in Domhoff (2017, p. 27)]; Schweickert, 2007: Walker & Stickgold, 2010), is likely to account for the perennially observed continuity between dream-life and awake-life (see Bell & Hall, 1971; Freud 1900/1953, pp. 1–13; Domhoff, 2017; Erdelyi, 2017; Hall & Nordby, 1972; Schredl, 2017, 2019). Dreams, however, may tend to access different regions of associative structure and thus yield discontinuities in specific probes. Thus, the associative structure of memory can accommodate continuities *and* discontinuities between dream consciousness and awake consciousness. Also, dreams, unlike awake consciousness, do not edit associations as much as awake consciousness and thus allow the expression of more distant (low-probability) associations. For this reason, they often strike us as "hyperassociative" (Hobson, 2011, p. 232).

7

OVERVIEW AND CONCLUSIONS

Dreams Have Meaning, and at More Than One Level

Before getting to first base on dream interpretation, we must first dispense with the question whether dreams actually have meaning; for if dreams were "mere froth" (a common dismissal of dream meaning cited by Freud (1900/1953, p. 634)), if they were only random, meaningless effusions of the night, there would not be much point in trying to interpret dreams. Nonsense would beget nonsense.

But is it not obvious that dreams have meaning? Unfortunately, the smart money has not always been on board on the subject. Already, as we saw in Chapter 1 (pp. 13–14), Cicero, some two millennia ago, in his "Argument Against Taking Dreams Seriously," was dismissive of the subject and disdained the "divination of dreams" as superstition and subject to "endless imbecilities." Academic psychology has been more circumspect in language but not much more encouraging conceptually. For several decades the impression has been given—it would be instructive to examine some of the leading introductory textbooks of psychology—that dreams are really random forms of cognition and so, one could conclude, meaningless noise. The focus has been on the neuroscience of sleep and dreaming, but not on the meaning of dreams. Astonishingly, more than half a century after the much ballyhooed cognitive revolution against behaviorism, cognitive psychology textbooks altogether avoid the subject of dreams, let alone the meaning of dreams, even though the phenomena of dreams intersect virtually all major topics of modern cognitive psychology. The flagship journals of psychology are similarly MIA on the subject.

Probably a part of the puzzle is Hobson and McCarley's extraordinarily influential 1977 publication of their *activation-synthesis hypothesis*, which was a neuroscience model of dreaming that provided an alternative to Freud's psychological approach. REM sleep, which at the time was thought to be coterminous with dreaming, was

DOI: 10.4324/9781003300441-8

not, according to the activation-synthesis model, provoked by wishes but by the cyclic activation, several times a night, of random firings from the pontine hindbrain (see our Chapter 4) that fanned outward to other regions, including frontal areas responsible for high-level cognition, where a synthesis of the incoming stimuli was attempted. Since some of the frontal brain areas involved in the highest levels of cognition (notably, the dorsolateral prefrontal cortex; see our Chapter 4) are substantially inhibited during dreaming, the debilitated frontal brain has to do "the best of a bad job" (Hobson, 2011, p. 151) in making sense of the random effusions originating from the pontine hindbrain. Not surprisingly, dreams are confusing and somewhat random—and not because of any defensive dream-work, as Freud would have it.

The Zeitgeist was just right for the activation-synthesis model, for it was both a neuroscience model, which was the right way to go for many scientific psychologists, and anti-Freudian, which was the accelerating ethos in psychology. Moreover, it was clearly on target on some of its criticisms of Freud's turn of the century venture. But the activation-synthesis model had problems of its own, as it gradually became evident. Some of its own facts and conclusions were not quite right and, actually, it was not altogether logical as a theory. As noted already in Chapter 4, the pons is not the necessary trigger of dreaming, which was then identified with REM sleep; the action is more frontal in the brain. According to neurological evidence marshalled by the "neuropsychoanalyst," Mark Solms, REM sleep and dreaming are not the same and, in fact, can be "doubly dissociated," in that there can be REM without dreaming and dreaming without REM—and so the "activation" component of the model was not quite accurate physiologically. To his credit, Hobson revised his theory (Hobson, Pace-Schott, & Stickgold, 2000; again, see Chapter 4), which became the three-factor *AIM model* (A = Activation; I = Input; M = Modulation), which fixed some of the problems but also introduced more degrees of freedom into the model. Also, Hobson (2011, p. 239; 2015, pp. 197–198) gave some ground on the question of dream meaning, claiming that he had been "misunderstood" (a question we have examined in some detail in Chapter 4, pp. 104–105). Finally, aside from the question of physiological locus, the activation-synthesis hypothesis was not logically tight. Even if it were the case that the instigator of dreams were random impulses (from wherever) it would hardly follow that dream contents had to be correspondingly random. Consider a TV remote control. One selects a channel by pressing a button that sends a control message to activate a particular TV program. The program can be deeply rich narratively and so in no way random, but the narrative does not reside in the signal that activated the program. The signal is merely a signal, not the narrative. This is an obvious but rarely noted point.

Whatever the neurological underpinnings of dreams, it actually is obvious that dreams have meaning. Just consider any of the dreams included in Chapter 3—or *any* published dream. Without exception they all have meaning, even if they are sometimes puzzling. What then is the problem? The sticking point is the issue of latent contents—deep as opposed to surface contents. Manifest (surface) contents have demonstrable meaning and are decidedly not random. Independent judges could read Freud's Irma Dream (pp. 63–67) or Hobson's Mozart Dream (pp. 71-74) and produce reasonable (and discriminable) paraphrases of each of the two dreams. Or, we could use recognition measures—for example, multiple-choice tests—to demonstrate that the meanings of the two dreams are clearly discriminated by the judges. This is all true—and obvious—but are we missing the point? Freud would have undoubtedly thought so and would have dismissed the meanings we have ploddingly sought to validate as vapid, mere superficial renderings of surface contents.

The interpretation of dreams that Freud introduced into psychology in *The interpretation of dreams* was the interpretation of deeper, latent contents, which, unlike the meaning of manifest contents, are not always obvious (or even, often, and not conscious). So, the question is not whether manifest contents have meaning—the vast quantitative content-analytic literature has incontestably shown that they do (see Chapter 4)—but whether latent contents have meanings that can be extracted through interpretation. The answer, again, is "yes," but this is not yet a settled issue in academic psychology. Certainly with jokes and with some paraphasias there can be little argument, but with more complex narratives like dreams, the matter is still apparently unresolved ("apparently" because of the silence of academic psychology on the subject).

Although the manifest-latent content distinction is fundamental, it does not constitute a dichotomy. Semantic depth is not all-or-none but more-or-less. Just as a river is uneven in depth over its rambling course, a dream narrative can also be uneven in semantic depth, calling for different levels of analyses for different segments of the dream. "The Picture Dream of Dolores P." illustrates this point. One component of the picture dream (Figure 3.1) is readily meaningful: a *bucket and a spouting hose*. Another component, *rectangles within a rectangle*, is puzzling, although with the author's contribution of necessary context, it acquires a clear additional meaning—it is the floor plan of the *professor's office complex*. We have now extracted a set of three meanings from this segment of the dream (a bucket and a spouting hose, some rectangles within a rectangle, and the professor's office). There are, however, additional layers of meaning that emerge with more context—for example, that Dolores P. had just finished a section of her *Introduction to Psychoanalysis* course that dealt with Freud's theory of sexual symbols. This additional information imparts a potential new meaning to the *bucket and spouting-hose* element of the dream. With the condensation of the two sets of elements (sex-office), an additional—and taboo—meaning emerges (sex in the professor's office).

Thus, in this simple and short dream, at least five meanings can be discerned, two surface layers of meaning (*rectangles within a rectangle, bucket and a spouting hose*), two latent meanings (*professor's office, sex*), which arose from the interaction of manifest contents with context, and a still deeper taboo wish, involving the interaction of interactions (conceived of as a "second-order interaction" in statistics). Thus, this simple, short dream features a mix of three semantic levels—two manifest contents, two latent contents, and a still more latent (deeper) latent content.

Context is the Key to Latent Meanings

The notion that context is a key to deep meanings has been a leitmotif of our book. We saw this in our discussions of Freud, who discovered latent contents in dreams—and, also, in other release-phenomena such as hysterical symptoms, jokes, fairy tales. In Freud's approach, the context is generated through free-associations, a preamble, and clinical queries. In Jungian approaches (see, e.g., the clinical demonstrations of Delaney (1979)), the context is generated through the clinician's elicitation of *amplifications*, which are focused elaborations by the patient of details regarding the nature, function, and feeling-tone of elements of a dream. In still other approaches, such as Gestalt Therapy, outlandish play-acting brings out new, sometimes unexpected contexts to clinical issues. All these approaches, and of other consciousness-raising (insight) therapies, are ultimately forms of context-generation meant to bring new meanings to problematic manifest contents.

The context can, of course, be "external," as in the case of perceptual illusions. The classic Ponzo illusion (see Figure 1.4) is quite compelling (everybody experiences the illusion, even if it is known aforehand that the perceived size differences are not objectively real). If, however, we remove the surrounding context, the fanning lines, the illusion collapses. Thus, the embedding of a manifest content in some context can yield new meanings (or new sizes, as in the Ponzo illusion).

Formalization of the Manifest-Latent Content Distinction: $m \neq m \times$ context

The common-sense idea that context may add new meanings to manifest contents is formalized in terms of a generally accepted statistical framework that every professional psychologist must master in a graduate course on ANOVA (*analysis of variance*). In this statistical framework, the manifest content, m, is an explicit event or feature—for example, a slip of the tongue, a dream segment, a detail in a work of art or poem. The latent content is the interaction of the manifest content with context ($m \times context$) which, by dint of the interaction, yields a novel meaning. Thus, the manifest-latent content distinction is defined by the inequality,

$$m \neq m \times context.$$

One advantage of this formalization is that it places the issue of manifest versus latent contents in the framework of well recognized and accepted statistical thinking—and practice. The manifest content, in ANOVA terms, is a *main effect* while the latent content is an *interaction*. When analyzing and reporting experiments for publication, the experimenter must provide analyses of *both* main effects and interactions. This practice is not a matter of mere convention but of scientific necessity, for the analysis of interactions often yields the important results of the experiment, results which might not be reflected in the analysis of main effects.

Consider the memory curves we have examined in Chapters 1 (pp. 23–26) and Chapter 6 (pp. 164–179) which dealt with the course of memory over time with repeated testing. What is this course? Is it amnesic (memory decreasing with time) or is it hypermnesic (memory increasing with time)? Suppose we tested two groups of subjects, one which had been exposed to a set of pictures and another to a list of nonsense-syllables. The overall main effect, which would be the average trend for the two groups, might be flat because the two groups would tend to cancel each other out, with the nonsense syllable group pushing the trend downward and the picture group tugging the memory curve upward. The main effect would suggest that memory stays constant over time. The statistical analysis of interactions, however, would get at the interesting results (missed by the main effect), revealing a significant interaction between stimulus and memory over time that showed that picture memory significantly trended upward whereas nonsense-syllable memory significantly trended downward. If we had not analyzed interaction effects, we would have been left with the false conclusion that memory was dead in the water and moved neither up nor down with time. Analogously, a failure to test for interactions in dreams or other narratives—which, actually, characterizes much of modern quantitative content-analysis—might miss the psychological action in the latent content.

The formalization of the manifest-latent content distinction demonstrates (as was done with the short dream of Dolores P.) that the manifest-latent content distinction comprises not a dichotomy but opposite poles of a grainy continuum of semantic depth. More complex materials may yield many layers of meaning arising from the interaction of interactions—"higher-order interactions" (second-, third-, fourth-, or still higher-order interactions). So, excepting some compact cognitive modalities, such as jokes (discussed further, below), complex narratives may not have just two levels of meaning but multiple layers of meanings.

The formalization of the manifest-latent content distinction also has the advantage of clarifying what may be murky or underdeveloped in informal treatments of the subject-matter. For example, Freud often used the term "latent" as a synonym for "unconscious" and this might suggest that latent contents are unconscious. But our formalization does not demand such a conclusion. Latent contents *can be* unconscious, just as manifest contents can be unconscious, but our formalization is agnostic on the issue. We lose nothing (and gain clarity) from resisting the forced fusion of "latent" and "unconscious." The latent content of jokes are not usually unconscious; the often unconscious latent content of a dream does not cease to be a latent-content upon the conscious understanding of the latent content (as when Freud gradually grasped some of the meanings in his own Irma Dream).

Although latent contents need not be unconscious they do require, as our formalization indicates, extra processing (not just of m but of $m \times context$). Without analysis of the interaction of context with the manifest content, the latent contents would fail to be extracted (and thus would fail to achieve consciousness). Such a failure to extract the latent content (which can be defensively motivated) is evident in real-life materials. We noted the very interesting fact in jokes that the taboo content is invariably relegated to the latent content (p. 58). This gives the receiver of the joke some psychological space (in case he or she wants to avoid its latent content) and to the joker, "plausible deniability," in case the latent content should turn out to be too unsettling (Groucho Marx didn't quite get away with it with his "I love my cigar too, but I take it out of my mouth once in a while" witticism (see pp. 54–55). (In general, the tendentious failure to extract correct but disturbing latent contents corresponds to the defense mechanism of *denial*—in common lay-parlance, "being in denial" (see Erdelyi, 1985).)

Dynamics: Weighting of Items in the Contextual Ecologyanoid

The formalization of the manifest-latent content distinction yields an unexpected dividend: the possible integration of two heretofore dissociated psychological domains, *cognition* and *dynamics*. Traditionally, psychodynamic phenomena, like the defense mechanisms, have been expressed through the metaphor of "force," following the model of classic physics. In the 19th century, however, there was a gradual recasting in physics of the force notion, especially with respect to magnetic forces, which resisted Newtonian force-vector analysis. The traditional "forces" were finally reformulated as "force fields" (by Michael Faraday) and given a deep mathematical treatment by James Clerk Maxwell (Einstein's favorite physicist). More recently, in 20th century physics, "force" notions, having also become highly mathematized, lost their anchoring in our subjective experience of "force" and were often recast as "interactions" (e.g., "strong interactions," "weak interactions").

Our formalization of the manifest-latent content distinction can also move us past the force metaphor to psychological interactions and yield a cognitive rendering of "dynamic" effects, including defense mechanisms, which traditionally have been framed in the old-fashioned language of psychological "forces." The key idea is that the biased selection by the subject of the operative context (which interacts with the manifest content), can produce radically different extracted meanings, as in the case of the "Paranoid N." or of "The Psychotic Dr. Schreber" (Chapter 3, pp. 89–92). The applicable context is not preset for us or logically defined and this freedom of context-choice opens the field of cognition to motivated warpings of meaning through the biased selection of context which can even reverse the meaning of surface contents (as in sarcasm) or outright eliminate them (the defensive repression of latent contents constituting, as noted, "denial"). Different subjects (or patients) might choose different contexts and weight them differently. Such individual differences, which are of interest on their own right (and deserve research attention) may explain why perfectly smart individuals may nevertheless see the world so differently.

N, the Magician

N is a star character in statistics; one would be hard pressed to find a formula in an introductory statistics textbook in which *n* does not play a role. *N*, of course, refers to *number*—the number of subjects used in an experiment, the number of dreams examined, and so on.

N is a crucial player in our work because it is a remedy for the "noise" that inevitably inheres in our data and often masks the phenomena of interest to us. This noise includes "error of measurement" (the errors we fallible humans cannot altogether avoid making when measuring even a simple dimension, like the length of our living-room), as well as the variability of our data resulting from the conceptual murkiness of the phenomena we are seeking to assess (e.g., "intelligence," "memory").

In the author's work on hypermnesia, for example, it is usually the case that subjects improve their recall of pictures from a first recall trial to a third recall trial, but it is also the case that not all subjects improve (only about 80–90% do) and, moreover, that the magnitude of the improvement is variable, the average being 3 to 4 items over the three trials. A minority of individuals fail to improve at all and a subset of these actually produce amnesia instead of hypermnesia, showing recall losses over the three trials. Hypermnesia for pictures is a powerful effect but it is subject, as it must be, to the depredations of noise. To capture our effect despite noise, we use a large enough *n*, which allows errors to cancel out, and show that *on the average*, recall goes up with time. With powerful effects (such as hypermnesia for pictures), a small sample, for example, $n = 10$, usually suffices for getting statistically significant outcomes. For weaker effects, for example, hypermnesia for a list of words (instead of pictures), the trend of memory is only weakly incremental and will often fail to be statistically significant until a substantially larger *n* is used. With extremely powerful effects, a very small *n*, even an $n = 1$, might suffice (as with a unique event). In most cases, however, noise will intrude, and so it is best not to be unduly frugal with *n*.

It is with weak effects that the magic of *n* especially shines: If there is a real phenomenon, even when it is masked by noise, *n* reveals it. As we increase *n*, facts emerge that were heretofore out of reach, or even invisible.

Subliminal Effects Can Be Detected in Large-n Free-Associations

In our Chapter 5 (pp. 119–122) we discussed the experimental corroboration of the claim that subliminal percepts emerge in the content of fantasy (and by extension, in dreams). A crucial detail was the use of a large enough sample of free-associations ($n = 120$) for each subject. To the naked eye the free-associations were a jumble of random responses. The systematic rating of each association and the aggregation of all the 120 ratings for each subject (for an average score for each subject for each stimulus item) showed, however, that the subjects, despite their disclaimers of awareness, nevertheless evidenced the registration of some of the subliminal contents. This finding at the time was quite surprising to some hard-nosed experimental psychologists although, on reflection, it turned out to be consistent with some classic earlier demonstrations that forced-guessing by putatively unaware subjects easily yields above-chance correct guessing. These highly reliable outcomes were incorporated later on (Erdelyi, 1970, 1972, 1996) into a Signal Detection Theory framework (see Chapter 5 and our APPENDIX) in which the stimulus recoveries were construed as the recovery of low-confidence percepts.

The crucial point for us is that an invisible (and highly doubted) effect turned out to be a reliable phenomenon once a sufficient number of free-associations were evaluated and averaged. Thus, *n* was doing its magic by rendering the invisible visible--and, in retrospect, obvious.

Regularities in Dream Content Are Revealed by Large-n Quantitative Analysis

Quantitative content-analysts are well versed in the use of large *n*'s to produce reliable dream data. For example, the Hall – Van De Castle norms in Chapter 5 (Table 5.2, p. 138) distinguish male and female dreamers in several respects. Hall made much of a 67% versus 48 % difference in the frequency of male characters in the dreams of male and female dreamers (which he designated "the ubiquitous sex difference"). Most students assume that males dream more about females and females dream more about males but the data reliably show that males dream more about males. There are other male–female differences in dream frequencies. For example, males dream more about *sex* than females (12% vs. 4%), more about *physical aggression* in social interactions (50% vs. 34%), and more about *animals* (6% vs. 4%). Thus, while any dream by itself cannot point to any regularities in dreaming, large-*n* probes easily turn up significant differences between male and female dreams.

Meaningful patterns with personal and, even, clinical implications can also be revealed by large-*n* data collected on a single dreamer over long time periods. For example, "Emma," a highly educated dreamer who had spent decades in Jungian therapy (see Domhoff (2003, pp. 103–195) had recorded her dreams over some three decades. An interesting pattern in Emma's dreams was their focus on two male figures, her husband (who engendered mostly negative dreams) and her pastor (who inspired mostly positive dreams). This emotional triangle pointed, of course, to an awake-life conundrum, though Emma denied any illicit relation with her pastor in awake-life. The Emma dreams also showed a changing pattern over the years. In the first decade of the dream sequences, Emma dreamt more about her pastor than about her husband (169 vs. 117 times). In the last decade-and-a-half, however, the pastor faded in dream frequency (70) as the husband gained ascendancy (201).

High-*n* probes of another dreamer, Barb Sanders (Domhoff, 2003, p. 116; see our Chapter 5, pp. 137–139) also yielded clinically suggestive frequencies which, in this case, were in accord with the dreamer's awake stances. For example, Barb Sanders reflected in her dreams her greater liking of her father than of her mother. Aggression scores ("Aggression to Characters" ratios, or the "A/C Index") was 0.70 for her mother but only 0.36 for her father. Concordantly, the Friendliness Index (F/C) was higher for her father (0.37) than for her mother (0.27). Note, no single dream (or even a few dreams) would reveal such valence differences. Her friendliness score for her father was, after all, only 37%, but with a large enough sample, this 37% was meaningfully higher than the 27 % score garnered by her mother (see pp. 137–139).

Barb Sanders' dream frequencies for other members of her family also corresponded to her awake valences. She had fraught relations with her middle-daughter (who may have been psychologically disturbed) and accorded her a very high aggression Index score (0.92), while her other two daughters elicited much lower scores (0.36 and 0.51). She had a favorite brother whose dream aggression index was only 0.27 (note, not 0, but lower than for any of her three daughters). There clearly is a pattern in the dream frequencies but the pattern can only be picked up with a large enough *n*.

Personality Emerges in Dreams, But Only (as in Awake-Life) with Adequate n's

The importance of large enough *n*'s is well known to research psychologists but sometimes gets lost in the shuffle. Both dream psychologists and academic personality psychologists managed to miss the emergence of personality in dreams and in awake behaviors by unwittingly stinting on *n* (see our discussion in Chapter 5, pp. 139–141).

Early efforts to show a correlation between the psychological trait dimension, *boundary thickness,* and *dream frequency* kept yielding reliable but low correlations (*r*'s of around .20). Hartmann and Kunzendorf (Hartmann, 2011; Hartmann & Kunzendorf, 2006–2007), sensing that "noise" might be undermining higher correlations, augmented *n* by correlating the scores not of individual subjects but of psychological *groups* (consisting of the aggregated scores of many individuals) that were presumed aforehand to vary in boundary thickness—for example, Naval Officers (thick boundaries), Museum School students (thin boundaries) (see pp. 140–141). The correlation for the groups between the trait and the behavior succeeded in breaking through to rarified levels (e.g., $r = 0.92$), which means that a personality trait, boundary thickness, could robustly predict a behavior of interest, dream frequency. We may assume that other traits—say, the "Big Five" of personality psychology (OCEAN, i.e., Openness, Conscientiousness, Extraversion, Agreeableness, Neuroticism) would also yield high correlations with awake scores, including awake behaviors. This research waits to be done. Actually, Hartmann's (2011) demonstration that boundary-thinness is correlated with Openness ($r = 0.73$) already suggests a positive outcome for Openness.

Interpretation Is Probabilistic

Complex Dreams Require Statistical n's But Jokes Work with n = 1

Our foregoing discussion of quantitative content analysis (pp. 192–193) showed plainly that the patterns that we can extract from dreams are probabilistic. Thus, the probability of a male dreaming about an animal is 6% while the corresponding probability for a female is 4%. Any single observation of animal content in a dream would not be particularly informative about the dreamer' gender. In the case of Barb Sanders' dream series (see above; also, pp. 137–139), a single aggressive dream toward her father would be uninformative. A large enough sample, however, would clearly show that she was more positively disposed toward her father than toward her mother, even if she sometimes had aggressive dreams involving her father.

Freud was not statistically minded and he was probably too definitive in some of his interpretations, as in the Irma Dream (pp. 65–68). Perhaps a few more dreams might have been required to confidently extract overall meanings such as his anger toward his medical friends. Nevertheless, the caution that applies to the *whole dream* need not apply to *parts of the dream*. Specific fragments of a broader dream may yield highly reliable interpretations even where the interpretation of the whole dream (involving higher-order interactions) is less certain. Imagine trying to extract the overarching meaning of *Don Quixote de la Mancha*, a narrative text that exceeds 1000 pages. It is possible (the author's college professor did), but the answer may not be reliable or complete. If, on the other hand, to return to Freud's Irma Dream, we were asked to interpret not the whole dream but only parts of the dream—for example, "trimethylamin" and "some remarkably curly structures ... modelled on the turbinal bones of the nose" (p. 65)—we could confidently discern the sexual latent content by dint of our contextual knowledge that this chemical and the anatomical structure played a special role in the theory of female sexuality of Freud's friend, Wilhelm Fliess. Thus, there may be enough *local context* to interpret a *local fragment* even when there is not enough *broader context* to interpret the *broader dream*. A dream, like any complex narrative, is not a homogeneous monolith. As in a picture-puzzle, parts may be solved before the whole is solved.

In conclusion, we might note that jokes, unlike complex whole dreams, easily yield reliable interpretations with an *n* of 1. Of course, jokes are designed to produce specific meanings economically, without undue statistical fussing. We need sufficient contextual information (we may fail to get the joke if we lacked some crucial context) but, as common sense suggests, along with research results (Bergstein & Erdelyi, 2008), the latent contents of jokes may be extracted with high reliability.

Context Reduces Degrees of Freedom in Interpretation

The semantic algebra game we considered in Chapter 2 (pp. 48–49) showed clearly—as would any cross-word puzzle—that as contextual information accumulates, the possible interpretations are correspondingly reduced until, at least in our example, only one correct solution worked. Not all context is informative. The first line of context for *x*, "I broke my *x*" excludes many interpretation of *x* but the second line of context, "I told Mary that I broke my *x*" adds no relevant information about *x* and therefore fails to reduce degrees of freedom.

It is the same with dreams. Some contextual elements, though not all, cumulatively help winnow plausible interpretations until only a few and, eventually, perhaps only one will serve. In general, as the number, *n*, of contextual elements increases, the degrees of freedom of possible solutions decreases, yielding increasingly reliable interpretations.

Symbolism

As noted in Chapter 2, the term "symbolism" was virtually absent in Freud's original *The interpretation of dreams* although "plastic representation" (concretistic representation), one of the original dream-work operations, turns out to contain the essential core of Freud's universal symbols. Influenced by works of Wilhelm Stekel, K. A. Scherner, and others, Freud began to enlarge the role of symbolism and gave the subject increasing prominence in the third (1911) and fourth (1914) editions of *The interpretation of dreams*, until the subject became a major component of the dream-work—and, therefore, of interpretation. It is, however, in *A general introduction to psychoanalysis* (1917/1963) (or, *Introductory lectures on psychoanalysis*, 1917/1961–1963), and not in the *The interpretation of dreams*, that Freud enumerates the roughly dozen-and-a-half universal symbols that have come to be known as "Freudian symbols" (of which a partial list is included in Chapter 2, pp. 44–45).

Academic psychology has little to say on "symbolism," although "metaphor," a conceptual first-cousin, has garnered some attention (Barrett, 2020; Glucksberg, 2001; Lakoff & Johnson, 1980). There certainly is cause for skepticism about the excessive deployment of symbolic keys to dreams, as in the five-volume work of Artemidorus of Daldis some two millennia ago (see p. 11).

In the case of Freudian symbols, it may be argued that less is more. If we focused on just a half-a-dozen or so of Freud's wider list of symbols, we could more confidently embrace the select subset. Consider two classic Freudian symbols and their referents: (1) "long and stiff objects," "revolvers," "sabers," etc. = *penis*, or *phallus*, and (2) "cupboards," "boxes," "ovens," etc. = *vagina* or the *uterus*. Could we not establish that the symbol-referent equivalences are reliable and, therefore, real? We might test a few naïve friends (who knew nothing about Freudian symbols) and ask them to match up the symbols (e.g., *spear, box*) with the correct referents (*penis, vagina*)—in our experiment we would randomize for each friend tested the order of the symbols and the order of the referents. If our expectations were met, and the referents reliably matched up with their symbols (as expected), we would have shown that the proposed symbolic system is grasped immediately by subjects without any training in the proposed symbolic system.

Universal Symbols and Universal Referents

An interesting feature of Freudian symbols is that they do not take much effort to memorize. Why is this so? The answer gives us a clue to the character of Freudian symbols: Freudian symbols typically resemble in physical appearance or in function the referents being represented or, at least, are associatively linked to them, and so are easy to recognize and remember. Thus, Freud's venture into symbolism seems to have been more terminological than conceptual since his symbolic representations remained true to his original notion that dream representations are "plastic," or concretistic.

As noted in Chapter 2 (pp. 44–45), some semioticists might object that what was being discussed here involves not symbols but *signs*. This nomenclatural issue is of little import for the basic ideas developed here. It really makes no difference whether we choose to speak of "Freudian symbols" or "Freudian signs," especially if, as discussed in Chapter 2, pp. 44–45, we distinguish between *primitive symbols* (e.g., II, ---), which would correspond to "signs," and arbitrary *abstract symbols* (e.g., *duo* [Latin], *san* [Chinese]). Thus, in Freudian (primitive) symbolism, objects that physically resemble a referent are often used to represent the referent.

For a while Freud toyed with the idea of using symbolism as the sole means of interpreting latent contents but eventually reconsidered and returned to the primacy of free-associations as conduits to deep meanings (see Chapter 2, p. 45; also, pp. 10–11, 195–196). Symbols, however, provide a first-blush glimpse of possible latent meanings which free-associations can more laboriously corroborate—or, sometimes, correct. In any event, Freud's universal symbols, even if valid, are probabilistic. A cigar is sometimes just a cigar.

Biologically Prepared Meanings (Darwin, Evolutionary Psychology, Ethology)

The hypothesis that "universal symbols" (e.g., "phallic symbols") are universal by dint of their physical or functional resemblance to referents that unquestionably are universal (a penis is a penis is a penis, regardless of race, creed, or nationality) transforms the problematic idea of universal symbols into an obvious relation between symbol and referent. In this new view, however, it is the referent that is universal and the symbol merely a rough copy of the referent.

There may be, however, more to universal symbols than physical or functional resemblances between symbol and referent, for it would be surprising, given the research trends of the last few decades, if biological factors did not also play a role in universal symbols (*archyetypes*, in Jung's terminology). Darwin and modern Darwinian psychologists ("evolutionary psychologists"), as well as ethologists, have been able to discover a limited number of *facial expressions* (some 7 ± 2 in number) and, also, symbolic *body postures*, which mammals manage to produce—and interpret—reliably (see pp. 18–20). In humans, a small set of universal facial expressions have been identified that cut across cultures. The findings are powerful but, still, probabilistic. As noted in Chapter 1 (see pp. 19–20), the expression for "happiness" is the most consistently recognized facial expression—ranging from 95% to 100% concordance for subjects from the five countries probed (USA, Brazil, Chile, Argentina, and Japan). "Fear," on the other hand, was not quite so uniformly interpreted from facial expressions (with concordances ranging from 54% to 85% for the subjects from the five nations). Since animals also show concordant understanding and production of facial expressions and postures it is not altogether unreasonable to consider that symbols might also have a biological underpinning.

Distortions—Bartlettian and Freudian: Implications for the Dream-Work Notion

As shown in our chapter on "Dreaming as Noisy Remembering" (Chapter 6, pp. 179–181), the now universally accepted class of cognitive distortions empirically demonstrated by Bartlett (1932) in his Cambridge University subjects turn out to be *identical* to those described earlier by Freud (1900/1953) in *The interpretation of dreams* and other (mostly clinical) works (1891/1953, 1901b/1960, 1905/1958, 1909b/1955, 1911/1958, 1917/1963; Breuer & Freud, 1895/1955). Remarkably, Bartlett, who had little interest or knowledge of Freud's work, made use of some of the very same terms as Freud did earlier to describe the characteristic distortions to be found in memory and perception (see Table 6.1 of Chapter 6, adapted from the author's 2006 target article, "The Unified Theory of Repression" in *BBS* [*Behavioral and Brain Sciences*]). Thus, Freud's "omission," "rationalization," "elaboration," "condensation," "symbolization," "reversal," "representation by triviality" found their counterparts in Bartlett's "omission," "rationalization," "elaboration," "condensation," "symbolization," "reversal," and "preserveration of the trivial." The distortions are the same but the posited *causes* of the distortions are different: For Freud, the distortions were a consequence of defense; for Bartlett, cognitive schematization. The author has already suggested (pp. 180–181) that Freud overemphasized defense as a cause of distortion while Bartlett—and modern cognitive psychologists—have correspondingly overemphasized cognitive factors while largely ignoring defense.

It becomes clear from the overlap of Bartlettian and Freudian distortions that the classic "dream-work" distortions are *not specific to dreams* but merely constitute an incomplete subset of the distortions that overtake *any* cognitive product, whether in awake states or in sleep—and for whatever reason (defense, cognitive schematization). Since they are not specific to dreams, the distortions found in dreams do not require the designation "dream-work," a term which we might choose to let lapse in favor of, simply, distortions, or *dream distortions* (when they involve dreams). Indeed, as already noted, since dreams are disinhibited, under-regulated states, they involve *diminished* work, and thus in any case would be better characterized as involving not "work" but "sub-work."

The plain fact that cognition—awake or dream cognition—is subject to a circumscribed set of some dozen-and-half distortions (summarized in Table 6.1 on p. 180)—which turn up in dreams, paraphasias, jokes, long-distance memory—suggests that we might be dealing with a counterpart of universal symbols, namely, *universal distortions*. Significantly, knowledge of such universal distortions helps in the interpretation of noisy, distorted cognition such as dreams.

Dreams are Hypermnesic (Sometimes)

As has been noted in our Chapter 6, "Dreaming as Noisy Remembering," Freud proposed in *The interpretation of dreams* (1900/1953, pp. 11–21, 589) that "dreams are hyperemnesic," by which he meant that "it is a very common event for a dream to give evidence of knowledge and memories which the waking subject is unaware of possessing."

In Chapter 6 (pp. 156–159) some evidence was presented for this claim. The evidence discussed comes from only a few dreams and so might be questioned by exacting methodologists. What makes the few hypermnesic dreams credible is that they involved the dreaming of technical terms which are highly unlikely to have been produced by mere chance. Thus, Zelda (pp. 156–158) had a dream about her deceased friend, Jean, who explained to Zelda (in Zelda's dream) that the culinary delight Zelda was enthusing about was "ratatouille." Zelda did not (consciously) know the term and had to check her cook books to discover its meaning (which she must have known unconsciously since the clever Jean was a figment of Zelda's dream). Similarly, in Freud's discussion of Delboeuf's dream about the fern, *applenium ruta muraria,* the dreamer did not recognize the term (which he slightly misreported as, *applenium ruta muralis*) and had to resort to some research to discover the specific meaning of the Latin name. Zelda was mystified by her dream about "CUTTY SARK" until weeks later she discovered its meaning from reading a billboard that advertised the whiskey; one of Freud's patients was similarly stumped by his dream about a mysterious *Kontuszówka*, which Freud was able to inform him was a Polish liqueur. The dreamers, obviously, possessed information that appeared in their dreams but not in their awake consciousness.

It does appear that dreams *can* be hypermnesic but the qualification "sometimes" seems justified since the *manifest contents* of most dreams—for example, those in Chapter 3—are already accessible to consciousness and are in no need of recovery. *Latent contents,* however, may be another story since they often are unconscious and purportedly are recovered (by design) in insight therapies. Thus, the preponderance of dream hypermnesias may involve latent contents. Systematic research on the subject is called for, including the estimation of spontaneous hypermnesias in awake narratives as controls for the frequency of hypermnesias in dreams.

In a different vein, Barrett (2001), the editor of the journal, *Dreaming,* provides some striking cases in which dreams appear to solve problems or puzzles that are beyond the reach of awake-cognition (see 86–88). Her psychiatrist friend, Morton Schatzman (who wrote an important book on *The Psychotic Dr. Schreber*) reported to her a poetic dream of a medical intern that solved a brain teaser—"What Word Starts with and Ends with 'He'? Sleep on a Brainteaser and Wake Up with a Headache." Dreams are sometimes reported to provide artistic contributions, for example, the tune for Paul McCartney's "Yesterday" or the music for Richard Wagner's opera, *Tristan and Isolde* (according to Wagner, "I dreamed all this, never could my poor head have invented such a thing purposely" [in Barrett, p. 73; see Chapter 3, p. 86]). In a more riveting kind of problem solving, a friend of Barrett's, Nancy Parsifal, claimed to have saved the life of her newborn baby by heeding a dream over the objection of two physicians and her husband (Barrett, pp. 131–134). Some of these claims, and there are many others and from disparate fields, are often astonishing but (as Barrett agrees) have not yet been mastered in standard, controlled studies.

Dreams as Leading, Lagging, and Concurrent Indicators

Indicators, as discussed in some detail in Chapter 6 (pp. 159–160), are objective correlates of events which are often "invisible"—invisible because the events of interest might be unconscious, because they may have occurred in the past or, significantly, because the events of interest, in the case of leading indicators, may not yet have come to pass. The claim, insufficiently corroborated so far, that dreams might be leading indicators of crucial future events (e.g., the outbreak of some somatic or psychological illness, one's likely recovery from such an illness, the course of a love relation) is a seminal question for dream psychology. Such dreams are sometimes referred to as *prodromal dreams, predictive dreams,* or, more dramatically, *prophetic dreams*. Academic psychologists, even dream researchers, have tended to give a wide berth to the question, presumably out of fear of becoming ensnared in paranormal claims (in this case, "precognition") which remain taboo in scientific psychology.

Without venturing past the perimeters of standard scientific psychology, we have noted that the fear of the paranormal has sometimes constrained dream science from dealing with the normal. Lagging indicators (memory measures), concurrent indicators (e.g., parasomnias), leading indicators (in economics and medicine) are standard fare in mainstream disciplines—we have devoted a full chapter (Chapter 6) to the subject—but the notion that dreams might be *leading* indicators has been notably avoided in dream research. This avoidance is an unfortunate mistake since a credible affirmative answer to the question of predictive dreams would be a ground-breaking development for scientific psychology—and also for neuroscience and everyday medicine. It is true that we might eventually end up with a negative answer—which in itself would be salutary, for we could then be able to assert justifiably that scientific research has discredited the long-held view that dreams could predict the future. This, however, is not a likely outcome.

As noted in Chapter 6, *there is nothing remotely unscientific about predicting the future,* as prediction is a bedrock feature of the scientific enterprise. Interestingly, mainstream psychologists, without in any way embracing parapsychological notions, have begun to underscore the "prospective" thrust of memory (Kvavilashvili & Rummel, 2020; Schachter & Addis, 2007; Seligman, Railton, Baumeister, Strirade, 2013). Thus, memory is not only about the past but also about the future, as the past tends to predict the future as well as to guide it. A similar future-orientation is beginning to develop in dream science with notions such as *predictive processing* and the view that the brain is a *Bayesian* or *inference machine* (Friston et al., 2011, 2018; Hobson, Hong, & Friston, 2014; Tuominen & Valli, 2019).

There is, moreover, some, although still insufficiently buttressed empirical evidence suggesting that prediction is possible for a variety of events, form "lexical leakages" predicting biopsy outcomes, to the prediction by dreams of one's chances of survival after surgery, to one's likelihood of developing Parkinson's disease 10 years after the outbreak of RBD (REM Behavior Disorder), or a dreaming woman's fluctuating treatment of males and females over the temporal course of her menstrual cycle. These research findings need to be replicated and elaborated but they certainly suggest that such events are not beyond the pale of the probable. We should note, however, that predictive dreams, if they are corroborated, are likely to be about information, biological or psychological, that is already ensconced in the dreamer, even if not in the dreamer's consciousness. It would be a completely different proposition to expect the dreamer to predict the outcome of some random external event (like tomorrow's winning lottery number).

Although the author has taken a conservative stance on paranormal effects in dreams, carefully staying within the confines of standard "normal" psychology, it is important to note that (a very small minority of) serious research psychologists (e.g., Cardeña, 2018; Child, 1985; Krippner, 2019; Ullman & Krippner, with Vaughan, 2002; Sherwood & Roe, 2003; Storm, Sherwood, Roe, et al., 2017) have argued, with research evidence, that some paranormal effects may be real. Just as modern physics has embraced what Einstein once termed "spooky effects," psychological science may yet change its stance toward some "paranormal" phenomena (in which case, these phenomena will, no doubt, be recast as "normal").

The Continuity between Dream-Life and Awake-Life

In many ways dreams tend to be different from awake cognition. Dreams, as noted in Chapter 2, are more primary-process in nature than normal secondary-process awake cognition: Dreams are disinhibited and prone to concretistic representation (in the form of pictures and behavioral enactments); they often abrogate reality-testing, linear time, logic; and frequently feature flagrant displacements and condensations. For example, in Allan Hobson's "Mozart Dream" (pp. 71–73), the long-dead Mozart appears in resplendent attire, beautifully plays a concerto—but with no orchestra and with the wrong instrument—and has noticeably gotten "overweight." Much of this does not make sense. Similarly, in Zelda's *Ratatouille Dream* (pp. 156–158), Zelda's friend, Jeannie, who has been dead for 15 years, appears in a dream and has a casual conversation with the dreaming Zelda about a special dish which she informs Zelda is called *ratatouille*.

One is tempted to conclude that dreams are very different from awake cognition. This actually tends to be true for the "formalistic" characteristics of dreams (Hobson, 1988, 2011, 2015; see Chapter 4, pp. 101–104), that is, their tendency to feature "primary-process" cognition (Freud, 1900/1953, 1901b/1960, 1915/1957, 1917/1963; see also our pp. 41, 101), but is not true of the actual *content* of dreams which is noisily continuous (correlated positively, if not perfectly) with awake cognition. In the first dozen pages of *The interpretation of dreams* (1900/1953) Freud reviews, under the heading, "The Relation of Dreams to Waking Life," the conclusion of several earlier authors to this effect, for example, "dreams carry on waking life" (Haffner, 1887, in Freud, p. 2), "the majority of dreams ... usually lead us back to ordinary life instead of freeing us from it" (Weygandt, 1893, p. 6, in Freud, pp. 7–8). Contrary to some treatments of Freud's position (e.g., Hall & Lind, 1970, p, 89; see also Chapter 5, 146–149), Freud matter of course embraced the basic continuity between dream-life and awake-life: "All of the material making up the content of a dream is in some way derived from experience, that is to say, has been reproduced or remembered in the dream... " (Freud, 1900/1953, p. 11).

Quantitative content-analysis has led to the same place. Mary Calkins, the first female president of the American Psychological Association, asserted in her 1893 article, "Statistics of Dreams," that there is "an essential congruity and continuity of the dream life with the waking life" (p. 323). This view, which has come to be known as the "the continuity hypothesis" (after Bell & Hall, 1971), has been taken up and pervasively confirmed by modern quantitative content-analysts, among them, Bell and Hall (1971), Hall and Nordby (1972), Hall and Van De Castle (1966), and Domhoff (2003, 2018a). Although there has been some recent debate about the specific nature and perimeters of this continuity (see the recent discussions in the journal, *Dreaming*, of Bulkeley (2018), Domhoff (2017, 2018b), Erdelyi (2017), Jenkins (2018), Schredl (2017); Chapter 5, pp. 146–149), there is general agreement about the continuity between awake and dream experiences. This continuity is statistical (often requiring large *n*'s for its demonstration) and, apparently, not uniformly applicable to all domains of awake-life (e.g., the three R's—reading, writing, and arithmetic (Hartmann, 2011, p. 43))—but is by now "an established generalization and therefore no longer a hypothesis" (Domhoff, 2018b, p. 358).

The continuity of content between sleeping- and awake-cognition has basic theoretical and applied implications. It suggests, for example, that the subject's associative-network structures (see pp. 34–40; 128–135; 181–184) subsume the cognitive products of both the sleeping and awake mind. Thus, dreams may yield much knowledge about awake cognition, just as awake-cognition may yield much knowledge about sleep-cognition. Crucially for dream interpretation, the continuity between dreaming and awake cognition provides contextual backdrops for dream contents that may on the surface appear puzzling or bizarre. For example, Alice V.'s strange dream about the struggling grey-elephant (pp. 69–70) is disambiguated by her memory of witnessing, at the age of four or five, her parents having sexual intercourse and her father, like the grey elephant in the dream, struggling to get up and raising his left leg (to hide his nakedness, in the case of her father). The elephant in the dream was, evidently, a stand-in for Alice's father.

Dreams are One Dialect from a Family of Release-Phenomena

Dream scholars tend, not surprisingly, to focus on their subject matter, dreams. Freud too concentrated on his subject in *The interpretation of dreams*, although he allowed himself, more than most, to wander off to grapple with other topics of psychology such as attention, inhibition, suppression/repression, perception, memory, sexuality, and, in his famous Chapter 7, to articulate what amounts to an information-processing model of the mind such as became popular more than half a century later (see Erdelyi, 1985, pp. 116–126). Freud was decidedly not a one-pointed thinker and he exuberantly explored a vast domain of psychology, and across many traditional borders. This restless, integrative energy yielded one of his most important, if largely unrecognized contributions to dream psychology, the treatment of dreams as just one dialect among a wide-ranging family of release-phenomena.

In his *Studies on hysteria* with Josef Breuer, published in 1895, just a few years before the appearance of *The interpretation of dreams*, Freud treats hysterical symptoms as puzzles with meaning, just as he was to treat dreams a few years later. A short time after the publication of his dream book he published one of his most popular works, *The psychopathology of everyday life* (1901b/1960), in which he dealt with what has come to be collectively called (in English translations) the "*parapraxes*," or, less formally, "Freudian slips," treating these misfired cognitive products the same way he treated dreams. Indeed, we began our consideration of Freud's technique of dream interpretation by illustrating Freud's approach not on a dream but on a *parapraxis*—in this case, the puzzling forgetting by an embittered young academician of the word *aliquis* in a failed quote from Virgil (*"Exoriar aliquis nostris ex ossibus ultor"*) (pp. 60–63). A few years later, in 1905, his book on jokes appeared. Only a little later, some of his famous monograph-length case-histories were published, for example, his 1911 case, *The psychotic Dr. Schreber,* which showed abundantly the overlaps between psychopathological symptoms and dreams. His popular, *A general introduction to* psychoanalysis (1917/1963) (aka *Introductory lectures on psychoanalysis,* 1917/1961–1963) systematically demonstrates through Freud's treatment of a succession of topics—dreams, daydreams, fantasy, the parapraxes, neurotic symptoms, regression, fixation, the power of "the sacred rule" (free-association)—that the principles applying to dreams are essentially the same as those that apply to a host of other release-phenomena.

We have here an integration on a vast scale of a sweep of superficially disparate phenomena—certainly a major theoretical achievement. But perhaps the most crucial yield of this integrative exuberance is methodological, for it turns out that a problem that is refractory in one dialect may turn out to be simple in another. This precept is familiar in mathematics and physics, though less so in psychology. It is, however, highly fruitful in dream science.

Sober scientific psychologists—or neuroscientists—may treat the manifest-latent content distinction as a nebulous and perhaps misleading notion (with Allan Hobson, for example, explicitly rejecting the manifest-latent content distinction, claiming that dreams are "transparent"). No one, however, worries about the notion of "getting a joke," which demonstrates the necessity of going beyond surface semantic structures to extract deeper-lying latent contents. Thus, jokes make obvious a basic claim that has been problematic for some dreams theorists. Jokes, however, also create (useful) problems for current dream science, pointing to a serious weakness in contemporary quantitative content-analysis (see our Chapter 5) which, out of concern for scrupulous objectivity, has focused so far on surface contents but cannot—at this juncture—achieve an elementary content extraction, the getting of the joke in a joke. It is highly likely that content counts, especially of fraught materials, are way off because of the neglect of latent contents—the author estimates that sexual dream content is undercounted by as much as 100%.

Our understanding of dream phenomena can yield a richness of meaning when applied to other complex narratives such as poetry or fairy tales. For example, is the choice of the color *red* a happenstance in the famous "Little Red Riding Hood" (or "Little Red Cap") fairy-tale or does it convey latent meanings touching on the coming of age of a young girl? There certainly is a loosening of reality-testing in fairy tales—in "Little Red Cap," the heroine and her grandmother are devoured by the wolf but manage to survive in his belly until their rescue by a hunter. Censorship is concretely instantiated in the revisions, over centuries, of the brutal oral-tradition version of the story, "The Grandmother Tale," which is much tamed in Perrault's "Little Red Riding Hood," although it still features the death of the heroine and her grandmother. The story is mitigated further in the Brothers Grimm's later, "Little Red Cap," which changes the ending to a happy outcome, with the miraculous saving of the heroine and her grandmother and the cathartic vengeance upon the "wicked wolf."

Thus, a wide-ranging palette of release-phenomena, seemingly unrelated to dreams, are enriched by our understanding of dreams. Conversely, ostensibly unrelated release-phenomena bring clarifications and methodological solutions to dreams. Science thrives on distinctions—but soars with unification.

Associative Structure Undergirds Meaning—As Well As Errors and Biases

Associative structure (see Chapter 6, pp. 181–184) is now widely accepted as a basic feature of all types of cognition, normal and abnormal, from memory to perception to aphasic errors to paranoid delusions to dreams and, now, as some social-cognition researchers have shown, "implicit" (unconscious) racial and gender biases. The emphasis of association is an old story, with Plato and his student Aristotle usually credited with introducing the notion. It became important in clinical neuroscience in the 19th century (e.g., with the breakthrough work of Broca and Wernicke on aphasia and with Freud's own contribution of 1891, *On aphasia,* as well as with Heinz Werner's later demonstration of "spheres of meaning" in aphasic errors (pp. 33–36).

Freud's free-association technique can be understood as a procedure for exploring the patient's associative structure with respect to problematic symptoms, thoughts, or, even, Freudian-slips. The "basic rule" of free-association (see pp. 59–60) is to say freely whatever comes to mind—anything whatsoever, without censorship or evasion. From a strictly logical standpoint, free-association is the simplest task one might conceive of since all responses are right and no response is wrong. Yet, from a psychological standpoint, the free-association task is impossible, for we humans can never be completely honest with another person, not even with ourselves. All of us inevitably cheat on the basic rule. Honesty carried too far is embarrassing, painful, and, even, dangerous.

There is, however, another reason than censorship why we cannot be truly free with our free-associations and this is the inescapable associative structure that underpins all our cognitive activities, including free-association, which both shapes and delimits our cognitive products and which we cannot overcome by a simple act of will. This shaping and limiting associative structure was put to practical use by two modern social psychologists, Tony Greenwald and Mahzarin Banaji, neither of them Freud enthusiasts, who developed (after Greenwald's original breakthrough in 1994 (see Banaji & Greenwald, 2013, pp. 32–38)), the famous Implicit Association Test (the IAT), which by now has seeped into popular culture. The IAT proves, through computer-administered multiple-choice testing of relevant association strengths, the existence of implicit, or unconscious racial and gender biases, even when the subject honestly feels free of such biases. There can be, apparently, a big difference between our conscious attitudes and our unconscious ones, especially about emotionally fraught issues. Notwithstanding the simple suggestion of Gordon Allport, the founder of personality psychology, that if you want to know something about a person, just ask the person, it turns out, as Freud insisted, that we are not conscious masters of our thoughts or emotional dispositions. Greenwald and Banaji learned from their own test that, despite their exemplary conscious stances, they nevertheless harbored racial stereotypes of which they were unaware and of which they disapproved. Taking the test again—and several times—Tony Greenwald did not solve the problem, as he kept flunking his own test (as most people do).

Freud also, already in his 1895 book with Breuer, found the same kind of disjunction between conscious and unconscious psychological stances. A female patient, for example, with exemplary loving feelings for her sister, was revealed, after some analysis, to harbor feelings of resentment, jealousy, and even hatred toward her sister—and an immoral hankering after her sister's attractive husband—all despicable sentiments to the patient's conscious mind.

Dreams, on account of their disinhibited nature, reveal more associative structure than awake cognition does (they are "hyper-associative," in Hobson's words) and can, for this reason, often uncover tawdry strands of our psychological make-up that are alien to our awake consciousness. It is for this reason that dynamic therapies are so painfully slow-moving, as they invariably make progress, if they make progress at all, against unremitting "resistance" that takes time and much emotional struggle to overcome.

Interestingly, Banaji and Greenwald, in their 2013 book, *Blind Spot: Hidden biases of good people*, as well as the present author in his 1985 book, *Psychoanalysis: Freud's cognitive psychology*, include the same quote from Fyodor Dostoyevsky's (1864) *Notes from underground*:

> Every man has reminiscences which he would not tell to everyone but only to his friends. He has other matters in his mind that he would not reveal even to his friends, but only to himself, and that in secret. But there are other

> things which a man is afraid to tell even to himself, and every decent man has a number of such things stored away in his mind.
>
> *(Dostoyevsky, 1864/1960, p. 27)*

It is the latter type of self-deception that is the focal point of psychodynamic therapies as well as the target of clever probes by social-cognition researchers such as Greenwald and Banaji in their Implicit Association Test. We have here, then, a convergence of views: Cognition is associatively structured and this fact both gives meaning to and robs freedom from our mental processes.

The Essential Fact about Dreams: They Are Confusing but Honest

We now come to the end of our book with a conclusion that has been weaving in and out of our discussions, from beginning to end: *Dreams are confusing but honest.* This is, of course, a relative assertion, for dreams are neither completely confusing nor completely honest. Like a tipsy man at a party who slurs his words and is hard to understand but lets slip some confidences, the dreamer also garbles his thoughts but reveals personal confidences that are withheld in awake life.

Not because of alcohol but because of the natural rhythms of our neurological substrates (see pp. 94–97), we experience nightly periods of disinhibition in which brain systems shut down and release primitive, hitherto inhibited contents and modes of thinking. For this reason, "*The interpretation of dreams is the royal road to the knowledge of the unconscious activities of the mind*" (Freud, 1900/1953, p. 608). This "unconscious" includes contents that would provoke distress were they brought out into the full glare of consciousness and, also, "primary-process" modes of functioning characterized by concretistic representation (e.g., pictorial representations, procedural enactments), break-downs of logic, reality-testing, and of linear time.

Knowledge of these various types of primary-process operations brings to light meanings that hide in plain sight. The cover of our book, Picasso's "The Dream," is an apt example for, with just a little familiarity with the notion of concretistic representation and the logic of condensation, we may discern—what most naïve viewers do not—what it is the young woman is dreaming about. Similarly, as we have noted for jokes, the taboo meanings are demonstrably relegated to latent contents (pp. 53–58; 188–190), which when interpreted, convey meanings, often prurient or nasty, that we would not allow ourselves to express publicly under normal circumstances. The wider set of release-phenomena, of which dreams are one dialect, are similar. Thus, jokes too are honest and (when not gotten) confusing. Fairy tales also, though often inscrutable to the consciousness of both adults and children, broach difficult subject-matters that adults usually feel uncomfortable discussing with their children (Bettelheim, 1974).

But not all of us are at home with jokes or concern ourselves with fairy tales or need to contend with the ravages of psychosis or aphasia. Dreams, however, are a universal phenomenon that all of us experience, and several times each night, which provide us with something like X-rays of the hidden innards of our murky mental life. For those of us committed to the Socratic imperative—"know thyself"—dreams are a great light that shines forth from the darkness of sleep.

APPENDIX[1]

Application of Signal Detection Theory to Narrative Recall, Including Dreams: The Technique, Rationale, and Empirical Grounding of Criterion-Controlled Free Recall (CCFR) (Erdelyi, Martin and Emily Orne, Dinges, Halberstam, Feigin-Pfau, Ionescu, Bergstein, Finks, Wong)

The basic problem addressed by signal detection theory (SDT) is how to separate two independent components of the detection (or memory) response, the subject's *sensitivity* to the stimulus and the subject's *criterion* for producing responses. In situations that involve uncertain detection or memory, as in dream recall (see, e.g., Hobson's or Zelda's dream in Chapter 3), the subject must decide whether to report or to hold back uncertain dream recollections.

Two subjects with the same detection level may produce highly discrepant detection *responses*. One subject may be very conservative and withhold uncertain

1 This Appendix is a revised and expanded version of an earlier Appendix published in Erdelyi (1996). Many individuals played a role in the development of the original criterion-controlled free recall (CCFR) method. The groundwork was laid in a collaborative venture with the Unit for Experimental Psychiatry of the University of Pennsylvania, headed by Martin and Emily Orne and David Dinges. Subsequently, a critical role was played by Michael Halberstam, then an honor student at Brooklyn College, who in collaboration with the author, developed the first working prototype of the method. Merryl Feigin-Pfau, a graduate student, followed up with critical empirical tests of the technique that justified a significant simplification of the procedure. Feigin-Pfau, along with fellow graduate students Marcos Ionescu and Jacqueline Bergstein and honor student, Joyce Finks, conducted successful validation studies of the CCFR, which Vermone Wong, an honor student, refined. [Adapted with permission of the University of Chicago Press. ©1996 by the University of Chicago].

responses, managing to get only a few hits but also only few false-alarms, while another subject may adopt a lax reporting strategy, achieving more correct detections ("hits") but, also, more incorrect detections ("false alarms"). Thus, the number of correct recalls, or hits, is an inadequate measure of stimulus detection—or dream recall. *Both* hit-rates and false-alarm rates must be considered, and *in tandem*, to assess sensitivity to the signal.

SDT provides this index of sensitivity in its famous "receiver operating characteristic" (ROC) curves, which plot hit-rates as a function of false-alarm rates. ROC functions are *isosensitive curves* (any given curve represents a single level of sensitivity) but each *point* on the ROC curve (representing a hit and false-alarm pair) corresponds to a different criterion level (laxer criteria being located toward the right side of the ROC plot—that is, high rates of hits and high rates of false alarms—and conservative criterions settings toward the left side of the curve—low hit rates, low false-alarm rates. The more bowed the ROC curve, the higher the sensitivity, a value that is measured mathematically by the index d' (among others).

The basic theoretical and procedural issues have been worked out by SDT and would seem to be ready for application to dream research—but for one problem. Classic SDT is based on *recognition* responses (e.g., saying "Yes" or "No" to *stimulus* items or to *distractor* items—a "Yes" response to a stimulus item being defined a *hit* and a "Yes" response to a distractor being defined a *false-alarm*—but dreams constitute *recalls* (see our Chapter 6, "Dreaming as Noisy Remembering"), which do not readily yield to standard SDT techniques.

The author and his colleagues have attempted to resolve this problem by developing the CCFR ("Criterion-Controlled Free-Recall") procedure for evaluating true dream-recall level that is independent of the dream recaller's response criterion. A noteworthy feature of the CCFR procedure is that it may be applied retroactively to narrative recall (including dreams) that have been already reported—or published.

Classic Signal-Detection Theory, ROC Functions, *d'*, P(A), and $H|F_c$

The essential idea behind the approach derives from a common sense reading of signal-detection theory's ROC (receiver operating characteristic) functions. Figure A.1 presents two such functions, *L* and *M*, in which *L* depicts an isosensitive function that is lower than *M* in sensitivity (or, discriminability) than the middle-level function, *M*.

The sensitivity difference between *L* and *M* can be explained by way of the mathematical superstructure of SDT, but also in quite intuitive terms: For any two isosensitive functions, *M* and *L*, for which $M > L$ in sensitivity (d'), it is the

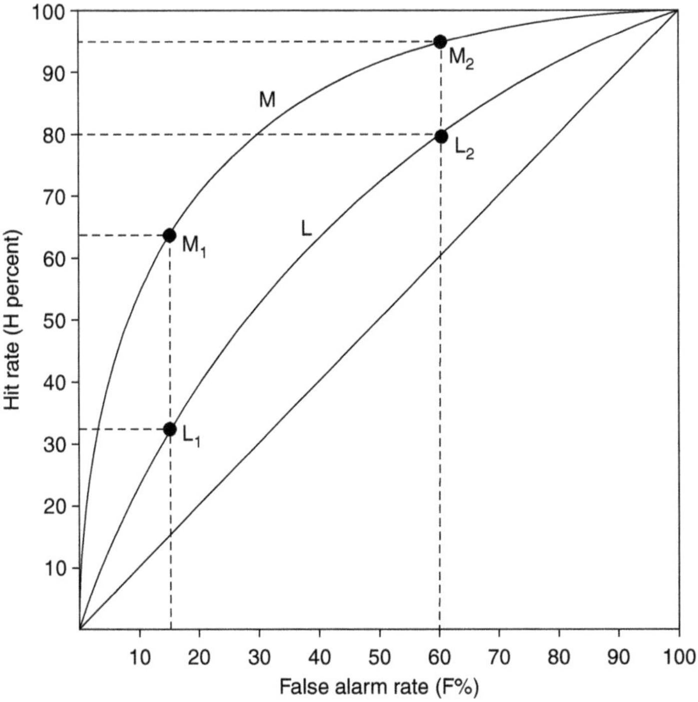

FIGURE A.1 Hypothetical ROC curves for two subjects, *L* and *M*, with low and middle levels of sensitivity *(d')*. Points on a particular curve represent different criterion placements but the same sensitivity level.

case (see Figure A.1) that for any particular false-alarm rate, F%, within the full range of 0% < F% < 100%, the hit rate, H%, of the more sensitive function will necessarily be higher. Thus in the example in Figure A.1, for a false-alarm rate of 15%, *M* yields a hit rate of about 63% while *L* yields a hit rate of only 33%. For another false-alarm rate, 60%, *M* yields a hit rate of 95% to *L*'s corresponding hit rate of 80%. If *M* and *L* represent the performance of two different subjects, then *M* is common-sensically more sensitive than *L* since, for any particular false-alarm rate within the full range of F%(0% < F% < 100%), *M* invariably garners a higher hit rate. Thus, if we defined the criterion-controlled hit rate H%′ as a hit rate conditionalized on a particular false-alarm rate $F\%_c$, that is, $H\%' = H\% \mid F\%_c$, it would follow that *M*'s H%′ > *L*'s H%′. Indeed, if the mathematical assumptions underlying SDT (Green & Swets, 1966; Swets, 1964) held, H%′ would be perfectly correlated with the sensitivity parameter *d′*. It should be also noted, since it plays a role in what follows, that the proportion of area, P(A), under ROC functions, often designated as a nonparametric counterpart of *d′*, would also be perfectly correlated with H%′. Macmillan and Creelman (1991) show, however, that most so-called nonparametric measures in SDT are actually parametric because of demonstrable implicit mathematical assumptions that may not be evident on the surface.)

Application of Classic SDT Notions to Recall: From ROC to roc Functions and Conditionalized Hits ($H|F_c$)

The proposed criterion-control technique applies the common-sense logic of SDT sketched out above, which is based on recognition measures, to free recall. The central idea is to conditionalize hit levels on a preset false-alarm level.

The term "level" instead of "rate" is used advisedly and calls for the interpolation of a technical point. In the standard ROC function, which is based on recognition, the subject makes decisions on items in a test set consisting of 50% stimulus items and 50% distractors. It is possible, therefore, to speak of "rates" because one knows the actual number of stimulus and distractor items to which the subject said "Yes." Thus, if a subject says "Yes" to 30 of the 50 stimulus items, his or her hit rate is 60%; if the subject says "Yes" to 10 of the 50 distractors, the false-alarm rate is 20%. In recall, however, we have no way of specifying the number of distractors, and so the notion of rates is inapplicable. Thus, in free recall, subjects can open-endedly vary their number of false alarms—10, 25, 50, 500—simply by varying their response productivity, and so no prespecified number of distractors can be used to calculate rate. Hence the ROC curves to be considered in free recall—*recall* operating characteristic curves—involve absolute levels, not rates of hits and false alarms. Our *recall* ROC curves, henceforth designated in lower case as *roc* curves, are defined as H = f(F), that is, number of hits as a function of number of false alarms, rather than the classic recognition ROC function, which is defined as H% = f(F%), namely, hit rate as a function of false-alarm rate. These roc curves are the basic isosensitive recall functions in the proposed criterion-controlled free-recall system. The $H | F_c$ index discussed up to now is simply the value of H for $F = F_c$.

How, in actual practice, can H be conditionalized on a fixed false-alarm level, F_c? Suppose a subject produces on one trial 25 hits and 15 false alarms, that is, 25 | 15, and on another trial, 101 hits and 105 false alarms, that is, 101 | 105. (These are the actual data of Maya for R_2 and R_{n+2}—see Chapter 6.) Obviously we cannot conditionalize on $F = 105$ since the subject did not produce that many false alarms (or responses, for that matter) in the earlier recall trial. Thus we can only conditionalize on the lower *F*, in this case, 15. We can pare-down but we cannot "pare-up."

Achieving the Target False-Alarm Level, F_c: Paring-Down Narrative Recall Texts

Confidence Ratings of Narrative Segments

Is there a rational way of paring down narrative recall text *post hoc* to suit our need? For the solution to this question, the author turned once again to techniques pioneered in classic SDT, in this case, the use of *confidence ratings* (Egan, Schulman, and Greenberg 1964; Pollack and Decker 1964). In recognition tests using this procedure, the subject is required to rate each of the test items for confidence that the item was part of the original stimulus set (rather than a member of the distractor set). Thus if a 0–3 rating scale is used, a 0 would designate no confidence; 1, low confidence; 2, moderate confidence; and 3, high confidence. The beauty of the approach is that at a later time and at the experimenter's leisure, the ratings can be collapsed to different binary ("Yes"/"No") decisions. Thus the experimenter can adopt a strict strategy on behalf of the subject and define only ratings of 3 as "Yes" and all the rest as "No." Or a laxer criterion can be adopted for the subject in which 2 or 3 responses count as "Yes" and only 0 and 1 as "No." The laxer criterion will produce more hits—but also more false alarms. By probing the full range of possible binary cuts, from most permissive to the strictest, the experimenter generates, on a post hoc basis, a set of "Yes"/"No" responses, which when evaluated against the items rated translate into hits ("Y" | stimulus) and false alarms ("Y" | distractor). From the pairs of H% and F% values thus generated for each binary cut, a standard ROC function can be plotted.

The tactic just described for recognition is applied to recall in the proposed criterion-control technique. After the subject has produced his or her narrative free recall, the experimenter requests that each segment—say, each sentence—be assigned a confidence rating. At a later time, once the false-alarm target, F_c, is defined (in Maya's example, $F_c = 15$), the experimenter sets out to prune the recall text of low-confidence segments until F_c is achieved. The logic of the procedure is that had the subject been asked to pare down the text, the subject would have cut out the segments of which he or she was least confident. Thus the experimenter would start by cutting 0-rated segments first, then move on to 1-rated segments, and so forth, until the pruned recall text reached the target F_c. The number of hits remaining in the adjusted text is H', that is, H | (F=15) for this recall text.

Scoring for Hits and False Alarms: Entrails Readings and Word Counts

Two practical issues remained to be resolved. The first is how to score narrative texts for hits and false alarms. This problem, worked out by Michael Halberstam and the author, has a surprisingly simple solution. We began with a decidedly unwieldy approach: a "clinical" (subjective) content scoring of recall protocols. The original, "War of the Ghosts" story (see Chapter 6) was segmented into 31 content units, each of which was scored for both hits and false alarms by the rater on a scale of 0–4 on the basis of the extent, in his judgment, that the narrative recall accurately rendered the contents of the unit (hit rating) and the extent the recall distorted it (false-alarm rating). The 0–4 ratings for both hits and intrusions for each of the 31 stimulus segments were summed to provide an overall H and F score. Halberstam (the judge) felt uncomfortable with the procedure, which, despite the author's repeated assurances based on past successes with subjective scoring (e.g., Haber & Erdelyi [1967]), Halberstam felt was unacceptably arbitrary—"like reading chicken entrails," he once complained. We had avoided more objective, "wooden-headed" approaches like word-counts because these would mindlessly miss the basic semantic structure, let alone the nuances of the narrative recall text.

Eventually, we decided to compare the "entrails readings" to the "wooden-headed" word counts. Perhaps there might be a significant correlation—the author had hoped for something in the 0.50 ballpark—which would sufficiently validate the subjective ratings until another judge could blindly rate the same material and permit calculations of interjudge reliability (which, based on past experience, the author expected to exceed $r = 0.80$). We randomly sampled 10 narrative recall protocols that had been already rated subjectively and carried out a straightforward word-count scoring of these recalls against "The War of the Ghosts." The 334 words in the story were alphabetically ordered in a scoring list that included word repetitions (see Table A.1). A copy of this list of 334 words was used for scoring each narrative recall. For each recall text, every word was checked, in order, against the alphabetized stimulus list and if the word was found it was underlined in the recall text to indicate that the recalled word was a hit. (Hence, all non-underlined words are false-alarms.) Every time a word correspondence was achieved, the word was crossed out from the stimulus list so that the subject would not get hits by repeating a word more often than it occurred in the story text. (Thus, "Indian" occurs one time in the story and the subject could garner a maximum of one hit by recalling the word "Indian" in his or her recall. If, however, the subject produced "Indian" two times, the first "Indian" would be counted a hit and the second one a false-alarm.) In sum, H, the number of hits, was defined as the number of word correspondences between recall text and story text.

We were astonished at the correlations found between the subjective scores and the word-count scores: For H, $r = 0.96$ and for F (number of false alarms), $r = 0.92$. Indeed, if an extremely short and an extremely long made-up recall protocol was added to the 10 recall narratives so as to increase variability in recall length, the correlations approached 0.99. Apparently, the subjective scoring—as done by Halberstam, at least—constituted an implicit word count. We naturally decided to drop the subjective scoring (which has poor face validity among experimentalists—and some scorers) in favor of the purely mechanical—indeed, computer scorable—word-count procedure. What would have been an inevitably suspect scoring scheme became the completely objective word-correspondence count.

The Circumvention of Confidence Ratings by Actual Per-Segment Hits and False-Alarms

The second problem, also tackled collaboratively by Halberstam and the author, was the intrusiveness and, even refractoriness of confidence ratings. How could one sensibly ask a 6-year-old to provide confidence ratings, when even college students often fail to grasp the idea? Moreover, in multitrial recall experiments such as we were conducting, early ratings almost surely influence later recall performance (and, of course, later ratings). Our solution—one of the most satisfying, if also most risky

TABLE A.1 "The War of the Ghosts" alphabetized into its 334 constituent words, with word repetitions included, used for word-count scoring of each of the narrative recalls

Order #	WORD	Order #	WORD	Order #	WORD
42	a	160	but	140	gone
53	a	198	but	235	had
174	a	231	but	216	has
256	a	30	calm	113	have
266	accompanied	57	came	139	have
303	all	184	came	143	he
93	along	317	came	220	he
127	along	69	canoe	226	he
21	and	80	canoe	234	he
29	and	120	canoe	259	he
36	and	56	canoes	300	he
50	and	240	canoes	305	he
59	and	70	coming	312	he
66	and	325	contorted	332	he
81	and	331	cried	33	heard
165	and	35	cries	61	heard
189	and	334	dead	203	heard
194	and	227	did	51	hid
245	and	296	did	252	his
254	and	85	do	320	his
258	and	134	do	322	his
262	and	14	down	218	hit
269	and	185	down	293	hit
280	and	314	down	164	home
294	and	12	egulac	213	home
304	and	244	egulac	253	house
330	and	46	escaped	19	hunt
95	are	261	everybody	112	i
117	are	323	face	123	i
224	are	229	feel	128	i
115	arrows	298	feel	138	i
116	arrows	313	fell	265	i
250	ashore	277	fellows	291	i
285	attacked	193	fight	295	i
242	back	273	fight	78	in
130	be	257	fire	118	in
27	became	76	five	215	indian
306	became	28	foggy	41	is
324	became	11	from	26	it
217	been	5	ghosts	302	it
236	been	225	ghosts	328	jumped
191	began	268	ghosts	181	kalama
52	behind	126	go	131	killed
264	behold	150	go	197	killed
316	black	212	go	279	killed
141	but	96	going	288	killed

(continued)

TABLE A.1 Cont.

Order #	WORD	Order #	WORD	Order #	WORD
136	know	162	other	108	the
210	let	178	other	119	the
54	log	276	our	147	the
255	made	318	out	156	the
101	make	65	paddles	161	the
202	man	44	party	166	the
248	man	105	people	171	the
195	many	183	people	177	the
274	many	327	people	182	the
281	many	199	presently	187	the
149	may	209	quick	200	the
39	maybe	307	quiet	206	the
10	men	133	relatives	239	the
77	men	163	returned	246	the
110	men	17	river	267	the
158	men	99	river	309	the
129	might	172	river	326	the
321	mouth	311	rose	73	them
132	my	83	said	152	them
7	night	111	said	31	then
114	no	122	said	25	there
63	noise	144	said	74	there
125	not	233	said	23	they
135	not	263	said	32	they
228	not	290	said	37	they
297	not	67	saw	45	they
55	now	208	say	60	they
219	now	20	seals	82	they
3	of	49	shore	121	they
64	of	237	shot	190	they
107	of	230	sick	223	they
155	of	299	sick	232	they
180	of	179	side	289	they
205	of	153	so	87	think
275	of	238	so	40	this
282	of	315	something	283	those
319	of	310	sun	38	thought
222	oh	91	take	221	thought
103	on	214	that	15	to
169	on	1	the	18	to
176	on	4	the	47	to
6	one	16	the	72	to
68	one	48	the	90	to
106	one	62	the	100	to
154	one	79	the	146	to
204	one	98	the	173	to
148	other	104	the	186	to

TABLE A.1 Cont.

Order #	WORD	Order #	WORD	Order #	WORD
192	to	102	war	278	were
243	to	167	warriors	287	were
251	to	207	warriors	84	what
272	to	292	was	308	when
260	told	333	was	137	where
301	told	188	water	22	while
175	town	88	we	284	who
145	turning	94	we	124	will
8	two	270	we	89	wish
58	up	13	went	151	with
71	up	159	went	86	you
97	up	168	went	92	you
170	up	241	went	142	you
329	up	249	went	9	young
211	us	271	went	109	young
286	us	24	were	157	young
2	war	75	were	201	young
34	war	196	were	247	young
43	war				

in the project—was to cut the Gordian knot, as it were, and dispense with overt confidence ratings altogether. We reasoned that the subject's actual performance in each recall segment (a line of recall in our study) would be correlated with the subject's confidence ratings for the segment.

Thus, recall performance on each line became the basis for pruning recall texts to a desired F_c. There are a number of ways of defining performance per line—for example, H, H – F, H/(H + F), F—but they all amount to the same relative measure as long as the number of words per line is approximately constant, which is easy to arrange with typed texts by setting left and right margins. (The measures mentioned would be perfectly correlated if the number of words per line were actually set equal.)

In our laboratory, we have usually taken F per line as an inverse indicator of recall quality (and presumed confidence rating). Thus, in lines averaging seven words (we usually allow few words per line), a line with F = 6 would be treated as poorer—and dropped earlier—than one with F = 5. In case of ties, we look at H to decide (for example, 5|3 is treated as superior to 4|3). (If both the H and F are equal, the line closest to the top is usually treated as better—a not altogether arbitrary rule since the first few lines typically are the best; more recently we have also given high priority to the last three lines to take advantage of both ends of the serial-position curve.)

Implementing the CCFR Procedure: Illustration of the Computation of $H|F_c$

The criterion-control procedure is illustrated with Maya's R_2 and R_n in Tables A.2 and A.3. Underlined words indicate correspondences between recall text and

TABLE A.2 Maya's R_2

		H	F
1	One night some men were	4	1
2	walking. They heard a crowd	3	2
3	scream. The men heard them	4	1
4	screaming. They rushed and	2	2
5	tried to find where the people	4	2
6	were screaming. At last, they	2	3
7	found them. They were on top	4	2
8	of the highest hill.	2	2
	Total H|F	25|15	
	Adjusted H: H| (F_c = 15)	25|15	

TABLE A.3 Maya's R_n (note, $R_n = R_{10}$)

		H	F	Order of line cut
1	One night three men heard	4	1	
2	a crowd scream for help. It	2	4	8
3	was the Indians calling for	3	2	
4	help. They were trapped from	2	3	14
5	the new hunting dog that came	4	3	
6	in town this morning. They	4	1	
7	rushed to find out what it	4	2	
8	was. They did not hear about	5	1	
9	the hunting dog. All they	3	2	
10	wanted to know is what was	3	3	15
11	happening. One man was near	2	3	13
12	by and the man told him what	4	3	16
13	was happening. The Indians	1	3	10
14	were in trouble because the	2	3	12
15	dog was not supposed to hunt	2	4	7
16	other animals besides rabbits	1	3	9
17	and deers. It was supposed to	2	4	6
18	hunt birds, tigers, and wild	1	4	4
19	bears. The three men wanted	2	3	11
20	to know what was this dog	1	5	2
21	business doing around here and	2	4	5
22	why was it hunting Indians.	0	5	1
23	They all cried. One of the	5	1	
24	men said, "I guess because the	4	2	
25	cooks needed more food."	0	4	3
	Total H|F	63|73		
	Adjusted H: H| (F_c = 15)	36|15		

stimulus text (hits); non-underlined words are errors (false alarms). First, each line of text is scored for H and F (see columns to the right of the text). For total H and F for the entire recall protocol, the per-line H's and F's are summed. Since the lowest total F was produced in R_2 (F = 15), the paring-down targets this F value. Thus, F_c = 15.

For R_n (Table A.3), the order of line-cuts is indicated in the rightmost column. The worst lines, defined by the highest F's per line, are, as explained above, cut first, and the cutting is continued (in this case up to 16 of the 25 lines) until F_c = 15. (In actual practice, one often cannot get the exact F_c because the dropping of the last line cuts F below the target F_c and the keeping of the line leaves the F value a trifle higher than F_c. This obviously is a small point. We have taken to dropping a fraction of a line when necessary and prorating F's and H's: A fraction of the F's in the line are cut so that the exact F_c is achieved and a corresponding fraction of the line's H's is then also cut.)

Empirical Validation of the CCFR

With the basic procedure outlined, empirical validation becomes the critical issue. The first set of studies evaluated the idea that performance does correlate with confidence ratings. In several probes conducted by Merryl Feigin-Pfau and the author, we correlated F's per line with confidence ratings per line for a number of subjects. The *r*'s varied substantially across subjects, averaging around a significant but not overly large $r = -0.30$. It was not clear whether the subjects, most of them taken from the subject pool, always understood the task or if they executed it seriously when they did. In any case, the relation becomes more impressive ($r = -0.60$ or better) when F's are aggregated (and averaged) for each confidence level. Thus, the average F for high-confidence lines tends to be low, and the average F for low-confidence lines tends to be high. From preliminary work, it appears that even higher correlations will be obtained when the notion of confidence is more optimally conveyed to the subject. But even at this juncture, the bypassing of the intrusive confidence ratings seems to be empirically justified.

A more basic issue is whether the $H|F_c$ measure is really a criterion controlled index of free-recall. Can we, for example, be sure that Maya's adjusted recall scores are in fact criterion controlled?

A very interesting, if inconvenient point arises in this connection: The procedure cannot be evaluated, as in recognition memory, by simply comparing the criterion-controlled recalls of two groups of subjects, one given lax and the other strict recall instructions. In classic (recognition-based) SDT tests, the subject's task is to decide whether to say "Yes" or "No" to a particular level of detection or memory. In recall-based analyses, the subject does not have a set level of detection or memory over the testing period as in recognition memory, since recall level (unlike recognition level) trends upward with retrieval time. Thus, as proposed by Erdelyi, Finks, and Feigin-Pfau (1989), two decision criteria are at play in recall: (1) At what point in time to *stop retrieval effort* and then (2) whether or not to *produce overt recall* for each more or less uncertain remembered item (this being the traditional criterion issue).

It is the latter, traditional type of criterion we wish to control, which concerns response productivity. Our specific experimental questions was whether a group of control subjects instructed to fabricate a large number of responses beyond those produced by a group of experimental subjects (ones actually recalling the story) and who, consequently, produce more hits and false alarms than the experimental subjects, will be successfully dealt with by the criterion control procedure.

Several studies have been carried out by the author and his students (Merryl Feigin-Pfau, Marcos Ionescu, Jacqueline Bergstein, Joyce Finks, and Vermone Wong) but only the most recent one (with Vermone Wong) will be summarized, although all of them proved successful. In this last study two groups of experimental subjects (the low- and high-memory groups) were first exposed to "The War of the Ghosts"—one of them once and the other twice—and then required to produce a narrative recall of the material. It is assumed that the group exposed to the story twice had better memory for the story, on the average, than the group expose to it only once. The recalls of both experimental groups were then transcribed and six blank lines were inserted in the middle and at the end of each recall text. Control subjects who had never been exposed to "The War of the Ghosts" were each yoked to one of the transcribed experimental recalls with interspersed lines. (Each of these recall texts, of course, varied in length.) These yoked subjects were instructed to fabricate story materials in the interspersed lines in such a way that when their interpolated fabrications were typed in, a blind judge would not be able to distinguish between the original recall narrative and the interweaved fabrications. The task was presented as a verbal game and (for once) the subjects found it both challenging and fun. The critical point is that the control subjects fabricated a large amount of extra material that fit in with the context of the original recall narrative and, consequently, as will be seen, produced many more hits as well as false alarms.

Thus, there were four groups in all: two experimental groups (X_1, X_2), which read the story once or twice, and two corresponding control group of subjects (Y_1, Y_2), who copied the recall productions of an experimental counterpart to whom they were yoked. Since the yoked subjects, as instructed, added a very large number of fabrications to the experimental subjects' recalls, they were bound to produce many more hits—but also many more false alarms—than the experimental subjects. The experimental question was whether the CCFR would "cure" the criterion "disease"—too many spurious hits, too many false alarms—without killing the true memory effect (the true memory difference between the high- and low-memory experimental subjects).

The average number of hits produced by the high-memory group (X_2) was 161 (with $F = 50$); the low-memory group (X_1) garnered 114 hits (with $F = 38$). Thus the raw, uncontrolled hit levels are consistent with the expectation that the experimental group exposed to the story twice would recall more story items than the group that was exposed to the story only once. But now let us consider the control subjects yoked to each of these two groups of experimental subjects. The Y_2 subjects (control subjects yoked to X_2 subjects) produced some 196 hits (and 132 false alarms); the Y_1 subjects (yoked to X_1 subjects) produced 157 hits (and 117 false alarms).

Now, we know that the yoked subjects could not have better memory for "The War of the Ghosts" than the experimental subjects since the yoked subjects never saw the story. Still, they substantially exceeded in hit levels the performance of their experimental counterparts (see Figure A.2) because of successful guessing—but at the expense of a binge in false alarms. The acid test of the CCFR procedure is whether it corrects for this excess of hits due to successful fabrications; that is, after the criterion control, the yoked subjects should not be substantially different in hit level from their experimental counterparts. If the CCFR succeeds in this basic goal, it is still crucial that the cure should not be too toxic to the true effects; that is, the criterion control should not destroy the true memory difference between the high- and low-memory experimental subjects. It turns out that the CCFR "medicine" was highly successful on both counts.

The conditionalized hits $(H|F_c)$, as noted earlier, represent only one point on an isosensitive roc function (the roc function being defined, simply, as the functional relation between hit level and false-alarm level, that is, $H = f[F]$). It may be desirable, especially if one worries about too much error variance being associated with a single point, to assess the criterion control's effect by plotting the entire roc functions for the four groups. These roc functions are generated by selecting a range of F's and determining the average H levels that corresponds to each of the F's probed. As shown in Figure A.2, for the X_1 group, a false-alarm level, F, of around

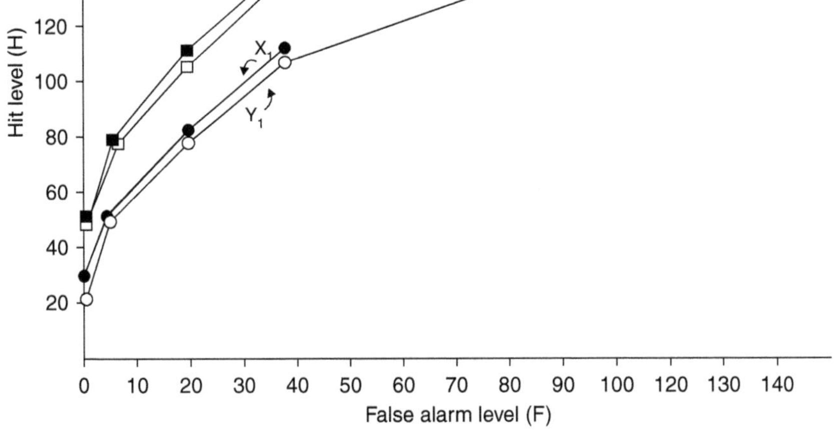

FIGURE A.2 The roc functions for the low- and high-memory experimental groups (X_1 and X_2) and their two yoked counterparts (Y_1 and Y_2).

38 is associated with a hit level, H, of around 114, and for the X_2 group, a false-alarm level, F, of around 50, is associated with a hit level of around 161.

The roc plots are very clear. The high- and low-memory experimental subjects produce two different isosensitive functions that distinguish the groups, as expected. For any false-alarm level chosen, $H|F_c$ is consistently greater for the high-memory subjects than for the low-memory subjects. Thus, the CCFR does not kill true memory effects. What it does do, apparently most effectively, is to eliminate illusory memory differences due to lax response criteria, that is, fabrications: There is no question, despite the substantial H difference between the yoked and experimental subjects that, in fact, the yoked subjects' recall scores are no different than their experimental counterparts'—they generate the same roc functions. Thus, for any F_c chosen, the yoked subjects have the same H as their experimental counterparts.

Alternatives to the $H|F_c$ Index of Criterion-Controlled Free Recall

The author will conclude this appendix with a few finer-grained issues. First, SDT experts may be jolted by the positive H levels associated with F = 0. This is neither an error nor a problem. We are not dealing with hit *rates* but with hit *levels*, and the positive H values for F = 0 simply mean that on the average subjects produced 2 or 3 perfect lines, that is, lines with only hits and no false alarms. Therefore, these lines—and the hits contained in them—did not have to be dropped when the target $F_c = 0$.

Another detail question, which may have already occurred to the reader, is which F target one should choose for the $H|F_c$ index. The smooth regularity of the roc functions suggests that it does not much matter. It is best to avoid extremely low F_c's (0, 1, maybe 5) because error variances associated with them might be high. (Also, high F_c's have to be avoided because not all subjects produce a large number of F's.) Still, a careful researcher might want to probe several F_c targets to ensure that the resulting $H|F_c$'s are consistent. Or better still, one could average $H|F_c$'s associated with different F_c's.

More Sophisticated Measures of CCFR: p(a)

The above averaging tactic suggests an even more desirable solution: Rather than average $H|F_c$'s associated with a handful of F_c's, why not average $H|F_c$'s for *all* F_c's? This, of course, would be infinitely tedious; the conceptual counterpart would be to take the area under the roc function in question. That is, integrate the roc function within a reasonable range of F (from F = 0 to $F = F_n$) and divide by A_{max}, the area that a perfect roc would produce (the area would be that of a rectangle, the maximum possible H multiplied by F_n). This measure ($\int f(F)dF/A_{max}$) is the counterpart of P(A) in classic ROC functions. With computers, each subject's data could be fitted with the appropriate roc function, integrated and then divided by A_{max}, for an index we may designate as p(a).

Of course, these programs have to be written and most researchers might prefer to avoid the complications of curve fitting and integration. A simple solution seems to have turned up. Vermone Wong and the author have found that when the H and F levels are transformed to logarithmic scales—when the roc functions are plotted on log–log graph paper—that the curvilinear functions straighten out into linear functions. Thus, if verified, log H = m(log F) + *c*, where *m* is the slope of the linear function and *c* the *y*-intercept (in this case, the H-intercept). The computation of the area under such a linear function reduces to the computation of the area of a triangle and the area of a rectangle. Thus for parsimonious purists, a fine index of true recall might turn out to be p(a) calculated on logarithms of H and F which we may designate $p_1(a)$.

Because of the impressive regularity of the roc functions, however, these alternative indices of true recall may turn out to be unnecessary, and the commonsensical conditionalized hit-level index, $H | F_c$, or H′, serve as the standard measure of CCFR.

Simplistic Alternatives to $H|F_c$ and p(a): Shortcuts to Dead Ends

This appendix concludes with a consideration of potentially simpler approaches to CCFR—and why they are not likely to be adequate:

1. *Why not use H – F as the criterion-controlled free recall?* The answer is that, because *roc* curves are not linear, hits minus false alarms, unlike $H | F_c$ or p(a), do not yield a constant estimate of sensitivity for different levels of productivity.
2. *Why not use some proportion measure, such as H | F or H | (H + F)?* The defect here is the same as that described above; these ratios would not remain constant with different levels of productivity, as $H | F_c$ does.
3. *Why not use standard SDT recognition techniques to evaluate memory level?* Because, as noted already, traditional SDT, which is based on recognition measures, is not equipped to handle narrative free-recall. Besides, recognition level is often not correlated with recall level, and phenomena such as hypermnesia that are robust with recall are hard or impossible to get with standard recognition (see Chapter 6; Bergstein & Erdelyi, 2008).
4. *Why not randomly drop responses until a desired response number is achieved?* Again, because the resulting H′ would not be constant for different levels of response productivity. This fact can be appreciated (again) from the fact that roc functions are not linear and dropping responses from an initial high number of responses (rightmost region of the roc functions) would result in a smaller loss of hits than dropping responses from an initially low number of responses (left-most region of the roc functions). Another way of putting it is that a conservative recall effort is likely to have a relatively high density of hits; an extremely lax recall effort, say one with 500 guessed words thrown in, would be relatively sparse in hits. To subtract randomly some constant number of responses would penalize the richer conservative recall text.

5. *Why not drop lines from the bottom of recall protocols until a desired number of recall responses is reached?* This would not be a bad idea if subjects reserved their poorest responses to the end. Serial position curves suggest that this is not likely, so that dropping lines from the bottom is bound to yield the loss of some of the better recalls. Dropping lines from the middle of the text might be a better idea, but not as good an idea as empirically evaluating the quality of lines and dropping the ones that are actually the poorest or least confident ones, which is what $H|F_c$ does.

It is possible that some other simple procedure will emerge. In that case it may replace the $H|F_c$ index. On the other hand, the $H|F_c$ index is simple enough and conceptually compelling.

REFERENCES

Abelson, R. (1995). *Statistics as principled argument. Psychological Press.*

Adams, J. K. (1957). Laboratory studies of behavior without awareness. *Psychological Review, 54,* 383–405.

Alessandria, M., Vetrugno, R., Cortelli, P., & Montagna, P. (2011). Normal body scheme and absent phantom limb experience in amputees while dreaming. *Consciousness and Cognition, 20,* 1831–1834. http://dx.doi,org/10.1016/j.concog.2008.01.005

Algee-Hewitt, M., Heuser, R., & Moretti, F. (2017).On paragraphs: Scales, themes, and narrative form. In F. Moretti (Ed.), *Canon/Archive: Studies in quantitative formalism from the Stanford Literary Lab* (pp. 65–94). n+1 Books.

Allport, G.W. (1937). *Personality: A psychological interpretation.* Holt, Rinehart and Winston.

Alkadhi, H., Brugger, P., Boendermaker, S. H., Crelier, G., Curt, A., Hepp-Reymond, M-C., Kollias, S. S. (2005). What disconnection tells about motor imagery: Evidence from paraplegic patients. *Cerebral Cortex, 15* (2), 131–140. https://doi.org/10.1093/cercor/bhh116

Allers, R., & Teler, J. (1960). On the utilization of unnoticed impressions in associations. In J. Wolff, D. Rapaport, and S. Annin (Eds. and Trans.), *Psychological Issues* (Vol. 3, pp. 121–154). (Monograph 7, Original work published 1924).

American Psychiatric Association. (2013). *Diagnostic and statistical manual of mental disorders* (3rd ed.). American Psychiatric Association/DSM-5.

Anderson, J. R. (1983). *The architecture of cognition.* Cambridge, MA: Harvard University Press.

Anderson, J. R., & Bower, G. H. (1973). *Human associative memory.* Washington, DC: Winston.

Andrews-Hanna, J. R. (2012). The brain's default network and its adaptive role in internal mentation. *The Neuroscientist, 18* (3), 251–270.

Andrews, M., Vigliocco, G., & Vinson, D. (2009). Integrating experiential and distributional data to learn semantic representations. *Psychological Review, 116,* 463–498.

Antrobus, J. (1991). Dreaming: Cognitive processing during activation and high afferent thresholds. *Psychological Review, 98,* 96–121.

Arieti, S. (1974). *Interpretation of schizophrenia.* NY: Basic Books.

Arnulf, I. (2011). Walking dreams in congenital and acquired paraplegia. *Consciousness and Cognition, 20* (4), 1425–1432. DOI: 10.1016/j.concog.2011.05.015

Arnulf, I. (2019, June 21-25). *Parasomnia: A window into [the] dreaming process.* [Keynote presentation]. 36th Annual International Dream Conference of the International Association for the Study of Dreams, Rolduc Monastery, Kerkrade, The Netherlands.

Aserinsky, E., & Kleitman, N. (1953). Regularly occurring periods of eye motility, and concomitant phenomena during sleep. *Science, 118*, 273–274.

Aserinsky, E., & Kleitman, N. (1955). Two types of ocular motility during sleep. *Journal of Applied Physiology, 8,* 1–10.

Ballard, P. B. (1913). Oblivescence and reminiscence. *British Journal of Psychology* 1 (Monograph supplement).

Banaji, M. R., & Greenwald, A. G. (2013). *Blindspot: Hidden biases of good people.* New York, NY: Delacorte Press.

Bandura, A. (1977). *Social learning theory.* Englewood Cliffs, NJ: Prentice-Hall.

Bandura, A., Ross, D., & Ross, S. A. (1963). Imitation of film-mediated aggressive models. *Journal of Abnormal and Social Psychology, 66*, 3–11.

Barrett, D. (2001). *The committee of sleep.* Crown/Random House.

Barett, D. (2020). *Pandemic dreams.* Middletown, DE: Oneiroi Press.

Bartlett, F. C. (1932). *Remembering.* Cambridge: Cambridge University Press.

Bell, A. P., & Hall, C. S. (1971). *The personality of a child molester: An analysis of dreams.* Chicago: Aldine and Atherton.

Berger, A. (1929). *Über das Elektrenkephalogramm des Menschen.* Archiv für Psychiatrie und Nervenkrankheiten, *87*, 527–570.

Bergstein, J., & Erdelyi, M. H. (2008). Recognition hypermnesia: How to get it. *Memory, 16,* 689–702.

Bettelheim, B. (1974). *The uses of enchantment: The meaning and importance of fairy tales.* New York, NY: Vintage Books.

Blagrove, M., Henley-Einion, J., Barnett, A., Edwards, D., Seage, C. H. (2011). A replication of the 5-7day dream-lag effect with comparisons of dreams to future events as control for baseline meaning. *Consciousness and Cognition, 20,* 384–391. DOI: 10.1016/j.concog.2010.07.006

Blagrove, M., Fouquet, N. C., Henley-Einion, J. A., Pace-Schott, E. F., Davies, A. C., Neuschaffer, J. L., & Turnbull, O. H. (2011b). Assessing the dream-lag effect for REM and NREM Stage 2 dreams. PLoS ONE 6(10): e26708. doi:10.1371/journal.pone.0026708

Broca, P. (1861). Perte de la Parole, ramollissement chronique et destruction partielle du lobe antérieur gauche du cerveau. *Bulletin de la Société Anthropologique, 2*, 235–238.

Brower, R. A. (Ed.) (1959). William Butler Yeats: 1865-1929. In G. B. Harrison (Gen. Ed.), *Major British Writers: Enlarged Edition II* (pp. 779–818). Harcourt: Brace and Company.

Boucetta S, Cissé Y, Mainville L, Morales M, & Jones B.E. (2014). Discharge profiles across the sleep-waking cycle of identified cholinergic, GABAergic, and glutamatergic neurons in the pontomesencephalic tegmentum of the rat. *Journal of Neuroscience, 34* (13), 4708–4727. DOI: 10.1523/JNEUROSCI.2617-13.2014. PMID: 24672016; PMCID: PMC3965793.

Bootzin, R. R., Acocella, J. R., & Alloy, L. B. (1993). Abnormal psychology: Current perspectives (6th ed.). McGraw-Hill. [Quoted from Sheehan S. (1982). *Is there no place on earth for me?* Houghton Mifflin].

Bosch H. (ca 1500). *The Garden of Earthly Delights.* Museo del Prado.

Bransford, J. D., & Franks, J. J. (1977). The abstraction of linguistic ideas. *Cognitive Psychology, 2*, 331–350.

Braun, A. R., Balicin, T. J., Wesenten, N. J., Carson, R. E., Varga, M., Baldwin, P., et al. (1997). Regional cerebral blood flow throughout the sleep-wake cycle: An $H_2{}^{15}O$ PET study. *Brain, 120,* 1173–1197.

Braun, A. R., Balicin, T. J., Wesenten, N. J., Gwadry, F., et al. (1998). Dissociated pattern of activity in visual cortices and their projections during human rapid eye movement sleep. *Science, 279*, 91–95.

Bregman, E. O. (1934). An attempt to modify the emotional attitudes of infants by the conditioned response technique. *The Pedagogical Seminary and Journal of Genetic Psychology, 45*, 169–198. https://doi.org/10.1080/08856559.1934.10534254

Breland, K., & Breland, M. (1961). The misbehavior of organisms. *American Psychologist, 16*, 681–684.

Breuer, J., & Freud, S. (1955). *Studies on hysteria.* In J. Strachey (Ed. and Trans.), *The standard edition of the complete psychological works of Sigmund Freud* (Vol. 2). Hogarth Press. (Original work published 1893–1895).

Bricker, P. D., & Chapanis, A. (1953). Do incorrectly perceived tachistoscopic stimuli convey some information? *Psychological Review, 60* (3), 181–188. https://doi.org/10.1037/h0054901

Brill, A. A. (1938). *The basic writings of Sigmund Freud.* New York, NY: Modern Library/Random House.

Broca, P . (1861). [Remarques sur le siége de la faculté du langage articulé, suivies d'une observation d'aphémie (perte de la parale).] (C. D. Green, Trans.). [Remarks on the Seat of the Faculty of Articulated Language, Following an Observation of Aphemia (Loss of Speech).] *Bulletin de la Société Anatomique, 6*, 330–357.

Brown, J. W. (1973). *Aphasia, apraxia, and agnosia: Clinical and theoretical aspects* Springfield, IL: Charles C. Thomas.

Brugger, P. (2008). The phantom limb in dreams. *Consciousness and Cognition, 17*(4), 1272–1278. https://doi.org/10.1016/j.concog.2008.01.005

Bulkeley, K. (2014). Digital dream analysis: A revised method. *Consciousness and Cognition, 29*. https://doi.org/10.1016/j.concog.2014.08.015

Bulkeley, K. (2018). The meaningful continuities between dreaming and waking: Results of a blind analysis of a woman's 30-year dream journal. *Dreaming,* 28 (4), 337–350. https://doi.org/10.1037/drm0000083

Buckner, R. L., Andrews-Hanna, J. R., & Schacter, D. L. (2008). *The brain's default network: Anatomy, function, and relevance to disease.* In A. Kingstone & M. B. Miller (Eds.), *Annals of the New York Academy of Sciences: Vol. 1124. The year in cognitive neuroscience 2008* (pp. 1–38). Malden: Blackwell Publishing.

Calkins, M. W. (1893). Statistics of dreams. *The American Journal of Psychology 5* (3), 311–343.

Cardeña, E. (2018). The experimental evidence for parapsychological phenomena: A review. *American Psychologist, 73* (5), 663–677. http://dx.doi.org/10.1037//amp0000236

Carroll, L. (1865; 1871). *Alice's adventures in wonderland; Through the looking glass.* In M. Gardner (Ed.). (1960). *The annotated Alice: Alice's adventures in wonderland* and *Through the looking glass*. New York, NY: Wings Books.

Castañeda, C. (1981). *The eagle's gift.* New York, NY: Washington Square Press.

Child, I. L. (1985). Psychology and anomalous observations: The question of ESP in dreams. *American Psychologist, 40* (11), 1219–1230. https://doi.org/10.1037/0003-066X.40.11.1219

Cicero, M. T. (1947). Argument against taking dreams seriously. In R. L. Woods (Ed.). *The world of dreams* (p. 199). Random House. (Original work published ca 45 BCE)

Christoff, K., Gordon, A. M., Smallwood, J., Smith, R., & Schooler, J. W. (2009). Experience sampling during fMRI reveals default network and executive system contributions to mind wandering. *Proceedings of the National Academy of Sciences of the United States of America, 2009*, 8719–8724.

Cicogna, P., & Occhionero, M. (2013). Such stuff as NREM dreams are made on? *Behavioral and Brain Sciences, 36* (6), 611–612. https://doi.org/10.1017/S0140525X13001246

Cicogna, P., & Occhionero. M. (2016). Phenomenal consciousness in dreams and in mind wandering. *Philosophical Psychology 29* (7), 1–9. DOI: 10.1080/09515089.2016.1213800

Claparède, É. (1911). Recognition et moite. *Archives de Psychologie Geneva, 11*, 79–90.

Cohen, B. D., Nachmani, G., Rosenberg, S. (1974, p. 11). *Referent communication disturbances in acute schizophrenia, 83* (1), 1–13. DOI: 10.1037/ h0036231.

Cohen, N. J., & Squire, L. R. (1980). Preserved learning and retention of pattern analyzing skill in amnesics: Dissociation of knowing how and knowing what. *Science, 210*. 207–210.

Cohen, J. (1998). *Statistical power analysis for the behavioral sciences* (2nd ed.). Hillsdale, NJ: Erlbaum.

Coenen, A. (2003). The divorce of REM sleep and dreaming. In E. F. Pace-Schott, Solms, M., Blagrove, M., & Harnad, S. (Eds.), *Sleep and dreaming: Scientific advances and reconsiderations* (pp. 133–135). Cambridge.

Collins, A. M., & Loftus, E. F. (1975). A spreading activation theory of semantic processing. *Psychological Review, 82*, 407–428.

Collins, A. M., & Quillian, M. R. (1969). Retrieval time from semantic memory. *Journal of Verbal Learning and Verbal Behavior, 8*, 240–247.

Conrad, K. (1948). Structural analysis of brain pathological cases: About Broca's motor aphasia. *Deutsche Zeitschrift für Nervenheilkunde, 159* (1–2), 132–87.

Craik, F. I. M. & Lockhart, S. (1972). Levels of processing: A framework for memory research. *Journal of Verbal Learning and Verbal Behavior, 11*, 671–684.

Cumming, G. (2012). *Understanding the new statistics: Effect sizes, confidence intervals, and meta-analysis*. New York, NY: Routledge.

Dang-Vu, T. T., Desseilles, M., Albouy, G., Darsaud, A., Gais, S., Rauchs, G., Schabus, M., Sterpenich, V., Vandewalle, G., Schwartz, S., Maquet, P. (2005). Dreaming: A neuroimaging view, *Schweizer Archiv für Neurologie und Psychiatrie, 156*, 415–425.

Darwin, C. (1859/1963). *The Origin of species*. New York, NY: Washington Square Press.

Darwin, C. (1871/1982). *The descent of man and selection in relation to sex*. Princeton, NJ: Princeton University Press.

Darwin, C. (1872; reprinted 1965). *The expression of emotions in man and animals*. Chicago: University of Chicago Press.

Delarue, P., Tenèze, M. -L. (1957). *Le conte populaire français* [The French popular tale]. Erasme.

Delaney, G. M.V. (1979). *Living your dreams: Using your sleep to solve problems and to make your best dreams come true*. San Francisco, CA: Harper & Row.

Delboeuf, J. R. L. (1855). *Le sommeil et les rêves*. Paris.

Dement, W., & Kleitman, N. (1955). Cyclic variations in EEG during sleep and their relation to eye movements, body motility, and dreaming. *Electroencephalography and Clinical Neurophysiology*, 9, 673–90. DOI: 10.1016/0013-4694(57)90088-3

Dement, W. (1976). *Some must watch while some must sleep*. Macmillan.

Dement, W., & Kleitman, N. (1957). The relation of eye movements during sleep to dream activity: An objective method for the study of dreaming. *Journal of Experimental Psychology, 53*, 339–346.

De Waal, F. (2007). *Chimpanzee Politics: Power and Sex among Apes* (Updated Edition). Johns Hopkins University Press.

Dittrich, L. (2016). *Patient H. M.: Memory, madness, and family secrets*. New York, NY: Random House.

Dollard, J., & Miller, N. (1950). *Personality and psychotherapy*. New York, NY: McGraw-Hill.

Domhoff, G. W. (1996). *Finding meaning in dreams: A quantitative approach*. New York, NY: Plenum Press.

Domhoff, G.W. (2003). *The scientific study of dreams: Neural networks, cognitive development, and content analysis*. Washington, DC: American Psychological Association.

Domhoff, G. W. (2011). Dreams are embodied simulations that dramatize conceptions and concerns: The continuity hypothesis in empirical, theoretical, and historical context. *International Journal of Dream Research, 4*, 50–62.

Domhoff, G. W. (2017). The invasion of the concept snatchers: The origins, distortions, and future of the continuity hypothesis. *Dreaming, 27*, 14–39.

Domhoff, G. W. (2018a). *The emergence of dreams*. Oxford University Press.

Domhoff, G. W. (2018b). Can Stimulus-Incorporation and Emotion-Assimilation Theorists Revive the Continuity Hypothesis they Deprived of Cognitive Meaning? A Reply to Jenkins. *Dreaming, 28* (4), 356–359. https://doi.org/10.1037/drm0000091

Domhoff G.W., & Fox, K. (2015). Dreaming and the default network: A review, synthesis, and counterintuitive research proposal. *Consciousness and Cognition, 33*, 342–353.

Domhoff G.W., & Schneider, A. (2008). Similarities and differences in dream content at the cross-cultural, gender, and individual levels. *Consciousness and Cognition, 17*, 1257–1265.

Dostoyevsky, F. (1960). C. Garnett (Trans.). *Notes from underground*. Dell. (Original work published 1864).

Dumay, N. (2015). Sleep not just protects memories against forgetting, it also makes them more accessible. *Cortex, 74*, 289–296. DOI: 10.1016/j.cortex.2015.06.007

Ebbinghaus, H. (1984). H. A. Ruger and C. E. Bussenius (Trans.). *Memory*. Dover. (Original work published 1885).

Edlow, B. L., Takahashi, E., Wu, O., Benner, T., Dai, G., Bu, L., Grant, P. E., Greer, D. M., Greenberg, S. M., Kinney, H. C., & Folkerth, R.D. (2012). Neuroanatomic connectivity of the human ascending arousal system critical to consciousness and its disorders. *Journal of Neuropathology & Experimental Neurology, 71* (6), 531–46. DOI: 10.1097/NEN.0b013e3182588293.

Egan, J. P., Schulman, A. I., & Greenberg, G. Z. (1964). Operating characteristics determined by binary decisions and by ratings. In Swets, J. A. (Ed.), *Signal detection and recognition in human observers*. New York, NY: Wiley.

Eichenlaub, J.-B., van Rijn, E., Phelan, M., Ryder, L., Gaskell, M. G., Lewis, P. A., Walker, M. P., & Blagrove, M. (2019). The nature of delayed dream incorporation ('dream-lag effect'): Personally significant events persist, but not major daily activities or concerns. *Journal of Sleep Research, 28* (1), 1–8.

Ekman, P., & Friesen, W.V. (1975). *Unmasking the face: A guide to recognizing emotions from facial clues*. Englewood Cliffs, NJ: Prentice-Hall.

Ellenberger, H. F. (1970). *The discovery of the unconscious*. Simon and Schuster.

Ellis, P. D. (2010). *The essential guide to effect sizes: Statistical power, meta-analysis, and the interpretation of research results*. Cambridge: Cambridge University Press.

Epstein, A.W. (1985). The waking event-dream interval. *American Journal of Psychiatry, 142* (1), 123–124. DOI: 10.1176/ajp.142.1.123.

Epstein, S. (1977). Traits are alive and well. In D. Magnusson & N. S. Endler (Eds.), *Personality at the crossroads: Current issues in interactional psychology* (pp. 83–98). Hillsdale, NJ: Erlbaum.

Epstein, S. (1979). The stability of behavior: I. On predicting most of the people much of the time. *Journal of Personality and Social Psychology, 37*, 1097–1126.

Epstein, S., & O'Brian, E. J. (1985). The Person-Situation debate in historical and current Perspective. *Psychological Bulletin, 98* (3), 513–537

Erdelyi, M. H. (1970). Recovery of unavailable perceptual input. *Cognitive Psychology, 1*, 99–113.

Erdelyi, M. H. (1972a). The recovery effect with a nonpictorial stimulus. *Psychological Record, 22*, 395–400.

Erdelyi, M. H. (1972b). The role of fantasy in the Pötzl (emergence) phenomenon. *Journal of Personality and Social Psychology, 24*, 186–190.

Erdelyi, M. H. (1974). A new look at the New Look: Perceptual defense and vigilance. *Psychological Review, 81*, 1–25.

Erdelyi, M. H. (1985). *Psychoanalysis: Freud's cognitive psychology*: Freeman.

Erdelyi, M. H. (1986). Experimental indeterminacies in the dissociation paradigm of subliminal perception. *Behavioral and Brain Sciences, 9*, 30–31.

Erdelyi, M. H. (1994). Hypnotic hypermnesia: The empty set of hypermnesia. In F. Frankel and C. Perry (Eds.), *Hypnosis and delayed recall [Special issue]* (Vol. 42, pp. 379–390). International Journal of Clinical and Experimental Hypnosis.

Erdelyi, M. H. (1996). *The recovery of unconscious memories: Hypermnesia and reminiscence*. Chicago: University of Chicago Press.

Erdelyi, M. H. (2004). Subliminal perception and its cognates: Theory, indeterminacy, and time. *Consciousness and Cognition, 13*, 73–91; 92–117.

Erdelyi, M. H. (2006a). The unified theory of repression. *Behavioral and Brain Sciences, 29*, 499–511.

Erdelyi, M. H. (2006b). The return of the repressed. (Response to commentaries.). *Behavioral and Brain Sciences, 29*, 535–551.

Erdelyi, M. H. (2010). The ups and downs of memory. *American Psychologist, 65*, 623–633. DOI:1037/a0020440

Erdelyi, M. H. (2012). Explicit and implicit memory. In B. Barth, P. Giampieri-Deutsch, & H. D. Klein (Eds.), *Sensory perception: Mind and matter*. Springer-Verlag.

Erdelyi, M. H. (2014). The interpretation of dreams, and of jokes. *Review of General Psychology, 18* (2), 115–126.

Erdelyi, M. H. (2017). The continuity hypothesis. *Dreaming, 27*, 334–344. http://dx.doi.org/10.1037/drm0000063

Erdelyi, M. H. & Goldberg, B. (1979). Let's not sweep repression under the rug: Toward a cognitive psychology of repression. In J. F. Kihlstrom & F. J. Evans (Eds.), *Functional disorders of memory* (pp. 355–401). Hillsdale, NJ: Erlbaum.

Erdelyi, M. H., & Kleinbard, J. (1978). Has Ebbinghaus decayed with time? The growth of recall (hypermnesia) over days. *Journal of Experimental Psychology: Human Learning and Memory, 4*, 275–289.

Erdelyi, M. H. & Stein, J. B. (1981). Recognition hypermnesia: The growth of recognition memory (*d'*) over time with repeated testing. *Cognition, 9*, 23–33.

Erdelyi, M. H., & Zizak, D, M. (2004). Beyond gizmo subliminality. In L. J. Shrum (Ed.), *Blurring the lines: The psychology of entertainment media* (pp. 13–43). Hillsdale, NJ: Erlbaum.

Fenollosa, E., & Pound, E. (1936). *The Chinese written character as a medium for poetry*. San Francisco, CA: City Lights Book.

Fisher, C. (1954). Dreams and perception. *Journal of the American Psychoanalytic Association, 3*, 5–48.

Fisher, C. (1956). Dreams, images, and perception: A study of unconscious-preconscious relationships. *Journal of the American Psychoanalytic Association, 4*, 5–48.

Fisher, C. (1959). The effects of subliminal visual stimulation on images and dreams: A validation study. *Journal of the American Psychoanalytic Association, 7*, 35–83.

Fisher, C. (1960a). Introduction (pp. 1–40). In J. Wolff, D. Rapaport, & S. H. Annin (Eds. and Trans.). *Preconscious stimulation in dreams, associations, and images: Classical Studies by Otto Pötzl, Rudolf Allers, and Jakob Teler. Psychological Issues, 2* (No. 3), Monograph 7 (pp. 41–120).

Fisher, C. (1960b). Subliminal and supraliminal influences on dreams. *The American Journal of Psychiatry, 116* (11), 1009–1017.

Fisher, C. (1988). Further observations on the Poetzl phenomenon: The effects of subliminal visual stimulation on dreams, images, and hallucinations. *Psychoanalysis and Contemporary Thought, 11,* 3–56.

Fisher, C., Gross, J., & Zuch, J. (1965). Cycle of Penile Erection Synchronous With Dreaming (REM) Sleep: Preliminary Report. *Archives of General Psychiatry,* 12 (1), 29–45. DOI: 10.1001/archpsyc.1965.01720310031005

Fisher, C., Cohen, H.D., Schiavi, R.C., Davis, D., Furman, B., Ward, K., Edwards, A., & Cunningham, J. (1983). Patterns of female sexual arousal during sleep and waking: Vaginal thermo-conductance studies. *Archives of Sexual Behavior, 12,* 97–122. https://doi.org/10.1007/BF01541556

Fleeson, W. (2001). Towards a structure- and process-integrated view of personality: Traits as density distributions of states. *Journal of Personality and Social Psychology, 80,* 1011–1027.

Fleeson, W. (2004). Moving personality beyond the person-situation debate: The challenge and the opportunity of within-person variability. *Current Directions in Psychological Science, 13,* 83– 87.

Foulkes, D. (1962). Dream reports from different stages of sleep. *Journal of Abnormal and Social Psychology, 65,* 14–25.

Foulkes, D. (1978). *The grammar of dreams.* New York, NY: Basic Books.

Foulkes, D. (1999). *Children's dreaming and the development of consciousness.* Cambridge, MA: Harvard University Press.

Fox, K., Nijeboer, S., Solomonova, E., Domhoff, G. W., & Christoff, K. (2013). Dreaming as mind wandering: Evidence from functional neuroimaging and first-person content reports. *Frontiers in Human Neuroscience,* 7 (Article 412), 1–18. DOI: 10.3389/fnhum.2013.00412.eCollection 0213

Frank, B., & Lorenzoni, E. (1992). Phantomerleben und Phantomschmerz. *Fortschritte der Neurologie und Psychiatrie, 60,* 74–85.

Freud, A. (1946). *The ego and the mechanisms of defense.* (C. Baines, Trans.). International Universities Press. (Original work published 1936)

Freud, S. (1953). *On aphasia.* (E. Stengel, Trans.). International Universities Press. (Original work published 1891)

Freud, S. (1950). *Psychology for neurologists* (completed in 1895), published posthumously as the project for a scientific psychology. In J. Strachey (Ed. & Trans.). *The standard edition of the complete psychological works of Sigmund Freud* (Vol. 1, pp. 283–397). Hogarth Press, (Original work completed 1905).

Freud, S. (1953). *The interpretation of dreams.* In J Strachey (Ed. & Trans.), *The standard edition of the complete psychological works of Sigmund Freud* (Vols. 4 & 5, pp. i-338 and pp. iii-627). Hogarth Press (Original work published 1900).

Freud, S. (1953). *On dreams.* (J. Strachey, Ed. and Trans.). *The standard edition of the complete psychological works of Sigmund Freud* (Vol. 5), pp. 631-685). Hogarth Press (Original work published 1901a).

Freud, S. (1938). *The psychopathology of everyday life.* In A. A. Brill (Ed., and Trans.). *The basic writings of Sigmund Freud* (pp. 1–117). Modern Library/Random House (Original work published 1901b).

Freud, S. (1958). *Jokes and their relation to the unconscious.* In J. Strachey (Ed. and Trans.), *The standard edition of the complete psychological works of Sigmund Freud* (Vol. 8, 1–258). London: Hogarth Press. (Original work published 1905).

Freud, S. (1963). The relation of the poet to day-dreaming (I. F. Grant Duff, Trans.). In P. Rieff (Ed.), *Character and culture: The collected papers of Sigmund Freud,* pp. 34–43. Collier Books. (Original work published 1908).

Freud, S. (1955). (A. Strachey and J. Strachey, Trans.). Analysis of a phobia in a five-year old boy. In J. Srachey (Ed.), *The standard edition of the complete psychological works of Sigmund Freud* (Vol. 10, pp. 1–149). London: Hogarth Press. (Original work published 1909a).

Freud, S. (1955). (A. Strachey and J. Strachey, Trans.). Notes upon a case of obsessional neurosis. In J. Strachey (Ed.), *The standard edition of the complete psychological works of Sigmund Freud* (Vol. 10, pp. 153–318). London: Hogarth Press. (Original work published 1909b).

Freud, S. (1963). *Psycho- analytic notes upon an autobiographical account of a case of paranoia (Dementia Paranoides)* [aka *The psychotic Dr. Schreber*]. In P. Rieff (Ed.), *Three case histories.* Collier. (Original work published 1911).

Freud, S. (1963). *From the history of an infantile neurosis* [aka The Wolf Man]. In P. Rieff (Ed.), *Three case histories.* Collier. (Original work published 1911).

Freud, S. (1958). (A. Strachey and J. Strachey, Trans.). Psycho-analytic notes upon an autobiographical account of a case of paranoia (Dementia Paranoides). In J. Strachey (Ed.), *The standard edition of the complete psychological works of Sigmund Freud* (Vol. 12, pp. 3–82). London: Hogarth Press, (Original work published 1911).

Freud, S. (1958). A Note on the Unconscious in Psychoanalysis. In J. Strachey, Ed.), *The standard edition of the complete psychological works of Sigmund Freud* (Vol. 12, 255–266). London: Hogarth Press. (Original work published 1912).

Freud, S. (1957). The Unconscious. (C. M. Baines and J. Strachey, Trans.). In J. Strachey, Ed., *The standard edition of the complete psychological works of Sigmund Freud* (Vol. 12, 159–215). London: Hogarth Press. (Original work published 1915).

Freud, S. (1963). *A general introduction to psychoanalysis. (J. Riviere, Trans.). Liveright. (Original work published 1917 and, in English, 1920). Also: Introductory lectures on psychoanalysis.* In J. Strachey (Ed. and Trans.). *The standard edition of the complete psychological works of Sigmund Freud* (Vol. 15 and 16). London: Hogarth Press, 1961 and 1963. (Original work published 1917 and, in English, 1920).

Freud, S. (1955). *From the history of an infantile neurosis.* (A. Strachey and J. Strachey, Trans.). In J. Strachey (Ed.), *The standard edition of the complete psychological works of Sigmund Freud* (Vol. 17). London: Hogarth Press, 1955. (Original work published 1918; revised 1924, 1925).

Freud, S. (1955). *Beyond the pleasure principle.* In J. Strachey (Ed. and Trans.). *The standard edition of the complete psychological works of Sigmund Freud* (Vol. 18). London: Hogarth Press. (Original work published 1920).

Freud, S. (1955). *Group psychology and the analysis of the ego.* In J. Strachey (Ed. and Trans.), *The standard edition of the complete psychological works of Sigmund Freud* (Vol. 17). London: Hogarth Press, 1955. (Original work published 1921).

Freud, S. (1961). *The ego and the id.* (J. Riviere and J. Strachey, Trans.). In J. Strachey (Ed.), *The standard edition of the complete psychological works of Sigmund Freud* (Vol. 19). London: Hogarth Press. (Original work published 1923).

Freud, S. (1964a). *New introductory lectures on psycho-analysis.* In J. Strachey (Ed. and Trans.), *The standard edition of the complete psychological works of Sigmund Freud* (Vol. 22). London: Hogarth Press. (Original work published 1933).

Freud, S. (1964b). *An outline of psycho-analysis.* In J. Strachey (Ed. and Trans.), *The standard edition of the complete psychological works of Sigmund Freud* (Vol. 23). London: Hogarth Press. (Original work published 1940).

Friston, K. (2018). Does predictive coding have a future? *Nature Neuroscience, 21,* 2019–1021.

Gabrieli, J. D. E., Corkin, S., Mickel, S. F., & Growdon, J. H. (1993). Intact acquisition and long-term retention of mirror-tracing skill in Alzheimer's disease and in global amnesia. *Behavioral Neuroscience, 107,* 899–910.

Giddan, N. S. (1967). Recovery of briefly flashed stimuli through images. *Journal of Personality, 35,* 1–19.

Giordano, A., Francese, V., Peila, E., Tribolo, A., Airoldi, M., Torta, R., Mutani, R., & Cicolin, A. (2012). Dream content changes in women after mastectomy: An initial study of body imagery after disfiguring surgery. *Dreaming, 22,* 115–123.

Goldiamond, I. (1958). Indicators of perception: I. Subliminal perception, subception, unconscious perception: An analysis in terms of psychophysical indicator methodology. *Psychological Bulletin, 55,* 373–411. DOI: 10.1037/h0046992

Goodglass, H. (1993). *Understanding aphasia.* San Diego, CA: Academic Press.

Gottesman, I. I., & Hanson, D.R. (2005). Human development: Biological and genetic processes. *Annual Review of Psychology. 56,* 263–86. DOI: 10.1146/Annurev.Psych.56.091103.070208

Graf, P., & Schacter, D. L. (1985). Implicit and explicit memory for new associations in normal and amnesic subjects. *Journal of Experimental Psychology: Learning, Memory, and Cognition, 11,* 501–518.

Graf, P., Squire, L. R., & Mandler, G. (1984). The information that amnesic patients do not forget. *Journal of Experimental Psychology: Learning, Memory, and Cognition, 10,* 164–178. DOI: 10.1037//0278-7393.10.1.164.

Gray, P. (2011). *Psychology* (6th ed.). New York, NY: Worth.

Grimm, J., & Grimm, W. (1812). Little Red Cap. (In Jack Zipes [1983, Ed and trans.]. *The trials and tribulations of Little Red Riding Hood* (pp. 123–126). Bergin and Garvey.

Green, D. M., & Swets, J. A. (1966). *Signal detection theory and psychophysics.* New York, NY: Wiley.

Haber, R. N., & Erdelyi, M. H. (1967). Emergence and recovery of initially unavailable perceptual material. *Journal of Verbal Learning and Verbal Behavior, 6,* 618–628. Also, in R. N. Haber (Ed.). (1968). *Contemporary theory and research in visual perception.* Holt, Rinehart and Winston.

Hall, C. (1951). What people dream about. *Scientific American, 184,* 60–63.

Hall, C. (1953). A cognitive theory of dreams. *Journal of General Psychology, 49,* 273–282.

Hall, C., & Van De Castle, R. (1966). *The content analysis of dreams.* New York, NY: Appleton-Century-Crofts.

Hall, C., & Lind, R. (1970). *Dreams, life and literature: A study of Franz Kafka.* Chapel Hill: University of North Carolina Press.

Hall, C. S., & Nordby, V. J. (1972). *The individual and his dreams.* New York, NY: Signet.

Hall, C., Domhoff, G.W., Blick, K., & Weesner, K. (1982). The dreams of college men and women in 1950 and 1980: A comparison of dream contents and sex differences. *Sleep, 5,* 188–194.

Hartmann, E. (1968). The 90-minute sleep-dream cycle. *Archives of General Psychiatry, 18,* 280–286.

Hartmann, E. (2011). *The nature and function of dreaming.* New York, NY: Oxford University Press.

Hartmann, E., & Kunzendorf, R. (2006-07). Boundaries and dreams. *Imagination, Cognition and Personality, 26,* 101–115.

Heuser, R., Moretti, F., & Steiner, E. (2017). Mapping London's Emotions. In F. Moretti (Ed.), *Canon/Archive: Studies in quantitative formalism from the Stanford Literary Lab* (pp. 223–250). n+1 Books.

Hilgard, E. R. (1962). What becomes of the input from the stimulus?: A symposium of research and interpretation? In C. W. Eriksen (Ed.), *Behavior and awareness.* Duke University Press.

Hineline, P.N, & Rachlin H. (1969). Notes on fixed-ratio and fixed-interval escape responding in the pigeon. *Journal of the Experimental Analysis of Behavior, 12,* 397–401.

Hobson, J. A. (1988). *The dreaming brain.* New York, NY: Basic Books.

Hobson, J. A. (2002). *Dreaming: An introduction to dream science.* New York, NY: Oxford University Press.

Hobson, J. A. (2005). *13 dreams Freud never had.* New York, NY: Pi Press.

Hobson, J. A. (2011). *Dream life: An experimental memoir.* Cambridge, MA: MIT Press

Hobson, J. A. (2012). In L. Oppenheim (Conference Organizer). *Minding the gap III: Dreaming: Psychoanalysis or neurobiology?* Conference at the New York Psychoanalytic Society and Institute, at Mt. Sinai Medical Center, New York, May 5, 2012. [To appear in *Contemporary Psychoanalyis.*]

Hobson, J. A., Pace, C. F., & Stickgold, R. (2000). Dreaming and the brain: Toward a cognitive neuroscience of conscious states. *Behavioral and Brain Sciences, 23.* 793–1121.

Hobson, J. A. (2015). *Psychodynamic neurology: Dreams, consciousness, virtual reality.* Hoboken, NJ: CRC Press.

Hobson, J.A., Friston, K.J., & Hong, C.C.H. (2014). Virtual reality in waking and dreaming consciousness. *Frontiers in Psychology, 5.*

Hobson, A., & Kahn, D. (2007). Dream content: Individual and generic aspects. *Consciousness and Cognition, 16,* 850–858. DOI: 10.1016/j.concog.2007.07.010

Hobson, J. A., & McCarley, R. W. (1977). The brain as a dream-state generator: An activation-synthesis hypothesis of the dream process. *American Journal of Psychiatry, 134,* 1335–1368.

Ingvar, D. H. (1979). "Hyperfrontal" distribution of the cerebral grey matter flow in resting wakefulness; on the functional anatomy of the conscious state. *Acta Neurologica Scandivanica.* https://doi.org/10.1111/j.1600-0404.1979.tb02947.x

Jenkins, D. (2018). When is a continuity hypothesis not a continuity hypothesis? Why continuity is now a problematic name for a continuity hypothesis. *Dreaming, 28* (4), 351–355. http://dx.doi.org/10.1037/drm0000089

Jacoby, L. L., & Witherspoon, D. (1982). Remembering without awareness. *Canadian Journal of Psychology, 32,* 300–324.

James, W. (1890). *The principles of psychology.* New York, NY: Holt.

Janet, P. (1889). *L'automatisme psychologique* [*Psychological automatism*]. Paris: Alcan.

Jockers, M. L. (2013). *Macroanalysis: Digital methods and literary history.* Urbana: University of Illinois Press.

Jones, B. E. (2000). The interpretation of physiology. *Behavioral and Brain Sciences, 23,* 955–956.

Jouvet, M. (1962). Recherches sur les structures nerveuses et mechanismes responsables des differéntes phases du sommeil physologique. *Archives Italiennes de Biologie, 100,* 125–206.

Jouvet, M. (1999). *The paradox of sleep: The story of dreaming.* London: MIT

Jung, C. G. (1968). *Analytical psychology: Its theory and practice.* (Originally presented at the Tavistock Lectures.) Pantheon.

Jung, C. G. (1974) (R.F.C. Hull, Trans.) *Dreams.* New York: MJF Books.

Kaplan-Solms, K., & Solms, M. (2000). *Clinical studies in neuro-psychoanalysis.* London: Karnac Books.

Kirk, R. E. (2003). The importance of effect magnitude. In S. F. Davis (Ed.), *Handbook of research methods in experimental psychology* (pp. 83–105). Blackwell.

Klasko, R. (2018, November 27). *The New York Times* (p. D5).

Klüver, H., & Bucy, P. L. (1939). Preliminary analysis of functions of the temporal lobes in monkeys. *Archives of Neurology & Psychiatry, 42* (6), pp. 979–1000. doi:10.1001/archneur psyc.1939.02270240017001

Kookoolis, A., Pace-Schott, E. F., McNamara, P. (2010). Dream content and memory processing: Dream lag effects within a single night and across several nights: A pilot study. *Dreaming, 20,* 211–217.

Kozbelt, A., & Nishioka, K. (2010). Humor comprehension, humor production, and insight. *Humor: International Journal of Humor Research, 23,* 375–461.

Kosslyn, S. (1994). *Image and brain: The resolution of the imagery debate*. London: MIT Press.

Kramer, M. (2000). Dreaming has content and meaning, not just form. *Behavioral and Brain Sciences, 23,* 959–961.

Krippner, S. (Ed.). (1990). *Dreamtime and dreamwork: Decoding the language of the night.* New York, NY: Putnam.

Krippner, S. (2019). History of anomalous dream research. In K. Valli & R.J. Hoss (Eds.), *Dreams: Understanding biology, psychology, and culture* (Vol. 1, pp. 317–324). Santa Barbara, CA: Greenwood.

Lakoff, G., & Johnson, M. (2003). *Metaphors we live by*. Chicago: University of Chicago Press.

LeDoux, J. E. (1996). The emotional brain: The mysterious underpinnings of emotional life. New York, NY: Simon & Schuster.

LeDoux, J. E. (2016). *Anxious: Using the brain to understand and treat fear and anxiety*. Penguin.

Landauer, T., & Dumais, S. (1997). A solution to Plato's problem: The latent semantic analysis theory of acquisition, induction, and representation of knowledge. *Psychological Review, 104,* 211–240.

Leuschner, W., & Hau, S. (1992). Zum Processing künstlich induzierter Tagesreste: Eine experimentelle Studie zum Pötzl-Phänomen. Sigmund-Freud-Institut.

Leuschner, W., Hau, S., Brech, E., & Volk, S. (1994). Dissociation and reassociation of subliminally induced stimulus material in drawings of dreams and drawings of waking free imagery. *Dreaming, 1994* (4), 1–27.

Llewellyn, S. (2020). *What do dreams do?* Oxford: Oxford University Press.

Llewellyn, S., and Commentators. (2013). Such stuff as dreams are made on? Elaborative encoding, the ancient art of memory, and the hippocampus. *Behavioral and Brain Sciences, 36*, 589–607. DOI: 10.1017/S0140525X12003135

Loftus, E., & Palmer, J. C. (1974). Reconstruction of automobile destruction: An example of the interaction between language and memory. *Journal of Verbal Learning and Verbal Behavior, 13,* 585–589.

Luppi, P.H., Clement, O., Fort P. (2013). Paradoxical (REM) sleep genesis by the brainstem is under hypothalamic control. *Current Opinion* in *Neurobiology, 23*, 786–792.

MacDonald, A. J. (1984). Dreams after amputation. *British Journal of Psychiatry, 145*, 669.

Macmillan, N., & Creelman, C. D. (2005). *Detection theory: A user's guide* (2nd ed.). Mahwah, NJ: Erlbaum.

Maggioloni, A., Cagnin, C., Crippa, F., Persico, A., Rizzi, P. (2010). Content analysis of dreams and waking narratives. *Dreaming, 20,* 60–76.

Malamud, W., & Linder, F. E. (1931). Dreams and their relationship to recent impressions. *Archives of Neurology and Psychiatry, 25* (5), 1081–1099. doi:10.1001/archneurpsyc.1931.02230050157008

Malinowski, J. (2021). *The psychology of dreaming*. Routledge

Maquet, P., Péters, J. M., Aerts, J., Delfiore, G., Degueldre, C., Luxen, A., et al. (1996). Functional neuroanatomy of human rapid-eye-movement sleep and dreaming. *Nature, 383,* 163–166.

Maquet, P., Schwartz, P. R. S., Albouy, S. L. G., Dang-Vu T., Desseilles, M., Boly, M., Melchior, G., & Peigneux, P. (2004). Regional organization of brain activity during paradoxical sleep. *Archieves Italiennes de Biologie, 142,* 413–419.

McNicol, D. (1972). *A primer of signal detection theory*. London: George Allen and Unwin.

Miller, N., & Dollard, J. (1941). *Social learning and imitation.* New Haven: Yale University Press.

Mineka, D. & Zinbarg, R. (2006). A contemporary learning theory perspective on the etiology of anxiety disorders: It's not what you thought it was. *American Psychologist, 61,* 10–26.

Mischel, W. (1968). *Personality and assessment*. New York, NY: Wiley.

Moretti, F. (2005). *Graphs, maps, trees*. London: Verso.

Moretti, F. (2013). *Distant reading*. London:Verso.

Moretti, F. (Ed.). (2017). *Canon/Archieve: Studies in quantitative formalism from the Stanford Literary Lab*. n+1 Books.

Moretti, F., and Pestre D. (2017). Bankspeak: The language of world bank reports. In F. Moretti (Ed.), *Canon/Archive: Studies in quantitative formalism from the Stanford Literary Lab* (pp. 195–221). n+1 Books.

Moskowitz, D. S. (1982). Coherence and cross-situational generality in personality: A new analysis of old problems. *Journal of Personality and Social Psychology, 43* (4), 754–768. https://doi.org/10.1037/0022-3514.43.4.754

Mulder, T., Hochstenbach, J., Dijkstra, P. U., & Geertzen, J. H. B. (2008). Born to adapt but not in our dreams. *Consciousness and Cognition, 17,* 1266–1271.

Neisser, U. (1967). *Cognitive psychology*. New York, NY: Appleton-Century-Crofts.

Nemiah, J. C. (1984). The unconscious and psychopathology. In K. S. Bowers & D. Meichenbaum (Eds.), *The unconscious reconsidered* (pp. 49–87). New York, NY: Wiley.

Newbern, J. W. (1971). *From sex to sexty # 2*, SRI Publishing Co.

Nielsen, T., Kuiken, D., Alain, G., Stenstrom, P., & Powel, R. A. (2004). Immediate and delayed incorporation of events into dreams: Further replications and implications for dream function. *Journal of Sleep Research, 13,* 327–336.

Nielsen, T. A., & Powell, R. A. (1988). Longitudinal dream incorporation: Preliminary evidence of cognitive processing with an infradian period. *Sleep Research, 17,* 112.

Nielsen, T. A., & Powell, R. A. (1989). The dream-lag effect: A 6-day temporal delay in dream content incorporation. *Psychiatric Journal of the University of Ottawa, 14,* 561–565.

Nielsen, T. A., & Powell, R. A. (1992). The day-residue and dream-lag effects: A literature review and limited replication of two temporal effects in dream formation. *Dreaming, 2* (2), 67–77. https://doi.org/10.1037/h0094348

Nielsen, T. A., & Stenstrom, P. (2005). What are the memory sources of dreaming? *Nature, 437*, 1286–1289. https://doi.org/10.1038/nature04288

Nir, Y., & Tononi, G. (2010). Dreaming and the brain: From phenomenology to neurophysiology. *Trends in Cognitive Science, 14* (2), 88–100. DOI:10.1016/j.tics.2009.12.001

Nofzinger, E. A., Mintun, M.A., Wiseman, M., Kupfer, D. J., Moore, R. Y. (1997). Forebrain activation in REM Sleep: An FDG PET Study. *Brain Research, 770,* 192–201.

Ohlmeyer, P., Brilmayer, H. & Hüllstrung, H. (1944). Periodische Vorgänge im Schlaf. *Pflügers Archiv, 248,* 559–560. https://doi.org/10.1007/BF01764449

Orenstein, C. (2002). *Little red riding hood uncloaked: Sex, morality, and the evolution of a fairy tale.* New York, NY: Basic Books.

Pace-Schott, E. F. (2007). The Frontal Lobes in Dreaming. In Barrett, D., & McNamara, P. (Eds.). *The new science of dreaming, Vol. 1* (pp. 116–154). Westport, CT: Praeger.

Pace-Schott, E. F., Solms, M.. Blagrove, M.. Harnad, S. (Eds.). (2020). *Sleep and dreaming.* Cambridge: Cambridge University Press.

Panksepp, J. (1998). *Affective neuroscience: The foundations of human and animal emotions*. Oxford: Oxford University Press.

Paul, I. H., & Fisher, C. (1969). Subliminal visual stimulation. A study of its influence on subsequent images and dreams. *Journal of Mental Nervous Diseases, 129*, 315–340.

Pavlov, I. P. (1960). Conditioned reflexes: An investigation of the physiological activation of the cerebral cortex (G. V. Anrep (Ed., and Trans.). London: Oxford University Press. (Original work published 1927).

Perrault, C. (1983). "Little Red Riding Hood," [*"Le Petit Chaperon Rouge"*]. In J. Zipes (Ed. & Trans.). *The trials and tribulations of Little Red Riding Hood: Versions of the tale in sociocultural context.* Bervin and Garvey. (Original work published 1697).

Plato. *The republic.* In B. Jowett (Ed.), *The dialogues of Plato (Book IX)* (pp. 280, 281). Clarendon Press.

Plato (360 B.C.E.). *The Timaeus.* B. Jowett (Trans.). p. 51 (Originally published 1892)

Pötzl, O. (1960). The relationship between experimentally induced dream images and indirect vision (pp. 41–120). In J. Wolff, D. Rapaport, & S. H. Annin (Eds. and Trans.). *Preconscious stimulation in dreams, associations, and images: Classical Studies by Otto Pötzl, Rudolf Allers, and Jakob Teler. Psychological Issues, 2* (No. 3), Monograph 7. (Original work published 1917)

Pribram, K. H. (1971). *Languages of the brain: Experimental paradoxes and principles in neurospsychology.* Englewood Cliffs, NJ: Prentice-Hall.

Pribram, K. H. (1991). *Brain and perception: Holonomy and structure in figural processing.* New Jersey, NJ: Erlbaum.

Pribram, K. H., & Gill, M. M. (1976). *Freud's 'Project' re-assessed: Preface to contemporary cognitive theory and neuropsychology.* Basic Books.

Propper, R. E., Stickgold, R., Keeley, R., & Christman, S. D. (2007). Is television traumatic? Dreams, stress, and media exposure in the aftermath of September 11, 2001. *Psychological Science, 18,* 334–340.

Ramachandran, V.S. (1998). *Phantoms in the brain: Probing the mysteries of the mind.* William Morrow.

Reber, A. S. (1993). *Implicit learning and tacit knowledge: An essay on the cognitive unconscious.* Oxford University Press.

Rechtschaffen, A., Verdone, P., & Wheaton, J. (1963). *Reports of mental activity during sleep. Canadian Psychiatric Association Journal, 8,* 409–414.

Raichle, M. E. (2015). The brain's default mode network. *Annual Review of Neuroscience, 38,* 433–447. doi: 10.1146/annurev-neuro-071013-014030.

Raichle, M. E., MacLeod, A. M., Snyder, A. Z., Powers, W. J., Gusnard, D. A., & Shulman, G. L. A default mode of brain function (2001), *Proceedings of the National Academy of Sciences, 98* (2), 676–682. https://doi.org/10.1073/pnas.98.2.676

Raichle, M. E, & Snyder, A. Z. 2007. A default mode of brain function: a brief history of an evolving idea. *Neuroimage. 37*:1083–90.

Revonsuo, A., & Valli, K. (2000). Dreaming and consciousness: Testing the threat simulation theory of the function of dreaming. *PSYCHE: An Interdisciplinary Journal of Research On Consciousness, 6.*

Rey, A. (2012). *Psychologie cognitive expérimentele.* puf.

Roediger, H. L., & McDermott, K. B. (1995). Creating false memories: Remembering words not presented in lists. *Journal of Experimental Psychology: Learning, Memory, and Cognition, 21,* 803–814.

Rosvold, H. E., Mirsky, A. F., & Pribram, K. H. (1954). Influence of amygdalectomy on social behavior in monkeys. *Journal of Comparative and Physiological Psychology, 47*(3), 173–178. https://doi.org/10.1037/h0058870

Rummelhart, D. E., McClelland, J. L., & the PDP Research Group (Eds.). (1986). *Parallel distributed processing: Explorations in the microstructure of cognition* (Vol. 1). Bradford.

Saurat, M.T., Agbakou, M., Attigui, P., Golmard, J.L., & Arnulf, I. (2011). Walking dreams in congenital and acquired paraplegia. *Consciousness and Cognition, 20* (4), 1425–1432. https://doi.org/10.1016/j.concog.2011.05.015

Schacter, D. L. (1987). Implicit memory: History and current status. *Journal of Experimental Psychology: Learning, Memory, and Cognition, 13,* 501–518.

Schacter, D. L., & Addis, D. R. (2007). The ghosts of past and future: A memory that works by piecing together bits of the past may be better suited to simulating future events than one that is a store of perfect records. *Nature, 445,* 27.

Schacter, D. L., & Graf, P. (1986). Effects of elaborative processing on implicit and explicit memory for new associations. *Journal of Experimental Psychology: Learning, Memory, and Cognition, 12*(3), 432–444. https://doi.org/10.1037/0278-7393.12.3.432

Schatzman, M. (1973). *Soul murder: Persecution in the family*. New York: Random House.

Schnessler, J. (2017). *The New York Times* (October 30).

Schredl, M. (2006). Repression and dreaming: An open empirical question [Peer commentary on the paper, "The Unified Theory of Repression" by M. H. Erdelyi]. *Behavioral and Brains Sciences, 29,* 531–532.

Schredl, M. (2017). Theorizing about the continuity between waking and dreaming: Comment on Domhoff (2017). *Dreaming, 27* (4), 351–359.

Schredl, M., Kleinfrechner, & Gell, T. (1996). Dreaming and personality: Thick vs. thin boundaries. *Dreaming, 6,* 219–223.

Schredl, M., Schäffer, F., Hoffmann, F., & Jacob, S. (1999). Dream content and personality: Thick vs. thin personalities. *Dreaming, 9,* 257–263.

Schredl, M., Dombrowe, C., Bozzer, A., & Morlock, M. (1999). Do subliminal stimuli affect dream content? Methodological issues and empirical data. *Sleep and Hypnosis, 1,* 181–185.

Schredl, M. & Piel, E. (2003). Gender differences in dream recall: Data from four representative German samples. *Personality and Individual Differences, 35,* 1185–1189.

Schwartz, S., & Maquet, P. (2002). Sleep imaging and the neuro-psychological assessment of dreams. *Trends in Cognitive Science, 6,* 2002.

Schweickert, R. (2007). Properties of the organization of memory for people: Evidence from dream reports. *Psychonomic Bulletin & Review, 14*, 270–276. https://doi.org/10.3758/BF03194063

Scoville, W. B., & Milner, B. (1957). Loss of recent memory after bilateral hippocampal lesions. *Journal of Neurology, Neurosurgery and Psychiatry*, 20, 11–21.

Seligman, M. E. P., Railton, P., Baumeister, R. F., & Striarde, C. (2013). Navigating into the future or driven by the past. *Perspectives on Psychological Science, 8* (2), 119–141. DOI: 10.1177/1745691612474317

Shakespeare, W. (1958). *Julius Caesar*. (P. Alexander, Ed.), pp. 334–387, Act II, p. 355. Collins. (Original work performed 1599–1600).

Shakespeare, W. (1951). *The Tempest*. (P. Alexander, Ed.), pp. 27–73, Act IV, p. 64. Collins. (Original work performed 1611).

Sheehan S. (1982). *Is there no place on earth for me?* Boston, MA: Houghton Mifflin.

Shevrin, H., & Luborsky, L. (1958). The measurement of preconscious perception in dreams and images: An investigation of the Pötzl phenomenon. *Journal of Abnormal and Social Psychology, 56,* 285–294.

Siclari, F. (2019, July 21-25). *The EEG correlates of dreaming*. [Invited presentation]. 36th Annual International Dream Conference of the International Association for the Study of Dreams, Rolduc Monastery, Kerkrade, The Netherlands.

Siclari, F., Baird, B., Perogamvros, L., Bernardi, G., LaRocque, J .J., Riedner, B.. Boly, M., Postle, B. R., Tononi, G. (2017). *The neural correlates of dreaming, Nature Neuroscience, 20* (6), 872–881. DOI: 10.1038/nn.4545

Siclari, F., Bernardi, G., Cataldi, J., & Tononi, G. (2018). Dreaming in NREM sleep: A high-density EEG study of slow waves and spindles. *Journal of Neuroscience, 38* (43) 9175–9185. DOI: https://doi.org/10.1523/JNEUROSCI.08556-18.2018

Skinner, B. F. (1938). *The behavior of organisms*. New York, NY: Appleton-Century-Crofts.

Smith, R. (1984). The meaning of dreams: The need for a standardized dream report. *Psychiatric Research, 13,* 267–274.

Smith, R. (1986). Evaluating dream function: Emphasizing the study of patients with organic disease. *Journal of Mind and Behavior, 7,* 206.

Snyder, F. (1967). *Experimental studies of dreaming.* New York, NY: Random House.

Solms, M. (1997). *The neuropsychology of dreams: A clinico-anatomical study.* Mahwah, NJ: Erlbaum.

Solms, M. (2003). Dreaming and REM Sleep are Controlled by Different Brain Mechanisms. In E. F. Pace-Schott, M. Solms, M. Blagrove, & S. Harnad (Eds.), *Sleep and dreaming: Scientific advances and reconsiderations* (pp. 51–58). Cambridge: Cambridge University Press.

Solms, M. (2012). In L. Oppenheim (Conference Organizer). *Minding the gap III: Dreaming: Psychoanalysis or Neurobiology?* Conference at the New York Psychoanalytic Society and Institute, at Mt. Sinai Medical Center, New York, May 5, 2012. [To appear in *Contemporary Psychoanalysis.*]

Solms, M., & Turnbull, O. (2002). *The brain and the inner world: An introduction to the neuroscience of subjective experience.* New York, NY: Other Press.

Spence, D. P. (1980). Lawfulness in lexical choice: A natural experiment. *The Journal of the American Psychoanalytic Association, 28,* 115–132.

Spence, D. P., & Holland, B. (1962). The restricting effects of awareness: A paradox and an explanation. *Journal of Abnormal and Social Psychology, 64,* 163–174.

Spence, D. P., Scarborough, H. S., & Ginsberg, E. H. (1978). Lexical correlates of cervical cancer. *Social Science and Medicine, 12,* 141–145.

Squire, L. R. (1987). *Memory and brain.* New York, NY: Oxford University Press.

Squire, L. R. (2009). The Legacy of Patient H.M. for Neuroscience. *Neuron, 61* (1), 6–9. DOI: 10.1016/j.neuron.2008.12.023

Stetter, E. (1950). Zür Phänomenologie des Phantomgliedes. *Deutsche Zeitschrift für Nervenheikunde, 163,* 141–171.

Stickgold R. (2005). Sleep-dependent memory consolidation. *Nature, 27,* 1272–1278. DOI: 10.1038/nature04286.

Stickgold, R., & Walker, M. (2005). Memory consolidation and reconsolidation: What is the role of sleep? *Trends in Neurosciences, 28* (8), 408–415.

Storm, L., Sherwood, S. J., Roe, C. A., Tressoldi, P. E., Rock, A. J., & Di Risio, L. (2017). On the correspondence between dream content and target material under laboratory conditions: A meta-analysis of dream-ESP studies, 1966-2016. *International Journal of Dream Research, 10* (2), 120–140.

Swets, J. A. (Ed.). (1964). *Signal detection and recognition in human observers.* New York, NY: Wiley.

Swets, J. A., Tanner, W. P., & Birdsall, T. G. (1961). Decision processes for perception. *Psychological Review, 68,* 301–340.

Tulving, E. (1983). *Elements of episodic memory.* Oxford: Oxford University Press.

Tulving, E. (1985). How many memory systems are there? *American Psychologist, 40* (4), 385–398. https://doi.org/10.1037/0003-066X.40.4.385

Tulving, E. (1989). Remembering and knowing the past. *American Scientist, 77,* 361–367.

Tulving, E., & Pearlstone, Z. (1967). Availability versus accessibility of information in memory for words. *Journal of Verbal Learning and Verbal Behavior, 6,* 175–184.

Tranel, D., & Damasio, A. R. (1985). Knowledge without awareness: An anatomic index of facial recognition by prosopagnosics. *Science, 228,* 1453–1455.

Tsu, J. (2022). *Kingdom of characters: The language revolution that made China modern.* New York, NY: Riverhead Books.

Tuominen J, Stenberg T, Revonsuo A, Valli K. (2019). Social contents in dreams: An empirical test of the Social Simulation Theory. *Consciousness & Cognition*, 69, 133–145. DOI: 10.1016/j.concog.2019.01.017.

Ullman, M., & Krippner, S., Vaughan, A. (2002). *Dream telepathy*. New York, NY: Macmillan.

Valli, K., & Revonsuo, A. (2007). Evolutionary psychological approaches to dream content: In D. Barrett & P. McNamara (Eds.), *The new science of dreaming: Cultural and theoretical perspectives.* (Vol. 3, pp. 95–116). Praeger.

Valli, K., & Revonsuo, A. (2009). The threat simulation theory in light of recent empirical evidence: A review. *The American Journal of Psychology 122* (1), 17–38.

Valli, K., & Hoss, R. J. (2019). *Dreams: Understanding biology, psychology and culture.* Greenwood

Van De Castle, R. (1971). *The psychology of dreaming.* Morristown, NJ: General Learning Press.

Van De Castle, R. L. (1994). *Our dreaming mind.* New York, NY: Ballantine Press.

Verdone, P. (1965). Temporal reference of manifest dream content. *Perceptual and Motor Skills, 20*(3, Pt. 2), 1253–1268. https://doi.org/10.2466/pms.1965.20.3c.1253

Walker M., & Stickgold, R. (2010). Overnight Alchemy: Sleep-dependent memory evolution. *Nature Reviews. Neuroscience. 11*, 218.

Wamsley E., & Stickgold, R. (2011). Memory, sleep, and dreaming: Experiencing consolidation. *Sleep Medicine Clinics, 6* (1), 97–108. DOI: 10.1016/j.jsmc.2010.12.008. PMID: 21516215; PMCID: PMC3079906.

Wang, B. (2018). *Forlorn in the rain: Translation and annotation of selected classical Chinese poetry and others.* Foreign Languages Press.

Watson, J. B. (1930). *Behaviorism*. Chicago: Chicago University Press.

Watson, J. B., & Rayner, R. (1920). Conditioned emotional reaction. *Journal of Experimental Psychology, 3*, 1–14.

Weisenberg, T., & McBride, K. E. (1935). *Aphasia: A clinical and psychological study*. New York, NY: The Commonwealth Fund.

Weiskrantz, L. (2002). *Blindsight: A case study and implications*. Oxford: Oxford University Press.

Werner, H. (1956). Microgenesis and aphasia. *Journal of Abnormal and Social Psychology, 52*, 347–353.

Wernicke, C. (1874) *Der aphasische Symptomencomplex: Eine psychologische Studie auf anatomischer Basis.* Breslau: Max Cohn & Weigert.

Williams, D. R. & Williams, H. (1969) Auto-maintenance in the pigeon: Sustained pecking despite contingent nonreinforcement. *Journal of the Experimental Analysis of Behavior, 12*, 511–20.

Wolf, F. A. (1995). *The dreaming universe: A mind-expanding journey into the realm where psyche and physics meet.* New York, NY: Touchstone. ISBN-13: 978-0-684-801159-9

Wolkstein, D., & Kramer, S. N. (1983), *Inanna: Queen of heaven and earth.* New York, NY: Harper & Row. ISBN 0-06-090854-8

Yeats, W. B. (1919). The Second Coming. In R. A. Bower (Ed.). (1959). *Major British writers: Enlarged edition* (p. 795). Harcourt, Brace & World.

Yip, W. (Ed. and Trans.). (1997). *Chinese poetry: An anthology of major modes and genres.* Durham: Duke University Press.

Zhang, J. (1992). *Psychoanalysis in China: Literary transformations—1919–1949.* Ithaca, NY: Cornell East Asia Series.

Zipes, J. (Ed. and Trans.). (1983). *The trials and tribulations of Little Red Riding Hood: Versions of the tale in sociocultural context.* South Hadley, MA: Bergin and Garvey.

Zizak, D. M., & Reber, A. S. (2004). Implicit preferences: The role(s) of familiarity in the structural mere exposure effect. *Consciousness & Cognition, 13*, 336–362.

AUTHOR INDEX

SUBJECT INDEX

For Product Safety Concerns and Information please contact our EU
representative GPSR@taylorandfrancis.com
Taylor & Francis Verlag GmbH, Kaufingerstraße 24, 80331 München, Germany

www.ingramcontent.com/pod-product-compliance
Ingram Content Group UK Ltd.
Pitfield, Milton Keynes, MK11 3LW, UK
UKHW020147200926
475702UK00016B/2597
* 9 7 8 1 0 3 2 2 9 2 2 1 2 *